CONCEPTS COMMON TO ACUTE ILLNESS

Identification and management

CONCEPTS COMMON TO ACUTE ILLNESS

Identification and management

Edited by

LAURA K. HART, R.N., B.S.N., M.Ed., M.A., Ph.D.
Associate Professor,
University of Iowa College of Nursing,
Iowa City, Iowa

JEAN L. REESE, R.N., B.S.N., M.N.
Associate Professor,
University of Iowa College of Nursing,
Iowa City, Iowa

MARGERY O. FEARING, R.N., B.S.N., M.A.
Clinical Nursing Specialist,
University of Iowa Hospitals and Clinics,
Iowa City, Iowa

Illustrated

The C. V. Mosby Company

ST. LOUIS • TORONTO • LONDON 1981

MOSBY

1906 75 1981
YEARS

A TRADITION OF PUBLISHING EXCELLENCE

Printed in the United States of America

The C. V. Mosby Company
11830 Westline Industrial Drive, St. Louis, Missouri 63141

Library of Congress Cataloging in Publication Data

Main entry under title:

Concepts common to acute illness.

Bibliography: p.
Includes index.
1. Nursing. I. Hart, Laura K., 1938-
II. Reese, Jean L., 1937- . III. Fearing,
Margery O., 1935- . [DNLM: 1. Acute disease—
Nursing texts. WY 154 C744]
RT41.C745 616'.0024613 80-28706
ISBN 0-8016-2117-8

C/D/D 9 8 7 6 5 4 3 2 1 02/D/223

CONTRIBUTORS

PAULETTE R. Di ANGI, R.N., B.S.N., M.A.

Assistant Professor, Mount Mercy College School of Nursing,
Cedar Rapids, Iowa

JOANN M. ELAND, R.N., B.S.N., M.A., Ph.D.

Assistant Professor, University of Iowa College of Nursing,
Iowa City, Iowa

MARGERY O. FEARING, R.N., B.S.N., M.A.

Clinical Nursing Specialist, University of Iowa Hospitals and Clinics,
Iowa City, Iowa

RITA A. FARREN FRANTZ, R.N., B.S.N., M.A., Ph.D.

Associate Professor, University of Iowa College of Nursing,
Iowa City, Iowa

ROSE MARIE FRIEDRICH, R.N., B.S.N., M.A.

Associate Professor, University of Iowa College of Nursing,
Iowa City, Iowa

LAURA K. HART, R.N., B.S.N., M.Ed., M.A., Ph.D.

Associate Professor, University of Iowa College of Nursing,
Iowa City, Iowa

CAROLYN K. DREESSEN KINNEY, R.N., B.S.N., M.A., Ph.D.

Assistant Professor, University of Iowa College of Nursing,
Iowa City, Iowa

SONJA I. LIVELY, R.N., B.S.N., M.A.

Assistant Professor, University of Iowa College of Nursing, Iowa City, Iowa

FRANCES K. MILDE, R.N., B.S.N., M.S.N.

Assistant Professor, University of Iowa College of Nursing, Iowa City, Iowa

PAULA CORNETT MOBILY, R.N., B.S., M.S.N.

Assistant Professor, University of Iowa College of Nursing, Iowa City, Iowa

SANDRA R. POWELL, R.N., B.A., M.Ed.

Associate Professor, University of Iowa College of Nursing, Iowa City, Iowa

JEAN L. REESE, R.N., B.S.N., M.N.

Associate Professor, University of Iowa College of Nursing, Iowa City, Iowa

CARMELA ANN REHTZ, R.N., B.S., M.S.

Assistant Professor, University of Iowa College of Nursing, Iowa City, Iowa

CAROL A. WATSON, R.N., B.S.N., M.A., Ph.D.

Assistant Professor, University of Iowa College of Nursing, Iowa City, Iowa

NANCY N. WYATT, R.N., B.S.N., M.A.

Lecturer, University of Minnesota School of Nursing, Minneapolis, Minnesota

PREFACE

During the past ten years nursing has emphasized the use of the nursing process to plan nursing care. However, it has been the process that has received attention while the identification of nursing knowledge has been relatively neglected. The purpose of this book, therefore, is to present the development of nursing concepts and their articulation with the nursing process.

The concepts addressed in this book have been limited to those frequently encountered in an acute care setting. We believe that nurses have an independent function regarding the identification, control, neutralization, and extinction of these problem phenomena. We also believe that nurses must identify those areas of function in which they have a primary responsibility for the provision of care and must articulate that care with the activities of other health disciplines.

The first chapter of this book explains the conceptual structure utilized in the development of each of the fifteen concepts presented. The goal of this work is to provide a clinical application model of a conceptual approach to nursing practice.

Laura K. Hart
Jean L. Reese
Margery O. Fearing

CONTENTS

CONCEPTS COMMON TO ACUTE ILLNESS

Identification and management

LAURA K. HART
JEAN L. REESE
MARGERY O. FEARING

Chapter 1

THE CONCEPTUAL MODEL AND THE NURSING PROCESS

Nursing as a profession maintains and increases its usefulness to society through innovations and enlargement of its knowledge base. The structures used to organize that knowledge influence how it is transmitted and expanded and guide the mode of its application.[3] Structures previously used to organize and transmit nursing knowledge have become burdened with ever-increasing scientific, technological knowledge and society's increased demands for health care expansion. Responding to these forces in the past, nursing moved from the organizational structure of the Nightingale health-hygiene model to the medical body-systems approach. Nursing is now moving to an integrated concept-process approach that uses concepts to structure knowledge and the nursing process to organize and guide it in practice.

The conceptual organization of knowledge allows a wide range of topics to be included under comprehensive ideas.[6] For example, the dynamics of the concept of inflammation provide a common structure for understanding events that occur with such diverse pathological problems as rheumatoid arthritis and carbuncle formation. Since patients with either of these problems experience inflammation, the principles used to guide their nursing care can emanate from the dynamics of this one concept.

Situations requiring the services of a professional are not necessarily characterized by the severity of the problem but by its degree of variability and its inherent predictive margin of error. The mark of a professional is the ability to accurately anticipate outcomes in variable, nonroutine situations.[12]

The diagnostic and management process referred to as the "nursing process" uses a systematic scientific approach to problem solution.[2] In nursing, this problem-solving process includes determining whether the client has a problem, the nature of the problem, the available interventions, and the effectiveness of the interventions used.

A conceptual organizing schema provides flexibility and generalization of nursing knowledge; when systematically used in the nursing process, it enhances predictive accuracy.[11] During the past 10 years nursing has emphasized the use of the nursing process to plan nursing care. However, the process has received the primary attention, while the other critical component of this approach, concept development, has been relatively neglected. The focus of this book therefore is the development of concepts and their articulation with the nursing process. The material presented here is based on the assumptions that (1) a conceptual organization of the body of nursing knowledge systematizes the phenomena for which nurses have primary responsibility, (2) such an organization of knowledge conveniently articulates with the scientific problem-solving nursing process, and (3) the systematic use of this type of categorization will facilitate the delineation of the foci of nursing care and suggest a logical scientific rationale for intervention approaches.

Concepts are developed by classifying two or more objects or events together and discriminating them from other objects or events on the basis of common characteristics. Since most attributes are on a continuum, their values can be infinite. As a result, the attributes specified to signify the presence of a concept, although actually arbitrary categories, are selected to reduce the ambiguity and complexity of communicating. Concepts are formulated because a constellation of attributes has meaning to the individuals interacting with that constellation.[6] For example, the Eskimos in the arctic use many nouns to denote the different types of snow. Since this substance is a major factor in their existence, it is of great importance that they be able to communicate about it as precisely as possible. The labeling the Eskimos have devised for the many types of snow is arbitrary, but meaningful to their existence. In like manner the categorizations, classifications, and terminology used by a profession should increase the precision of the practitioners' communication.[13]

Some concepts are formulated by designating that it is necessary for all attributes of that concept to be present in order for the concept to be recognized. An example of this type of concept is the specific color canary yellow. The exact light waves associated with this color must be present in order to have canary yellow. However, an example of a different type of concept is chair. According to *Webster's New World Dictionary*, a chair is a seat for one. However, chairs come in many sizes, shapes, and colors. They can be wood, glass, plastic, metal, or rock. They may or may not have a back, arms, or legs. The existence, then, of some of the concept's attributes, in a variety of subsets, is sufficient to designate an instance of this "either or" type of concept.[1,4,8,9] The more latitude a concept has in its allowable subset variance, the more difficult it becomes to determine the presence of that concept. Professional nurses are faced with this problem. The concepts they most frequently deal with are of this "either or" arrangement. An additional difficulty posed by this type of concept is that two or more concepts may share attributes, that is, their attribute subsets may be composed of the same characteristics. For example, one may consider when a chair can be called a bench, and when a bench is labeled a couch. The point at which the label for the characteristics on this continuum changes appears arbitrary, but distinctions can be made on the basis of the function of the object. So it is with concepts such as hypoxia, ischemia, and shock. The decision regarding which concept is dominant in a given situation is based on the number and arrangement of the characteristics present. Distinguishing between concepts having similar attributes requires the ability to discriminate attribute subtleties and their function. This identification of the concept being confronted or determination of the nature of the problem is the most critical and perhaps most difficult aspect of problem solving. It involves not only awareness that a problem exists, but also suspension of judgment regarding the nature of the problem until an adequate data base has been collected.[7] The more encompassing the problem, the larger the data base and the more critical its scrutiny must be.[5]

It is in the assessment phase of the nursing process that data collection, classification, and analysis should occur. During this assessment both objective and subjective data must be collected about the client, the environment, and existing support systems. Objective data are behaviors or events that are observable and/or measurable by a person other than the client. Subjective data are information obtained from the client regarding a symptom or condition that can be perceived only by the client, not by the examiner.

The concept that categorizes, or labels, the nature of the problem provides an organizational structure to the data clusters. In the assessment phase of the nursing process data must be collected and analyzed to (1) determine whether the criteria that designate a specific concept have been fulfilled, (2) identify the stressor(s) that has/have precipitated the concept, and (3) identify the constraints, capabilities, and/or resources available to the client. In conceptual phraseology the stressors, whether physiological, psychological, or sociological in origin, are referred to as the antecedent condition. The constraints, capabilities, and resources available to the client are called intervening variables.

A concept is deemed present if its criteria are present. The concept's structure provides an explanation of the dynamics of the presenting problem. The presence of the concept's criteria is what stimulates the initiation of nursing intervention. However, it is the antecedent condition and intervening variables that direct the approaches used to correct, neutralize, resolve, and/or assist in coping with the deficit or problem. The purpose of nursing intervention is to alter the antecedent condition and/or the intervening variables. The number and type of alternative interventions viable as solutions to the presenting problem are affected by the intervening variables present and the limitations imposed by the antecedent condition. For example, if a client is hypoxic because of emphysema, the physiological changes cannot be altered. The interventions will have to be directed toward controlling intervening variables such as rate of metabolism or level of activity.

Actualization of the concept of pain might be verified by the client's verbal statement of its presence and by concomitant signs of restlessness. The intervention used to alleviate this pain is not directed toward the verbalization or the restlessness, but rather toward the cause of these behaviors. The intervention selected must be guided or modified by the antecedent condition (e.g., a surgical incision) and intervening variables (e.g., time since operation and the person's pain perception). Changes in the concept's criteria, the verbalization and restlessness, are simply indicators of the intervention effectiveness. The outcomes of the intervention can be gauged by the change in degree or number of the criteria. These changes may be so great that the concept ceases to exist.

Components of this conceptual model and their relationships to the nursing process are depicted in Figs. 1 and 2.

The antecedent condition is the physiological, psychological, or sociological stressors that precipitate the concept. The concept's actualization is verified by the

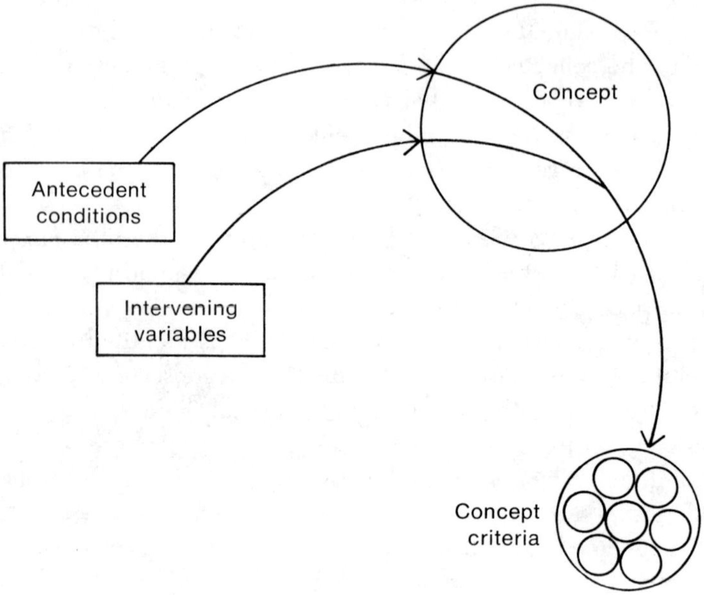

FIG. 1. Components of the conceptual model.

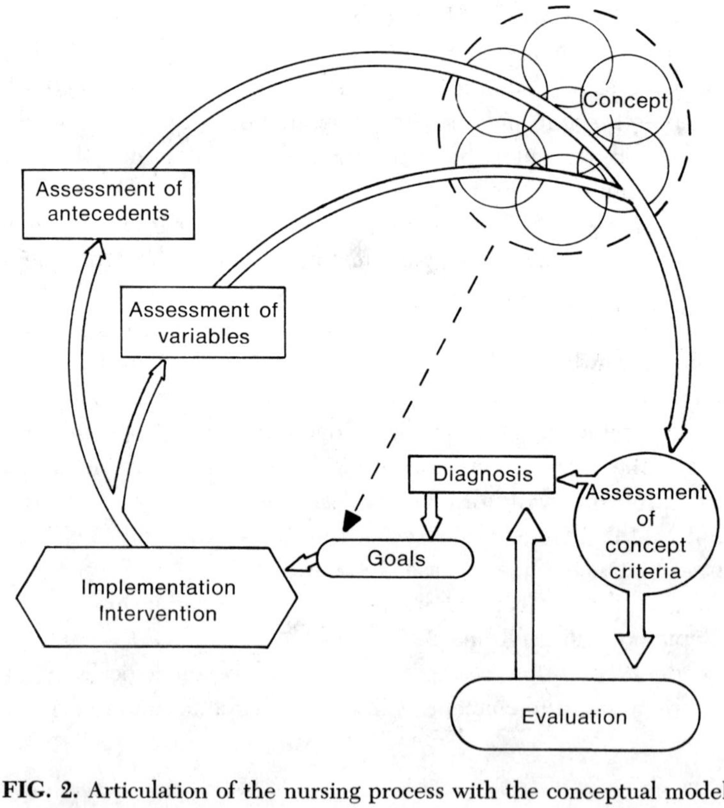

FIG. 2. Articulation of the nursing process with the conceptual model.

presence of its criteria. The intervening variables are the constraints, capabilities, and/or resources available in the client or in the environment that may amplify or reduce the degree of the concept's impingement on the client or alter the concept's complexion. The antecedent condition and intervening variables not only influence the concept's presentation, but are the factors that the nursing interventions must address. Changes in the concept's presenting behavior provide evaluation criteria regarding the interventions' effectiveness.

Success in the intervention phase of the nursing process is directly related to the accuracy of the concept assessment as well as to the planning of interventions that articulate with the concept structure. The power in this conceptual model is that although the specific techniques used to intervene in problem situations may be singular to each instance of the concept and directed at affecting the particular antecedents and/or intervening variables, the underlying principles used in intervention decision making evolve out of the concept's dynamics and remain constant for all instances of the concept.

The first step in the planning phase is to identify the goals, or nursing care objectives, to be achieved. The principles that assist in the identification of goals pertinent to the nursing care of the patient emanate from the concept's dynamics. Goal statements that are written in a client-oriented format and that specify desired behavioral changes provide criteria for the evaluation of the effectiveness of the selected interventions. These behavioral objectives, or goal statements, should specify (1) the person who is to exhibit the behavior, (2) the desired behavior, and (3) the degree of the behavior required. In certain instances the condition imposed on the performance of the desired behavior would also be included. For example, in the goal, "Mr. W. will sleep at least 6 hours every night without the aid of sleeping medication," the condition "without medication" enhances the specificity of the criterion measure.[10]

When goals are short term, it is often helpful to the evaluation process if the behaviors to be changed are described in detail. Also, the length of time available for goal achievement should influence the degree of change expected in the behavior.

The concept discussions in this book address the generality of each concept rather than singular instances of the concept. Therefore the goals advanced in the intervention discussions are of a general, long-term nature. Suggestions regarding specific short-term goals that might be used in singular instances of the concept are found in the discussions of the specific behavioral outcomes that might be expected as the results of successful intervention. For instance, one of the criteria for determining the presence of the concept of psychological immobility could be lack of interest in personal appearance. Hence a short-term goal could relate to the client carrying out parts of daily personal hygiene without prompting.

Evaluation of the achievement of intervention goals must consider the process in total. The plan's design is influenced by the abstractive abilities of the nurse, but the process will not be a success unless the nurse's communicative and psychomotor skills are equal to the task. The interventions must be adjusted when the criteria depicting a concept fade or increase and/or when another intervening variable or antecedent condition is discovered.

Each chapter in this book addresses a specific concept that frequently is experienced by persons with acute illness. These concepts are first explored at an abstract level, in which the structure and dynamics of the concept provide a conceptual definition. The concept is then operationally defined by identifying the behaviors relevant and critical to instances of that concept. It is this operational, or behavioral, definition that provides the criteria to be used in determining whether a concept is present. Antecedent conditions are explored to identify the possible variations for concept initiation. Discussion of the intervening variables is directed toward how they change the complexion or impact of the concept.

Goal statements are based on principles evolved from the concept's structure and dynamics, and the intervention specifically attempts to modify the antecedent condition or intervening variables. At the end of each goal and intervention discussion, behavioral outcomes that can be used as evaluation criteria are identified.

REFERENCES

1. Archer, E. J.: The psychological nature of concepts. In Klausmeier, H. J., and Harris, C. W., editors: Analysis of concept learning, New York, 1966, Academic Press, Inc.
2. Bailey, J. T., and Claus, K. E.: Decision making in nursing, tools for change, St. Louis, 1975. The C. V. Mosby Co.
3. Bell, D.: Notes on the post-industrial society. I. Public Interest **6**:24, 1967.
4. Berlyne, D. E.: Structure and direction in thinking, New York, 1965, John Wiley & Sons, Inc.
5. Beveridge, W. I. B.: The art of scientific investigation, New York, 1961, Vintage Books.
6. Bourne, L. E., Jr.: Human conceptual behavior, Boston, 1966, Allyn & Bacon, Inc.
7. Dewey, J.: How we think, Boston, 1910, D.C. Heath & Co.
8. Haygood, R. C., and Bourne, L. E., Jr.: Attribute-and-rule-learning aspects of conceptual behavior, Psychol. Rev. **72**:175, 1965.
9. Henderson, K. B.: Logical model for conceptualizing and other related activities. In Komisar, B. P., and MacMillan, C. J. B., editors: Psychological concepts in education, Chicago, 1967, Rand McNally & Co.
10. Higgins, N., and Sullivan, H.: Writing worthwhile objectives, Tempe, Ariz., 1978, Teaching for Competence.
11. Mitchell, P., and Walter, J. B.: A conceptual framework. In Walter, J. B., Pardee, G. P., and Molbo, D. M., editors: Dynamics of problem oriented approaches: patient care and documentation, Philadelphia, 1976, J. B. Lippincott Co.
12. Scott, W. R.: Some implications of organizational theory for research on health services, Milbank Mem. Fund. Q. **44**:35, 1966.
13. Worff, B. L.: Linguistics as an exact science. In Carall, J. B., editor: Language, thought and reality, Cambridge, Mass., 1956, M.I.T. Press.

LAURA K. HART

CAROLYN K. DREESSEN KINNEY

You "admit" me

You receive
my disclosure
of self

You border me
with terms

You limit me
with words

And smugly
measure me
with comparisons

You relate to the
me
you have created
not
the me
I am.

PAULETTE R. Di ANGI

Chapter 2

LOSS OF IDENTITY CONTROL

CONCEPTUAL DEFINITION

Loss of identity control is the experience of major or minor alterations or uncertainties regarding self-definition and efficacy in maintaining control over one's life situation. More generally, this state might be described as a problem of self-definition in relation to external reality.[1] Such a state evolves out of conflicts between the two aspects of identity; self-realization and social definition.[33]

Tabachnick[34] defines identity as the capability of formulating personal goals with the organizational ability of attaining those goals. He believes that the functions of this dynamic control evolve from the integration of self-realization and social definition. Self-realization refers to adherence to one's values, and social definition refers to continuity in social relationships.[34] Inherent in this perception of identity is the maintenance of an inner autonomy that provides the power to control one's social destiny.

Erikson[9] suggests that if a person does not have a sense of ego identity, that person does not have a feeling of being alive. He states that this feeling is so vital that a child will resist any attempts to eliminate the opportunity for the development of an ego identity with a strength similar to that of an animal defending its life. The sense of identity is developed from a confidence that (1) an inner continuity can be maintained and (2) this inner continuity matches one's meaning to others. A sense of identity evolves from the awareness that the manner in which one controls one's experiences is as successful as that of others, and that others recognize this success.[9]

Greenacre[14] stresses that the inner and outer faces of identity contribute to identity formation. Self-image, or sense of identity, is based on the awareness of how one's form and functioning articulate with the desired appearance and function. She also recognizes that developments in and beyond adolescence modify this sense. Athough Erikson[7,8] suggests that an identity pattern is crystalized mainly during adolescence, this does not imply that problems with identity do not occur at other times. However, identity problems usually occur in relation to tasks that are specific to the particular life period. Identity problems result from disequilibria between self-realization and the social definition pertinent to the specific developmental period or to the specific situational experience in which the individual is currently engaged.

Mahler[20] and Jacobson[17] state that the self-feelings that evolve from the psychic differentation process, that of differentiating "me" from "not me," make up the young child's sense of identity. Spiegel[30] proposes that an individual's past experiences form an inner frame of reference against which new experiences can be compared. This frame of reference provides the basis for a continuing personal identity. Ideas such as Spiegel's suggest that the sense of identity has a social dimension that relates to external reality, vacillates, and is modified throughout the life cycle.

The socially defined aspect of identity is developed and expanded through social roles. A person's memory, sense of time, perceptions of self and others, and psychological functions are shaped by the role configurations expected by society. An individual's regular methods of acting are therefore the result of consistent confrontations by significant others.[13]

The definition of one's social role flows from many levels of social structures. Formal organizations or bureaucracies bestow universal and impersonal identity norms. Symbolic institutions such as religion legitimate particular life contingencies. However, it is the family structure that provides a socially and personally defined reality. The family structure usually provides intense and frequent interactions with behavior norms based on cumulative and implicit background expectations.[35] This social sense of identity relates to perceptions about one's place among others. It is the link between an individual and the individual's environment. It is the way by which a person is established in the world.[5]

A socially ascribed identity outlines expectations related to the social catagories one falls into without choosing them. Examples are the expectations attached to age, sex, and race. Achieved identity outlines expectations attached to age, sex, and race. Achieved identity outlines expectations of members of the specific groups to which the person belongs such as a profession or vocation. An adapted social identity evolves out of the complementary characteristics of a role transaction and is often attached to future expectations. Examples of adapted social identities are the roles of a superior, a helper, or a person being helped.[31] The social expectations attached to the role assist in structuring the identity of the person fulfilling the role.

The person's identity is the central organizing principle that accounts for the unity, self-sameness, and continuity of the personality and its shared sameness with the community.[23] This self-sameness relates the persistence of certain behavior patterns and appearance. The private and interpersonal aspects of the personality intertwine and become interdependent aspects of the identity. However, a person may have many social selves. The differences in the person's behavior often evolve from the varying demands of each social situation.

Erikson[10] traces the roots of identity to the infant's development of a sense of trust. This forms the basis of identity because trust evolves gradually to a feeling of being "all right."[8] As feelings of autonomy develop, so do self-awareness and feelings of control. One's basic identity pattern is gradually established by successive ego synthesis throughout childhood.[6] Comfort with self, knowledge of one's direction, and anticipation of recognition from significant others are concomitant to a sense of identity. This sense is constantly lost and regained as one moves through life.[8]

When social demands change abruptly, the personality system is faced with the challenge of resynthesis. These demands may necessitate major redefinitions of self and perspectives of life.[23] Although perceptions of self change many times during a person's life, it is when the sense of inner control is altered that perceptions of identity begin to change. When questions arise in an individual's mind such as "Who am I? Will such a disrupted body grow together again? Do I really know what I want to be? Will I be able to make the right decisions?" and "Am I comfortable with the way others perceive me?" the person is experiencing a state of uncertainty regarding identity. When such uncertainties escalate and threaten identity control, they may be equivalent, psychosocially, to a threat to life. When others are not available to, or do not, recognize the person's positive characteristics, the individual's identity control begins to dissipate. As self-esteem is lowered, feelings of continuity, or being directed toward the future, are interrupted. The person may perceive a loss of human capacities, functions, and dignity. Perceptions of indignities may strip and disfigure the victim's self-perception.

ANTECEDENT CONDITIONS

Identity control is lost to some degree for every patient who is admitted to an acute care institution. Hospitalization implies the presence of an illness so serious it cannot be treated on an outpatient basis.[26] the individual is abruptly confronted by the reality of personal mortality. The person's usual social responsibilities must be abandoned, and the dependent identity of a hospitalized patient accepted. Often this transactional role differs decidedly from the individual's usual adult role.

Measurable physical changes associated with the stress of hospitalization have been identified by many research studies. Newly admitted patients have exhibited increased urine corticosteriod levels that decreased to normal during the first week of hospitalization.[21] Another patient group was found to have higher urine potassium levels on the day of admission than on the second day of hospitalization. Also, the amount of decrease seen on the second day was greatest in those patients who received nursing intervention designed to reduce the stress of hospitalization.[25] In a third study platelet aggregation time was faster and systolic and diastolic blood pressures were higher shortly before hospitalization than just prior to surgery or discharge.[12]

Although many situations can threaten a person's identity control, this chapter will be limited to examination of the impact of hospitalization. Threats to the continuity between past self, anticipated self, and perceptions of significant others can stem from loss of control in the following four dimension of one's hospital experience: physical, environmental, cognitive, and psychological.[26]

Loss of physical control

Prior to the illness the person's body provided mobility and accommodated physical comfort. The body usually performed as it was directed. During illness a person begins to lose control over physical functions. The body is unable to stop phenomena such as pain and hypoxia. There seems to be no way to physically control cancer growth, an internal hemorrhage, or an inflammatory process. Energy may not even be available to transport the body through space. The body may no longer be able to perform even the simple, everyday acts of walking to the bathroom or taking a bath, much less ingesting solid food. Therapeutic measures and devices such as anesthesia, traction, intravenous therapy, catheters and nasogastric tubes provide additional physical constrictions.[26,28] Such changes in physical control directly influence perceptions of one's body image.[11]

Body image is basic to continuity between the past self and the anticipated future self. Perceptions of disfigurement and/or loss of physical function may be experienced as psychological or social role losses. The degree of identity control lost in this dimension depends on the extent to which the individual's patterns of adaptations are interrupted. If the focal point of the person's past social role or status evolved primarily from a physical attribute such as strength, mobility, or attractiveness, the loss of physical control will have a great influence on the individual's sense of anticipated identity.

Loss of environmental control

Most hospitals have administrative policies to regulate environmental management. These policies are established to assure at least a minimal level of safety for patients and their possessions. Usually hospitals strongly suggest that patients keep only a minimal number of possessions and clothing with them. Patients are cautioned against keeping money or valued possessions in their rooms. Although these policies are intended to protect patients, it almost appears that the patients are being systematically stripped of the environmental props that identify their social status.

Patients usually have little control over decisions such as which room or bed they will be assigned, or who their roommate is to be. They don't even control such basics as their cleaning, drinking, eating, and medication schedules. An additional dimension of this loss of schedule control evolves from the lack of clock or calendar in the average hospital room. Time is such an important feature in our culture that Americans seem to "live by the clock," yet hospitals seldom provide patients with time cues for schedule orientation.

Environmental powerlessness invades even the territory that has been specifically assigned to the patient: the bed, nightstand, table, chair, and call light. The top of the stand or table is often taken over by the nurse for such things as dressings, trays, and bottles, and the patient's glasses, cards, books, toilet articles, and watch are placed into the drawer. After giving care, the nurse may forget to reposition the furniture and possessions so that the patient has access to them. The glass of water is 10 feet away, the chair is positioned so the patient is not able to get up without help, and the call light is out of reach. Such oversights regarding the call light can eliminate the patient's control in almost every dimension.[26,28]

The question still remains unanswered as to whether humans have a genetically determined capacity for territoriality. Behaviors of claiming and defending an area do suggest, however, that the territoriality drive arises from the need for security and identity. Relinquishing a claim to one's territory or the invasion of one's territory can threaten the identity definition that evolves from territory.[3,19]

Body territory includes the space encompassed by the body, whereas personal space is the area immediately surrounding the body.[18] As perspectives about identity become narrowed by limitations to mobility, territorial drive may intensify. Hospital staff members often must enter both the territory and the personal space of hospitalized persons to carry out activities on the patients' behalf. At times these activities become so routine that hospital personnel may forget that the activity involves intrusion. However, the patients may interpret these nonverbal communications as indifference to their comfort and/or dignity. Because patients have so little control over territorial and personal space in the hospital, such intrusions may be a source of loss of status and identity.[24]

In a study of intrusions of territory and personal space of hospitalized patients, Allekian[2] found that patients were less upset by intrusion into their body space than into their personal or territorial space. The patients perceived contact with body parts as necessary to treatments that had to be done. although the patients in this study reacted with annoyance when personnel moved the furniture in their space without asking, they were less annoyed when the objects moved were less related to their sense of identity. They had greater annoyance regarding the moving of their bedside table than removal of their chair, and even stronger reactions to the handling of their personal belongings without permission. However, even the raising or lowering of windows or shades without the patient sharing in the decision and the interactional intrusion of loud voices were sources of annoyance. Allekian[2] concluded that intrusions of territorial and personal space were perceived by the patients as reducing their personal evironmental control and their identity.

Loss of cognitive control

One of the most devastating losses hospitalized patients experience is that of knowledge.[28] In every new, stressful, or crisis situation the person involved attempts to assess the meaning of the things and events encountered and, if possible, determine possible consequences. The situation must be understood before coping strategies can be devised. Usually the necessary cues for comprehending what is occurring arise out of the social context of a situation. Similarities with past experiences help one understand and interpret the new experience. However, when the situation encountered is an uncommon event such as acute illness and hospitalization, a person has much greater difficulty defining what is being experienced, understanding implications of the event, and knowing how to respond in order to survive.[22]

A patient who perceives serious symptoms will attempt to identify the prognosis of the problem. However, the patient is at a loss to make such judgments when the needed formation is lacking. Most people interpret the withholding of information by the hospital staff as negative. Imaginations run rampant, and the patient envisions even the most innocuous events to have dreadful and dire consequences. For example, every new piece of equipment brought into the environment takes on personal significance and constitutes a threat. People who have not previously had such illness experiences tend to think that their reactions and feelings are unique. When patients do not receive adequate information about their progress or current situation from the health team, they attempt to obtain benchmarks of their progress by gathering information about others in similar situations.[27] Patients are often surprised and relieved to know how typical their symptoms are to the illness.

Although the lack of knowledge about physical progress may carry a greater threat, the lack of knowledge about even the simplest and most mundane aspects of one's experience can accentuate feelings of loss of control. Not knowing how to turn on the television or how to get another cup of coffee may be as frustrating as not knowing when the next pain pill is due or when the physician will make rounds.

No test or procedure is perceived as routine by the person who is to receive it. Even the taking of a temperature is not routine. This is not only because of the information these measures provide, but also the lack of infomation the patient may have about what is going to be done, when, how, and why. The situation appears to be one in which everyone knows what is going on within and around the patient except the patient.

Loss of psychological control

Variables that precipitate feelings of loss of psychological control during hospitalization can be divided into two categories. The first evolves from the routines and administrative structures of hospital. Many aspects of the system communicate to patients that they are not seen as individuals, but as objects, numbers, or diagnoses. The routines that direct the admission process, the waiting periods at clinics, and the hospital ward or room provisions are examples of aspects of the hospital system that can have a dehumanizing impact on patients. The long waiting periods at the clinics connote a form of abandonment.[4,32] Admission questions concerning financial arrangements, religious affiliation, and even marital status and age may seem to question the patient's value system and social status. The usual procedure of assigning a bed as the patient's place of residence in the hospital and directing the patient to remove clothes, don the hospital gown, and assume a horizontal position between white sheets can be perceived by the patient as being reduced to anonymity. The patient may not yet feel like a patient and may certainly not feel like going to bed. However, these factors are directed impersonally toward all persons served by the institution.

The accouterments of hospitalized patients deprive them of rights, privileges, satisfactions and status symbols that they may have spent years acquiring, and these losses may be intensified when the patients perceive that dehumanizing actions are being directed toward them personally.[15] It is a shock to find that one's name is not known and that in the eyes of the hospital staff one's identity resides in one's disease or bed location. Patients may find themselves referred to as "the G.I. bleeder in bed 3" or "Dr. Smith's surgical wound infection." When physicians and nurses on rounds talk over and about patients but never talk to or with them, there is no doubt in the patients' minds that they are viewed by the staff as objects of action rather than as people. The view that the patient is simply an acute problem or an extension of a machine may be particularly true of personnel attitudes in intensive care units. The comatose, heavily sedated, or irrational patient is easily seen as an extension of tubes, respirators, or signaling devices. Hospital personnel may spend much more time adjusting and tending the parts of machines than attending the patient as a person. Patients feel depersonalized when they are treated as inanimate, unhearing, unfeeling objects or as machines to be manipulated, addressed as fragmented problems, and treated with detachment. Self-expression, self-respect, affection, empathy, and social intercourse are almost as important as food, water, sleep, and elimination.

Feelings of psychological control evolve from feelings of trust and autonomy. When hospital personnel exclude the patient from discussions about the patient's condition, they convey that they do not view the patient's input as important. When nurses do not carry out even simple safety measures such as checking identification bands before administration of medication, they communicate disinterest in the patient's well-being. When nurses exclude the patient from decisions about even the most basic activities such as bathing and eating, it seems that the patient's ideas and desires are not important. The overall message sent is that patients are to be "done to" and not to be included in the "doing." Such omissions strip the patient of feelings of autonomy and destroy or prevent the development of feelings of trust.

BEHAVIORAL DEFINITION

The behaviors that characterize individuals whose identity control is being threatened or who perceive that it is being lost pertain to either the area in which control is being lost or to the area the person is using to compensate for the control loss.

Objective data

Loss of physical control. Patients frequently use two methods to avoid the shame, embarrassment, and humiliation that often accompany losses of body parts and/or functions. The person may become much less active and avoid social interactions, and/or the person may refuse to participate in or even acknowledge the care the changed body requires.

The patient may become quiet and withdraw from conversations. Requests to allow only family members to visit may be given to the nurse, or a sign may appear on the door of the patient's room commanding "keep the door closed." The patient may refuse to leave the hospital room or to get out of bed.

Individuals may aso refuse to become involved in physical care activities. This lack of involvement may range from passively allowing others to do what is required, such as dressing changes or appliance applications, to actively refusing even to look at the affected part. The individual may reverse all mirrors in the room or move the dresser so the body's reflection will not be seen. The patient who refuses therapy that is designed to improve lost function may be denying the loss. Yet this same person may acknowledge how helpful such therapy was for other patients. An example is a patient who has had a stroke and refuses to continue physical therapy as soon as a minimal amount of function returns. It is as if the patient were saying that if one does not notice or focus on the limp arm or dragging foot with therapy, these disabilities will not be there.

Another common denial technique is refusal to talk about the body change or loss. The patient may not allow conversation to focus on anything about the patient's physical being.

Loss of environmental control. The concreteness and maneuverability of the environment may provide the additional control needed to compensate for other control losses. An example of this is the patient's insistence that a specific piece of furniture or possession be kept in exactly the same place at all times or that each possession and piece of clothing be folded or arranged in exactly the same way each time it is used. These behaviors are similar to a young child's bedtime routine. Although the sequence of the routine is not in itself particularly functional, the sameness of the routine provides the security that the person has control over at least one sequence of events.

Loss of cognitive control. When feelings of loss of cognitive control persist, patients use a number of avenues to try to obtain information. The nurses may be sent on frequent reconnaissance missions to find out things such as whether the laboratory reports are back, whether or when the patient is to go to the x-ray or physical therapy department, and when the physician is coming.

In addition, there may be questions about other patients, for example, "How long has it been since Mr. J. had his surgery? How long did his surgery take? Who is his doctor? Did he have the same thing I do?" The answers to such questions provide information that can be used to compare the individual's situation with that of others.

Patients also frequently ask each other about their experiences. Symptoms, treatments, and outcomes may be compared in detail. Stories gathered in this manner are often retold to each new visitor as if they were a litany. Such ruminations help patients become more aware of progress parameters.

Loss of psychological control. Behaviors indicative of feelings of psychological control loss pertain to the narrowing of the perceptual focus that accompanies increased feelings of anxiety and ego disturbances. Individuals who have lost psychological control have difficulty using ideas and adapting to reality. Their attention span may be shortened; they may be unable to concentrate long enough on a task to complete it. These tasks could range from tasks as difficult as a colostomy irrigation to simply writing a letter. Disturbances in idea selection and specific drive preoccupation may accompany this shortened attention span. The same themes may be repeated in all conversations, and not uncommonly they contain a combination of unrelated or even opposing ideas. External stimuli are ineffective in breaking such idea cycles.

If feelings of psychological control loss escalate, a diffusion of orientation perspectives can occur, with the patient demonstrating confusion regarding time, place, and person referents.

Subjective data

Loss of physical control. Deteriorations in physical status are frequently accompanied by discouragement and depression as the individual perceives a decrease in the ability to maintain independence and social attractiveness. Sadness regarding the lost abilities, functions, or body parts is accompanied by shame, embarrassment, and/or humiliation that the body is now inferior. When despair and discouragement are the dominant feelings, the individual may appear passive. Verbalizations regarding the loss often include statements of condescension or resignation about what are perceived to be the inevitable results of the change in status, for example, "I suppose my wife will be wearing the pants in the family now," or, "As soon as I go home, I suppose I should try to sell the farm. A farmer can't farm without both hands."

When the dominant feelings are shame and humiliation, the individual's verbalizations most often carry anger or hostility. Postures of passive withdrawal may suddenly change as hostile statements project the patient's shame as anger at others. For example, when the physicians are on rounds, the patient may ask them, "Have you come to see the freak?" At times the patient may express anger through sarcastic humor. An example is the burn patient's statement, "Well, I can always get a job in a side show. They'd put me right next to the two-headed calf."

Giving a name to the support device, prosthesis, or appliance being used provides an avenue for making fun of the device without acknowledging that it is an extension of the individual. The hemodialysis patient's referral to the dialysis machine as Susie Bell and question, "Is Susie Bell ready for me today? You know we really have a thing going between us," show how jest can be used to cover true feelings and fears.

Loss of environmental control. Annoyance, indignation, and anger are precipitated by intrusions into a person's territory. However, the expression of such feelings may not be directed at the party perceived to be the source of the affront. When the intruder is thought to be powerful or in control of the patient's physical destiny, the frustration and anger are often displaced to other personnel. Anger may be expressed about such safe subjects as the food (e.g., "It is bad and always cold; there is never enough coffee"), the other patients (e.g., "They are always noisy at night"), or the personnel (e.g., "Why can't the other nurses be as good as you are? No one but you ever pays any attention to what I need").

Loss of cognitive control. The patient who is left in ignorance about what is to happen is highly susceptible to reality distortion and fantasy activation. The anxiety associated with the new and the unknown places the person in a state of constant vigilance. Prolonging such a state can result in a sense of fatigue. The patient may be unable to rest because of worry about what is happening or is going to happen. The patient may make statements such as "I am so tired, but I just can't rest because I'm worried about. . . ."

Loss of psychological control. The process of human reduction, or dehumanization, results from one's perception of being treated as a thing or object of action. Doubts, confusion, and uncertainty develop regarding encounters with others. The person begins to question what is really being experienced. Feelings of numbness, strangeness, and unreality precipitate the belief that life is just happening, is not being lived. Heightened feelings of isolation, loneliness, and alienation develop. The patient may believe that others are indifferent to the private feelings being experienced and that it is useless to try to communicate. These feelings may increase to the point that the individual is unable to describe what is being experienced. The patient may make statements regarding anticipated negative criticisms such as "There is no use to talk to anyone here; they don't listen; they won't believe you anyway. They don't really care what happens to a person. They don't even know your name."

INTERVENING VARIABLES

A patient's responses to the identity threats and control losses that occur during hospitalization are accentuated by social expectations and modified by the social support system.

Social expectations

The social expectations that influence identity control evolve from the mastery of previous developmental tasks and the status of current developmental tasks. In addition to developmental expectations, the social definition of illness identifies social sick-role expectations.

Developmental expectations. At each stage of growth the individual self exists in relationship to others. Therefore the definition of self hinges on the ability to interpret and respond to social cues. Erikson's developmental model speaks to the interaction between self and others at each stage of growth. The family composes the society for the child during the first two developmental stages. The idea of "me" gradually develops during infancy. Feelings of trust develop as the child's behavior evokes responses that help meet the child's needs. The feedback the child receives during the second developmental stage forms the foundation of the child's self-concept. The self experiences different degrees of being "good me," "bad me," and "not me." If the tasks of these two stages, the development of trust and autonomy, are not adequately mastered, the potential is high for recurring identity confusion throughout life. Each of the successive developmental tasks of initiative, industry, identity, intimacy, generativity, and integrity add new dimensions to and demand resynthesis of the self. Each task must be adequately mastered to allow success in future tasks. The earlier the stage in which a task is not mastered, the more involved the effect on the individual's ability to maintain identity control. In addition, the task that is currently in the process of completion is the most vulnerable area of identity. If the threat to identity involves the realm of the current developmental task, the individual will have much less adaptive flexibility. The person in the midst of developing intimate relationships may be devastated by things that threaten intimacy. For example, such a person may find death preferable to a colostomy. However, a farmer facing generativity mastery may find the loss of a hand much more devastating than having a colostomy. Such a body change should not necessarily drive his wife away, but it may be seen as something that will decrease or destroy his productive capacity, force him to sell his farm, and change his social identity.

Sick-role expectations. Society defines illness in terms of the social role the individual is expected to fulfill. A person is perceived to be ill when unable to fulfill the responsibilities of that role. From this perspective, disease, or pathology, is not synonymous with illness. For example, although a broken leg does present pathological changes, it is not perceived as an illness unless it prevents the person from fulfilling role responsibilities. This definition of illness focuses on the condition's consequences to society. Social expectations regarding the sick role arise from this perspective. Illness will exempt a person from role responsibilities. However, accompanying this exemption is the social requirement that the person seek help and that the person follow the advice and accept the help received. In addition, as an outgrowth of the person's need for help, the community recognizes the person's need to be dependent in the areas related to the illness. These social expectations regarding illness and sick role are especially pertinent to those who are acutely ill. Unfortunately, most hospital systems are structured to treat the patient as if the dependency were not limited to those areas related to the illness. The hospital structure encourages and rewards passivity and dependence. Too often the ideal patient is the docile person who surrenders a measure of self-integrity.

Strength of social support system

During times of stress a person depends heavily on the support and assistance of others. The continuance of a sense of efficacy depends on the extent of the individual's social network and the strength of attachment to that network. When a person perceives identity threats, the need for affiliation increases.[29] When affiliations or social supports are sufficiently strong, they can provide central meaning to a person's life. When the interaction of affiliations involves nurture, empathy, encouragement, information, material assistance, and, most important, sharing, the affiliation diminishes the perceived impact of almost any adversity. Often the mere knowledge that this type of support is available if needed is enough to give a person the confidence required to cope with the given situation.

NURSING INTERVENTION—GOALS AND EVALUATION CRITERIA

Since hospitalization generates some degree of threat to every patient's perceptions of control, the nursing management of this concept is important to the progress of all patients, regardless of the presence of other concepts. Other psychological concepts are often precipitated by threats to an individual's identity. Therefore the nursing care designed to strengthen and/or restore the individual's identity control can often forestall more extreme coping strategies such as agitated, destructive, and bizarre behavior and psychological immobility.

Nursing activities directed at reducing or neutralizing the threat to identity control brought about by the hospitalization have two primary goals. The first is to help the hospitalized individual maintain feelings of autonomy or control over the social situation. The second goal is to allow the patient's energy to be directed toward healing and restoration. The development of a trust relationship is interwoven with the maintenance or return of the patient's feelings of control. As trust increases and feelings of control are strengthened, the addition of this new support structure reduces the patient's need for constant vigilance. The subgoals that assist the achievement of these primary goals are either to neutralize the effects of the antecedent control loss or to compensate for the loss by accentuating feelings of control in a different dimension.

Increase psychological control

Strengthening an individual's sense of identity control begins with provisions directed at increasing the psychological control felt by the person. This involves personalizing nursing care and relating to the patient as unique and important. Some simple approaches that can assist in achieving this goal are the use of common courtesy such as introducing oneself, learning and using the patient's name, including significant others in introductions, identifying other staff members by name, and making sure patients in close proximity are acquainted with one another. These measures convey the message that the patient is perceived as having a personal identity. In addition, the exchange of names through introductions is a sharing of oneself and an opening to continued and expanded sharing. The nonverbal message of such courtesy is that the patient is seen as an individual.

An admission nursing history can also reinforce the message that the patient's nursing care will be personalized. Inquiries regarding the patient's usual life patterns and methods used to meet basic needs convey interest in the person's comfort. The nursing history not only helps the nurse identify problem areas and develop plans for needed assistance, but also helps the patient develop self-awareness in areas that may not commonly be addressed. The identification of the patient's strength and control in the meeting of certain basic needs can strengthen feelings of security regarding ability or function. In addition, such discussions can convey the nurse's interest in the person. It often is an unusual experience to discuss one's sleeping, eating, and/or elimination habits with another. If the other person not only willingly listens to such information, but in fact encourages the discussion, the clear nonverbal message is that the nurse is interested in the person as an individual. It should, of course, be made clear to the patient why such information is being gathered. Identification of the patient's significant others, the part they play in the patient's life, whether and how often they will be visiting, their involvement in the patient's care, and the degree of their understanding and knowledge of the patient's condition can help the nursing staff develop a plan supportive of the patient's needs. A nursing history that includes this type of information as well as data regarding basic needs and usual patterns conveys to patients that they have a voice in decisions regarding their care.

However, if such information is gathered but never used in the nursing care, the patient may soon feel betrayed and/or may be mistrustful when subsequent overtures are attempted.

Since no one nurse can provide care 24 hours a day, it is necessary to keep up-to-date written plans regarding the patient's progress and preferred patterns of care. This enables the staff to coordinate efforts and provide continuity to the message of personalized interest. When patients must re-explain each day their preferences regarding morning care, they soon have no doubt that they are not and will not be heard regarding more important matters. If the nurses cannot remember when a dressing is to be changed, how can the patient trust them to remember such a thing as an allergy to penicillin?

Limiting the number of persons assigned to the patient's care can also assist in maintaining continuity. In addition, reducing the number of persons with whom the patient must validate trustworthiness reduces demands on the patient's vigilance.

Meeting commitments made to the patients also contributes to the patients' sense of psychological control. Certain institutional commitments relating to the medical management of the patient, including such things as administration of medication and treatments, must be met. When the nursing staff consistently administers ordered treatments on time, safely, and in a skilled, comfortable manner, patients become more secure in the belief that the staff knows how to and will care for them. If these commitments are neglected, the care and safety of the patients are undermined.

A second area of commitment relates to the independent functions of the nurse. For example, the recognition of a comfort need and the implementation of comfort measures indicate the nurse is alert to the patient's interests. If a patient does not receive a breakfast tray and the nurse promises to find out why, a commitment has been made. If the nurse does not return with the tray or an explanation of its absence, the commitment has not been met.

The nurse's recognition of a need of the patient, making a commitment to assist with that need, and fulfillment of the commitment can indicate to the patient that the nurse is watchful regarding the patient's interests even without prompting. For example, the nurse might observe, "It seems a little cool tonight. Would you like another blanket available for your use?" The nurse noticed the need, identified it, and allowed the patient to make the decision. Of course, if the patient agrees and the blanket or an explanation of its absence does not appear, trust will be eroded.

A third type of commitment relates to the patient's right to be knowledgeable about things of concern. The patient who is informed in advance about rules, procedures, schedules, and the physical and social environment of the hospital is more emotionally prepared for the upcoming experiences. Advanced preparation may not always be possible, particularly when plans are changed, but explanations after the fact are better than none at all.

Nonverbal communication is very influential in conveying the nurse's concern and interest in the patient. The nurse who takes time to sit at the patient's bedside to talk, even if only for a few minutes each day, indicates interest and willingness to listen. Eye contact during these conversations sends the nonverbal message that the nurse is willing to become involved in the patient's interests and concerns. This can be particularly important with patients who have a physical deformity or disfiguring illness. People who feel uncomfortable about themselves look to see how they are received by others. If acceptance is conveyed by the nurse through facial expressions and eye contact, the individual can begin to develop self-acceptance and gain an increased sense of psychological control. Touch can also be a powerful means of nonverbally communicating personal interest and acceptance, but it must be used judiciously and with a careful reading of how the patient is responding. Whereas some people find touch reassuring, others view it as a threatening personal invasion.

As can be noted in the previous discussion, the strengthening of control feelings in any of the dimensions of the hospital experience will facilitate the development of a trust relationship. Feelings of psychological control are strengthened through personalization of care and acceptance of the patient as a person of worth.

Increase in the patient's feelings of psychological control can be measured by behaviors that represent trust development. Behavioral cues such as looking at the nurse and making eye contact, allowing the nurse close physical proximity, referring to the nurse by name, introducing the nurse to significant others, and/or asking the nurse questions concerning care indicate the patient is developing a trusting relationship with the nurse.

Increase environmental control

Hospitalized patients often feel at the mercy of the environment. The hospital schedule is foreign to them, the equipment brought into the room is often ominous looking, and even the arrangement of the furnishings of the room may not meet their needs. Giving patients as much control as possible over the environment often allows them to believe they have some influence over what is happening. Having patients decide such matters as where the bedside table is placed, whether the privacy curtain is drawn or open, the most convenient location for the call light, when they would like a bath, or what they would like for dinner can convey to patients that not only are they allowed to make decisions but that it is expected they will do so.

Since nursing care often involves intrusive procedures, it is important to recognize and respect the patient's personal space and territory. Patients should be asked for permission before their privacy is invaded, and whenever possible they should be allowed to state the most convenient time for that invasion. Permission should always be sought when handling patients' personal belongings, and the patients should be included in decisions regarding the storage and/or location of their possessions. When possessions are relocated to make room for administration of a treatment, the nurse should explain why the objects are being moved and whether they can be returned after the procedure.

When possible, patients should be allowed to use and display possessions as they wish. The nurse should determine whether the patient desires such things as a particular arrangement of toilet articles, a display of family pictures or cards, or the use of personal clothing. When possible, patients should be given as much space as they appear to need to be comfortable. Often the more threatened a person feels by a situation, the greater the needed "buffer area."[16] The personalization of territory, the acknowledgment of it as the patient's territory, and the patient's right to control its use should assist in strengthening the individual's environmental control. Often this increase in control over concrete and familiar items or events can compensate for control losses in other dimensions. Mrs. D. provided a dramatic example of this. This 90-year-old woman had been hospitalized with a fractured hip. When her granddaughter visited a few days after admission, Mrs. D. confided that the community hospital was certainly providing much poorer service than it used to: "I don't know why, but all they bring on the meal trays is bread and milk." When the granddaughter expressed surprise at this, Mrs. D. insisted that it was so. After their visit the granddaughter asked the head nurse about the meal trays, explaining what Mrs. D. said. The nurse said that complete meals were being served, but all the woman would eat was bread and milk, and that this was of considerable concern to the staff. On the next visit two major changes were found. The furniture in the room was completely rearranged. Grandma explained, "I talked the aide into moving the furniture. It's much better this way." Later she noted, "The sisters must be back on top of things. I'm starting to get meat, potatoes, and desserts on my trays." Giving this woman some control over her environment had reduced her anxiety about the hospitalization to the point where she could again perceive events realistically.

Since excessive environmental control demands by the patient often indicate that other needs are not being met, it can be expected that as other areas of control are enhanced, environmental demands will lessen. A decrease in the patient's projection of angry feelings (e.g., complaints about room temperature or cold coffee) or a decrease in a compulsive need for room arrangements can indicate an increase in the patient's feelings of control.

Increase cognitive control

Knowledge and information are necessary for people to gain a sense of cognitive control over what is happening to them. Pointing out progress that is being made and providing patients with benchmarks of further progress enable cognitive preparation for the future. Telling patients about similar experiences of other patients helps them know they are not the only ones in their situation. Such explanations, however, should not minimize the patient's concerns. For example, the statement "Oh, all our patients here have had similar experiences during the recovery phase," does not convey the same message as do examples of common experiences of other patients and indication of recognition of the patient's individual responses, such as "I can see how you might be concerned about what is happening to you. This experience is to be expected at this phase of your recovery. Most people find the third day after surgery a difficult day."

Information regarding events that will occur, sequences and timing of treatments or tests, the meanings behind procedures, and even why a procedure is done a certain way provides control through cognitive understanding. However, a patient may appear disinterested or even increasingly anxious as explanations are given. Such responses need to be examined to determine whether the patient understands the terminology being used or whether other fears or concerns are interfering with the patient's ability to focus on what is being said. The patient's anxiety level may be interfering not only with ability to comprehend, but also readiness to learn.

It may be difficult for a patient to understand explanations about coming events because the items and/or events being discussed are not familiar. For example, the patient may have no idea what a cardiac monitor or a piggyback I.V. is, much less a cystoscope. If the real item is not available, pictures are useful in familiarizing the patient with its size, shape, and use.

Children particularly need concrete interaction regarding events and equipment before they are ready to encounter them. One of the primary ways children gain feelings of control over the events in their life is through play. During play children can assume the position of being in charge. They are able to manipulate objects and events and observe the results. Feelings can be safely expressed through action, and roles can be understood through practice. Play therapy is a valuable method for desensitizing children to the hospital and the events that are to occur there. Allowing children to see the rooms they will be visiting, to handle the equipment they will encounter, and to don such things as the physician's surgical clothes helps desensitize them to these things. Treatments such as dressings and injections are much less threatening to children if the children have first been allowed to administer them to their dolls.

Including significant others in information-sharing sessions provides the patient with someone who can validate the message. Also, significant others can help the patient identify predicted progress. Asking the patient what previously had been explained and articulating the new information with the previous explanation can help the patient structure the newly acquired knowledge as well as provide an opportunity to dispel misperceptions.

Interaction with support groups composed of patients with similar problems can also strengthen cognitive control. Hearing others identify problems they have encountered and explain how they have handled them not only provides examples of how to cope but also helps dissipate the fear of the uniqueness and unmanageableness of the situation.

Criteria indicating an increase in cognitive control include increased understanding of explanations provided by hospital personnel (manifested by ability to repeat information correctly) and decreased data-gathering behavior such as continued asking of questions and repetitive comparing of situations. Decreased vigilance and the ability to rest and relax are further verification of increased cognitive control.

Increase physical control

Gradually increasing a patient's involvement in care activities and consistently benchmarking recovery progress increase the patient's awareness that return to health is occurring and return to physical self-sufficiency is a possibility. When patients are not consistently informed of healing progress, they often attach negative interpretation to observed events. For example, a surgical incision can be a disquieting sight. If dressing changes are performed under a cloak of silence, the patient may perceive that the incision is something to disdain. However, if the nurse notes how nicely it is healing and how healthy the tissue looks, the patient is provided with a realistic, specific appraisal of healing progress. Such focusing on specific physical functioning assists the patient in the redevelopment of a sense of physical powerfulness. Such appraisal should include not only identification of the current status, but also, when possible, comparisons with usual progress and with past functioning levels. The following conversation provides an example of this:

Patient: I don't seem to be getting my strength back very fast.
Nurse: You do seem a little shaky, but that's not unusual. Remember, yesterday you were only able to sit on the edge of the bed for a few minutes. Today you made it to the chair and back. That's a big improvement. Tomorrow I'll help you walk over to the door.

When the change in the patient's physical self involves the loss of a function or body part, the individual must adapt body image perceptions to incorporate the changes. Although it would be unrealistic to propose that the body change was a positive occurrence, perceptions regarding the patient's body should be advanced with a neutral or a positive attitude. For example, when a patient's dysfunctioning leg is continually referred to as the bad leg, it is more difficult for the patient to adopt a body image that accepts the changed limb.

The attitudes of hospital personnel during initial adjustment periods can be very influential. This group of people provides a segment of society that the patient can use to judge social reactions to the bodily changes. Since body image is developed in a large measure through the social reinforcement provided by others, the reactions of significant others are also relied on during periods of body image reconceptualization.

The patient's family and friends compose a second group of reacting significant others. Although the patient may feel accepted by those who provide care in the hospital, the ability to face the future depends a great deal on the reactions and understanding of the people who will play an important part in that future. Many of the patient's adaptive changes depend on the family's interaction. Explaining to the patient's close significant others the physical changes that have occurred and the progress that has been accomplished and that can be expected better prepares them to provide the reactions and reinforcement needed by the patient during the reconceptualization period.

A third level of support during this process can be provided by other patients who have had similar disruptions. Resource people from such groups as the United Ostomy Association or Reach to Recovery often help patients understand that the physical problem can be mastered. Group meetings can be an important means of mutual support in which patients begin to reformulate their body image by identifying with, learning from, and helping others in similar circumstances.

Patients who have experienced very traumatic or extreme body disturbances and those who had negative body images prior to the body part loss may require extended assistance in the reconceptualization process. The hospitalization period may be too brief to allow for the needed resolution of feelings toward the body change. In such instances coping strategies such as agitation, psychological immobility, and/or destructive behavior may be exhibited. These persons need continued support while making the required societal adjustments, and they should be referred to external sources that can provide this support (e.g., public health nurse agencies, community mental health clinics, rehabilitation centers, psychiatric hospital outpatient departments, private psychologists, and psychiatric nurses).

Behavioral criteria that indicate the patient is experiencing increased feelings of physical control and reconstruction of body image include identification of physical changes and verbalization of plans to accommodate to the changes (e.g., the patient might say, "I've found that I can't get out of bed on the right side, but with the chair placed on the left side of the bed I can move from the bed to the chair in one motion", acceptance of an appointment with a resource person to join a patient support group, and interest in rehabilitation or physical therapy.

CONCEPT OUTLINE

I. *Conceptual definition:* Loss of identity control is the experience of major or minor alterations or uncertainties regarding self-definition and efficacy in maintaining control over one's life situation.

II. *Antecedent conditions*
  A. Loss of physical control
  B. Loss of environmental control
  C. Loss of cognitive control
  D. Loss of psychological control

III. *Behavioral definition*
  A. Objective data
    1. Loss of physical control
      a. Avoidance of social interaction
      b. Refusal to participate in or acknowledge care body requires
      c. Refusal to leave hospital room or bed
      d. Avoidance of looking at body changes
      e. Avoidance of talking about physical functioning
      f. Refusal of rehabilitative therapies
    2. Loss of environmental control
      a. Insistence on sameness in routines of care
      b. Rigid routines of use and placement of possessions
    3. Loss of cognitive control
      a. Sending of nurses on reconnaissance missions
      b. Asking about progress of other patients
      c. Exchange of information with other patients about illness experiences
    4. Loss of psychological control
      a. Shortened attention span
      b. Disturbances in idea selection and preoccupation
      c. Diffusion of orientation perspectives
  B. Subjective data
    1. Loss of physical control
      a. Shame, embarrassment, and humiliation
      b. Despair and discouragement
      c. Condescendence and resignation
      d. Projection of anger at others
      e. Sarcastic humor
      f. Assignment of names to support devices
    2. Loss of environmental control
      a. Expression of anger regarding safe subjects such as food, noise, other patients, and other staff
    3. Loss of cognitive control
      a. Fatigue
      b. Statements regarding worries
    4. Loss of psychological control
      a. Feelings of numbness, strangeness, and unreality
      b. Feelings of isolation and alienation

c. Anticipation of negative criticisms
d. Difficulty describing feelings

IV. *Intervening variables*
A. Social expectations
1. Developmental expectations
2. Sick-role expectations
3. Strength of social support system

V. *Nursing interventions—goals*
A. Increase psychological control
1. Use of common courtesy
2. Use of patient's name
3. Use of nursing history to identify usual life patterns
4. Explanation of reason such information is being gathered
5. Identification of knowledge level of patient and significant others
6. Communication with staff via written plan for patient
7. Assignment of limited number of persons to care for patient
8. Fulfillment of commitments
9. Use of nonverbal actions to communicate concern and interest
a. Touch
b. Eye contact
c. Sitting at bedside

B. Increase environmental control
1. Patient allowed to decide furniture placement when possible
2. Encouragment of patient's participation in decisions regarding basic care when possible
3. Permission requested to invade patinet's privacy
4. Permission requested to handle patient's personal possessions
5. Patient allowed to make decisions regarding use of or display of personal possessions when possible

C. Increase cognitive control
1. Provision of benchmarks of progress
2. Provision of information regarding sequence and timing of events
3. Exposure of patient to concrete and/or pictorial examples of equipment
4. Use of play therapy with children
5. Inclusion of significant others in information sessions
6. Use of patient support groups for sharing of perceptions and problems

D. Increase physical control
1. Provision of realistic, specific appraisal of progress
2. Focus on physical functioning ability
3. Referral to body change in neutral or positive terms
4. Increase of patient's involvement in care of body
5. Provision of social reinforcement of acceptance through personnel, family, significant others, and patient groups
6. Referral to external support services when assistance with adjustment is required after hospitalization

VI. *Evaluation criteria*
A. Use of names of personnel
B. Introduction of personnel to significant others
C. Freely asking questions of personnel
D. Decreased incidence of angry projections
E. Decreased need for maintenance of specific routine
F. Increased ability to correctly explain reason for and sequences of therapeutic measures
G. Increased ability to relax and rest
H. Willingness to talk about physical changes
I. Verbalization of plans to accommodate for changes
J. Participation in discussions of patient groups
K. Acceptance of rehabilitation or physical therapy
L. Acceptance of appointments with external resource persons

REFERENCES

1. Abend, S. M.: Problems of identity: theoretical and clinical applications, Psychoanal. Q. **43**(4):606, 1974.
2. Allekian, C.: Intrusions of territory and personal space: an exploratory study of anxiety-inducing factors in hospitalized patients, Int. J. Psychiatry Med. **5**:27, 1974.
3. Ardrey, R.: The territorial imperative, New York, 1966, Atheneum Publishers.
4. Carnoy, J. M.: Kaiser, you pay your money and you take your chances, Ramparts **9**:26, 1970.
5. DeLevita, D. J.: The concept of identity, translated by I. Finlay, New York, 1965, Basic Books, Inc., Publishers.
6. Erikson, E. H.: The problem of ego identity, J. Am. Psychoanal. Assoc. **4**:56, 1956.
7. Erikson, E. H.: Identity and the life cycle, selected papers, New York, 1959, International Universities Press, Inc.

8. Erikson, E. H.: Childhood and society, ed. 2, New York, 1963, W. W. Norton & Co., Inc.
9. Erikson, E. H.: Identity versus identity diffusion. In Mussen, P. H., Conger, J. J., and Kagen, J., editors: Readings in child development and personality, New York, 1965, Harper & Row, Publishers, Inc.
10. Erikson, E. H.: Identity, youth, and crisis, New York, 1966, W. W. Norton & Co., Inc.
11. Fisher, S., and Cleveland, S. E.: Body image and personality, ed. 2, New York, 1968, Dover Publications, Inc.
12. Fleischman, A. I., Bierenbaum, M. L., and Stier, A.: Effect of stress due to anticipated minor surgery upon in vivo platelet aggregation in humans, J. Human Stress **2**:33, 1976.
13. Gerth, H. H., and Mills, C. W.: Character and social structure, the psychology of social institutions, New York, 1964, Harcourt, Brace, & World, Inc.
14. Greenacre, P.: Early physical determinants in the development of the sense of identity, J. Am. Psychoanal. Assoc. **6**:612, 1958.
15. Henderson, A. R.: Psychology of hospitalized patients, J. Natl. Med. Assoc. **68**:378, 1976.
16. Horowitz, M., Duff D., and Stratton, L.: Body buffer zone, Arch. Gen. Psychiatry **2**:650, 1964.
17. Jacobson, E.: The self and the object world, New York, 1964, International Universities Press, Inc.
18. Little, K. B.: Personal space, J. Exp. Soc. Psychol. **1**:237, 1965.
19. Lyman, S. M., and Scott, M. B.: Territoriality: a neglected sociological dimension, Soc. Problems **15**:236, 1967.
20. Mahler, M.: Panel on problems of identity, J. Am. Psychoanal. Assoc. **6**131, 1958.
21. Mason, J. W., Sachar, E. J., Fishman, J. R., Hamburg, D. A., and Handlon, J. H.: Corticosteroid responses to hospital admission, Arch. Gen. Psychiatry **13**:1, 1965.
22. Mechanic, D.: Illness behavior, social adaptation, and the management of illness, a comparison of educational and medical models, J. Nerv. Ment. Dis. **165**:79, 1977.
23. Paranjpe, A. C.: In search of identity, New York, 1975, John Wiley & Sons, Inc.
24. Plutchik, R.: The emotions: facts, theories, and a new model, New York, 1962, Random House, Inc.
25. Pride, L. F.: An adrenal stress index as a criterion measure for nursing, Nurs. Res. **17**:292, 1968.
26. Roberts, S. L.: Behavioral concepts and the critically ill patient, Englewood Cliffs, N.J., 1976, Prentice-Hall, Inc.
27. Roth, J. A.: Timetables, structuring the passage of time in hospital treatment and other careers, Indianapolis, 1963, The Bobbs-Merrill Co., Inc.
28. Saylor, D. E.: Understanding patient's feelings of loss, Hosp. Progr. **58**:88, 1977.
29. Schacter, S.: The psychology of affiliation: experimental studies of the sources of gregariousness, Stanford, Calif. 1959, Stanford University Press.
30. Spiegel, L. A.: The self, the sense of self, and perception. In: The psychoanalytic study of the child, Vol. 14, New York, 1959, International Universities Press, Inc.
31. Spiegel, L. A.: Identity and adolescence. In Lorand, S., and Schneer, H., editors: Adolescents: psychoanalytic approach to problems and therapy, New York, 1961, Paul B. Hoeber, Inc.
32. Sussman, M. B., Caplan, E. K., Haug, M. R., and Stern, M. R.: The walking patient: a study in outpatient care, Cleveland, 1967, The Press of Case Western Reserve University.
33. Tabachnick, N.: Three psycho-analytic views of identity, Int. J. Psychoanal. **46**:467, 1965.
34. Tabachnick, N.: Self-realization and social definition, two aspects of identity formation, Int. J. Psychoanal. **48**:68, 1967.
35. Weigert, A. J., and Hastings, R.: Identity loss, family and social change, Am. J. Sociol. **82**:1171, 1977.

disorganized scattering
ideas
teter-toddles
on the edge
of some dark threat
jumble-tumble
disconnected present
resurrected past
singing
with bubbling laughter
sobbing with muted tears
jet spray of wanton words
say
what is best
forgot.

PAULETTE R. Di ANGI

CAROLYN K. DREESSEN KINNEY

Chapter 3

AGITATION

CONCEPTUAL DEFINITION

Agitation involves the expression of feelings through actions or body language rather than verbal descriptions of inner anxieties, fears, and conflicts.[7,18,20] Agitation is an action state in which body movements are irregular, continuous, rapid, or vigorous; the mind and/or feelings are excited or disturbed; and speech is excited and/or in earnest.

When a person experiences a threat to self-esteem, anxiety is evoked. The individual's physiological response to this anxiety stimulates the autonomic nervous system and increases production of epinephrine, preparing the person to fight or flee from the perceived threat.[7] Whether an individual proceeds to a fight or a flight response depends on a combination of factors from the person's past experiences and the present situation. Until an internal, unconscious decision is made concerning whether to fight or flee, the individual experiences ambivalence, which may be manifested outwardly as agitated behavior.

Agitation does not represent retreat from a stress-producing situation, but is an individual's unconscious attempt at diversional activity that, in effect, postpones the fight or flight decision. The increase in physical activity functions both as a stopgap measure for release of pent-up energy and as a means of communicating needs of which the agitated individual may not even be aware. Often an agitated person appears to be overtly communicating one message, whereas the primary message is less obvious. For example, a man who was hospitalized on a psychiatric unit while he underwent tests to determine whether he had a brain tumor repeatedly approached the ward's locked door and vigorously shook and rattled it. The psychiatric aide who was caring for him interpreted this behavior to mean that the patient was angry and wanted to leave. The aide attemped to find out why he was angry and to explain why he could not leave the area. Later, when the nurse talked with the man, it was found that he was not angry but simply did not think he belonged there.

Agitation occurs in most people at one time or another in varying degrees. Agitated behavior becomes a problem or is maladaptive only when it consistently prevents the individual from dealing with the present.

Agitation may escalate until it reaches an extreme, diffuse form of manic behavior or hyperactivity. Kalkman[18] believes that such behavior is an escape into action rather than facing or attempting to understand problems. During this period of escalated activity the person's threshold to both internal and external stimuli is lowered. The person becomes very responsive to all the surrounding stimuli; yet, at the same time, the individual can be selectively inattentive almost to the point of being nonresponsive to another's attempts to communicate.[16] The short attention span and the inability to focus on important details of the environment can create a continued need for activity in the individual. The response of others in the environment and the amount of incoming stimuli can be the ultimate factors that influence whether an individual becomes agitated and the degree to which agitation is manifested. Although hyperactivity usually lacks obvious goal direction, it may be a means of attempting to gain control of self and others.[18]

Acting out behavior is a type of agitated behavior; it demonstrates the cyclical nature of agitation.[20] A person may have an unsatisfied need for attention. If unable or unwilling to express this need verbally, the person may use acting out behavior as a means of attaining attention. If the agitation does gain the desired attention, the behavior may be reinforced and repeated. If, instead, fear and anger are precipitated in others and they react in a punitive or restrictive way, the person's desperation for the desired attention may be aggravated. The person's hostility, resentment, or confusion may perpetuate and accentuate the agitated behavior. Agitation can accelerate to the type of aggressive, destructive behavior described by Clack[8] as a forceful verbal, nonverbal, or symbolic abuse of self, another person, or thing either in actual or attempted actions. This phenomenon of destructive behavior is discussed in Chapter 6.

Generally the psychodynamics involved in the process of agitation are as follows:

1. An individual experiences a situation in which certain expectations are not satisfied or met. This is perceived as a threat to or loss of self-esteem.
2. The resultant feelings of anger, fear, and/or anxiety increase available energy with the increase of epinephrine.
3. If the individual is unable or unwilling to express the feelings verbally, body activity may be used to dissipate some of the energy or to communicate the feelings.
4. If this behavior does not result in satisfaction of the individual's need, the behavior may escalate.
5. This escalation may change the agitated behavior to violent destructive behavior. The behavior may also move into a diffuse form of agitation wherein the individual becomes oversensitive and overresponsive to all stimuli, which supports a continued state of hyperactivity. If the hyperactivity does not help the individual escape the omnipresent depressive thoughts associated with the loss of self-esteem or if exhaustion results from a continued and unabated physiological and psychological depletion, psychological immobility can occur. This concept is discussed in Chapter 4.

ANTECEDENT CONDITIONS

A threat to or loss of self-esteem associated with one or more of the following conditions is a common antecedent to agitation.

Developmental arrest

Genesis of some agitated behaviors such as acting out has been placed by some authors in the late infancy to toddler stage.[11,14] However, the general behavior patterns seen in agitaton more closely resemble those in the preadolescent to adolescent developmental stage. The effect of earlier development on the adolescent period must be recognized, since mastery of each succeeding task depends on previous accomplishments. If earlier developmental tasks have been unsuccessful, the individual lacks resources for later developmental crises.[10] This is particularly so during adolescence because at this stage all accomplishments of previous development form an integrated whole. The personality reorganization that should occur during these phases of growth involves not only the development of identity but of autonomy as well. Problems may arise as emancipation from parents and childhood is sought.[26]

Acting out types of behavior can be expected especially in preadolescence and adolescence, since this age is marked with fantasy and impulses expressed in action rather than symbolic thinking.[27] This behavior often represents a cry for help from an individual who senses a loss of inner control.[3] The child is faced with a conflict between desire for independence and need for dependence. Adolescents seek freedom and at the same time are fearful of it. They frequently appear to reject external authority while wishing for external forces to limit their expression of freedom. When reasonable limits are imposed, the adolescent feels more confident to explore avenues of expression within those limits.[17]

Verbal communication helps establish individuation, form body image, and develop a sense of identity. The ability to use speech also provides a means for testing reality. When wants and wishes consistently remain unexpressed verbally, actions tend to become a form of wordless communication.[4] If this inhibition persists during the adolescent developmental phase, defective word-symbol formation results. The individual then tends to show what is being felt or thought rather than express it verbally.

If the individual is unable to master the adolescent developmental tasks, an impasse or arrest in the development of the behavior repertoire may occur.[5] Individuals with this problem tend to rely on nonverbal, action-oriented, or agitated behavior to help them cope with each new challenge. This behavior may become so much a part of the individual that past unmastered stressful experiences may dominate perceptions of present situations.[5] The individual ineffectively relives past conflicts rather than face each new situation as a unique encounter. Unresolved past conflicts prevent the person from directing energy to present situations to comprehend the current reality.

Environmental uncertainties and inconsistencies

The reactions of a person who has been repeatedly exposed to an uncertain environment, in which it is impossible to know what is expected of oneself or what in turn can be expected from others, will be tentative and uncertain. Rexford[30] found that in families in which the parents did not provide consistent warmth and appropriate limits the children were more likely to act out their conflicts and anxieties. The ambivalence and inconsistencies that predominate in the relationship between such parents and their children seem to encourage the children to demonstrate rather than verbalize their feelings.

When individuals confront inconsistency and/or ambivalence in a situation in later life, the adolescent, action-oriented behavior may again emerge. For example, when admitted to an acute care setting, a person is placed in a situation in which conflict of dependence versus independence is often experienced. The person is faced with the need to be cared for by others, while at the same time perhaps desiring to remain independent and self-sufficient. When health care providers do not allow a client the opportunity to express needs, wants, and desires verbally, the individual is likely to resort to communicating nonverbally through body actions. In addition to these stresses, the acute care setting is fraught with uncertainties regarding such elements as diagnostic procedures, unfamiliar surroundings, ambiguous requirements and demands on the patient, life-threatening prognoses, and painful treatment procedures. Individuals may attempt to gain some sense of security by using action or activity to control this uncertain situation, which contains many elements typical of those experienced during adolescence.

Catecholamine levels

The catecholamine hypothesis proposes that depression is associated with a deficiency of the brain neurotransmitter norepinephrine and that manic behavior is associated with an excess of norepinephrine. The hypothesis regarding this catecholamine's effect on mood has evolved from three sources of observation. Animal research has found that norepinephrine is associated with the firing frequency at synapses. A second source of data regarding the effects of neurotransmitters on humans has come from observations of the effects of psychoactive drugs. Drugs that elevate mood also increase the level of norepinephrine at synapses, whereas those which depress mood reduce the level of this biochemical.[33] In research with psychiatric patients low levels of norepinephrine have been found in the urine of persons experiencing depression, whereas high levels have been found in manic patients.[19,23] Although this evidence lends support to the catecholamine hypothesis, the causes for these variations are not yet known. It has been shown only that these variations in norepinephrine levels exist and that they are associated with affect.

BEHAVIORAL DEFINITION

Objective data

Motor-behavioral response. The earliest indicators of agitation are the behavioral cues that the person is beginning to experience increased anxiety. From the hierarchical levels of anxiety it can be seen that as anxious feelings increase, so does the possibility that agitation will occur.[28] Mild anxiety is behaviorally manifested as restlessness, finger tapping, or foot bobbing. This degree of anxiety poses few behavioral problems but can be a warning that some of the individual's needs are not being met and that the potential for agitation is increasing.

As anxiety progresses to the early-moderate level, motor responses such as periodic pacing or increase in muscle tension such as fist clenching or facial muscle tension may be used to control the need for movement. The physiological preparedness for action will become more observable, and the person may be increasingly unable to sit for any length of time. When sitting, the person may be perched on the edge of a chair in apparent readiness to respond to whatever may happen.

At times behaviors during this moderate stage may indicate that the agitated individual is beginning to act out hidden or unconscious feelings. The individual may react impulsively to what is happening and use attention-seeking behaviors such as loud, boisterous, grandiose talk. Limit-testing behaviors such as threats of elopement or warnings that control will soon be lost are examples of behavioral manifestations indicating that needs are still unsatisfied and that agitation is continuing to escalate.

For example, John had been pacing most of the morning but briefly sat down in the hospital corridor to talk with another patient. He said in a voice that could be heard down the hall at the nurses' station, "You know, I don't think my business back home can get along much longer without me. I'm the only one who can keep it going. If I don't find out pretty soon what these doctors think, I'm just going to pack up and leave."

As the person enters the late-moderate to early-severe stages of anxiety, the agitated behavior will become increasingly obvious. Constant movement will be seen most of the time, and argumentativeness will often become the mode of relating to others. Negative responses to other patients or health personnel or overreactions to minor frustration or irritants may occur more frequently.

For example, Laura had been pacing back and forth in front of the nurses' station for 5 minutes. She would glance through the window toward those sitting at the desk as she walked by, her head tucked down and her hands in tight fists. She finally knocked on the door of the nurses' station. A nurse indicated there was a conference in progress and asked her what she wanted. Laura responded, "I want to talk to Dr. S." The nurse said the physician would be out soon and shut the door. Laura continued to pace with increasing speed and began to kick the wall and bang on the window as she walked by. This time she was ignored. Then she walked toward the exit door at the end of the hall and shouted, "I'm going to leave this damn place; these people are going to be sorry."

Eye contact may be only sporadic, or, if anger is beginning to be present, the person may stare piercingly at others. Open hostility may be seen, and in advanced stages the agitated individuals may come close to striking out or throwing or hitting things. Such actions represent movement toward the fight response and border on or overlap with the concept of destructive behavior. (See Chapter 6.)

The late-moderate to early-severe stages of anxiety can also mark movement toward the flight response. The individual may become so hyperactive that almost all obvious goal-related behavior is absent. The behaviors seen can be interpreted as symbolic attempts to flee in body and mind the anxiety-provoking situation through repetitive, time-filling, and mind-clouding activities. The individual may be unceasingly preoccupied with changing clothes, adorning self or surroundings with bric-a-brac and brightly colored objects, or becoming involved in the business of others.

Ultimately, if the anxiety is not relieved, the individual may withdraw from interactions with the environment (see the discussion of psychological immobility in chapter 4) or adopt the unreality of bizarre behavior (see Chapter 7).

Cognitive response. The progressive levels of anxiety seen in agitation cause narrowing of the individual's cognitive functioning. In the initial stages of agitation the perceptual functioning coincides with that which can be seen in mild anxiety states, in which the cognitive abilities are heightened and the narrowed focus is beneficial for problem solving and decision making.

As the person moves to a more advanced state of agitation, which corresponds with a moderate anxiety level, perceptions may still be narrow, but the person will begin either to focus on many isolated thoughts or to fly from one thought to another with only limited connections. The following conversation provides an example of this:

Nurse: Henry, how do you like it at the hospital?
Patient: Fine, fine, good. . .good place to be, me that is, good place for me. Place. . . win, place, show. First place in the race.

These rapid associations of thought may include expansive ideas, ambitious goals, and expectations. The individual may appear to attend to selectively chosen thoughts and comments and to ignore all unpleasant ideas and negative responses. Decisions may be made quickly, but they may also be immediately altered. If desires are thwarted, the agitated individual may attempt to persuade or ridicule whoever is standing in the way. The individual may be quick to find fault in others and often will take advantage of perceived weaknesses, as the following example illustrates.

Jean was busy straightening and restraightening her room when the nurse came in to talk with her. Unable to convince Jean to sit down for a few minutes, the nurse suggested they go for a walk to get away from the distractions of the room. Jean responded, "Well, you could certainly use the exercise, you are putting on a little weight. But I'm not interested in talking with you. I don't have any problems and I don't need your help, so just go on the walk by yourself, Fatso."

Agitated individuals may alternate from an outward facade of self-sufficiency and decisiveness to a demanding attitude that others provide them with advice and answers to their problems. As agitation progresses to the severe anxiety level, the individuals' may be able to focus only fleetingly on any particular topic. Reality testing will be poor and generally will be influenced by the present mood. Severely agitated persons may express present perceptions of reality by such comments as "That doctor really doesn't like me. Nobody likes me. Even my mother has hated me all my life!" or "I'm really here in this hospital to help entertain the patients. There's nothing wrong with me!"

Subjective data

Affective response. The affect of the agitated individual often is an indication of internal ambiguity. Emotional lability reflects the rapid changes in mood as the person's affect swings quickly from euphoria to anger to diversional laughter. The agitated individual may one minute express extreme self-assurance and the next expound depressive and derisive ideas.

As agitation progresses, individuals may verbalize anxiety and fear, or they may only describe themselves as being unable to sit still or as having excess energy. Some patients will be concerned about these restless feelings, whereas others will deny the problem, as exemplified by the following conversation:

Nurse: You seem to be having some trouble sitting still this morning. Tell me how you are feeling.

Patient: Oh, I'm feeling fine, just fine. I just have so much energy today I want to get as much done as I can. Don't want to waste time, you know.

INTERVENING VARIABLES

Environmental support

Support from the environment and from individuals in that environment can have a major influence on whether a person becomes agitated, whether agitation is sustained, and the degree to which the cycle of agitation escalates. A supportive environment can enable even the agitation-prone individual to handle stressful situations successfully, whereas a nonsupportive environment can add enough burden on the individual that agitation may be precipitated.

Social environment. Relationships with significant others are often the crux of the agitated individual's problems. Family members can communicate that they value the patient; thus reinforcing the patient's continued contribution to the family, or they can negate or minimize the patient's input, further threatening the patient's self-esteem. Often in the family background is a constellation of relationships that have placed many high expectations on the patient.[12] Continued pressure to meet these expectations can aggravate the movement toward agitation.

The social role and life situation of the patient and the impact of the illness and/or hospitalization on these factors can be very influential on whether a patient becomes agitated. The individual who has always been "in charge" and has been relatively successful in this approach is likely to want to handle the circumstances surrounding hospitalization much the same way.

Physical environment. Paradoxically, the hospital milieu can provide a protective environment and be overly stimulating at the same time. Relief from daily demands of a job or other responsibilities can decrease the individual's sense of threat to self-esteem. However, the hospital experience, with concomitant emotional and cognitive stress resulting from diagnostic procedures, the impact of diagnosis, and the subjective meaning of the illness, can promote agitation.

An agitated individual responds readily to external stimuli. The noisy, unsettling atmosphere of a hospital, with the constant bombardment of people asking questions and requesting to examine the patient, can elevate the person's potential for becoming agitated.

Current developmental level

The chronological developmental level of individuals and the developmental tasks with which they are presently dealing influence whether coping strategies have been developed for dealing with stresses such as hospitalization. Adolescents struggling with inherent acting out tendencies are far more likely to become agitated than are adults, since they may not have learned alternative mechanisms for dealing with stress. In addition, if the person's cognitive development has advanced to the point that the individual is capable of abstract thinking, learning can be more readily transferred from one situation to another.

The following example capsulizes the various intervening variables that can impinge on a patient and precipitate an episode of agitated behavior. Had any one of the variables been modified, the ultimate outburst might have been averted.

Karen, a 16-year-old high-school student, was admitted to the hospital for a complete examination to determine whether any physical changes could explain recent school truancy and outbursts of anger. During the day Karen was examined twice by a team of physicians and underwent several diagnostic tests. She exhibited some resistance but appeared to be attempting to comply with the requests of those around her. Late in the afternoon Karen appeared to be having trouble making herself comfortable in the quiet isolation of her room. She was in the bed one minute, the chair the next, and mumbled to herself through clenched teeth. At this time Karen was approached by a young, male medical student who insisted on talking with her and examining her again. Karen's response was a definite, "No, I don't want to go through that again!" The young physician-to-be persisted, only to be shouted at and thrown out of the room. As he left, he said to his supervisor, "She doesn't belong here, she should be transferred to the psychiatric ward."

NURSING INTERVENTIONS—GOALS AND EVALUATION CRITERIA

Nursing goals for patients experiencing agitated behavior follow a continuum of care from the immediate safety needs of the patient to the more self-actualizing needs of increased self-awareness and verbal expression of feelings. The specific areas of nursing intervention that stem from these goals correspond with the hierarchy of needs outlined by Maslow.[25] As each succeeding need is met, the likelihood of success in the next is increased. Although these patient-care approaches do follow a hierarchical structure, it must be recognized that the hierarchy is not invariant. The scheme is a flexible representation, and several of the levels may need to be dealt with concurrently. The intervention goals most appropriate for a given patient depend on the degree of agitation exhibited.

Provision of safe environment

Since agitated individuals' cognitive functioning is often diverted and restricted, the patients' concern for safety may be limited. The impulsivity of agitated patients may place them in situations that are dangerous for themselves or others. Some patients may need to be protected from the accessibility of sharp objects such as scissors and knives because their potential for harm increases as agitation escalates. It is also necessary to police the environment for potential safety hazards such as obstacles in doorways, table corners protruding into walkways, and broken glass on the floor since agitated individuals may be unable to focus on such details. This is particularly true of individuals in the more advanced stages of agitation, when their ability to concentrate is substantially reduced. Asking patients to help identify potentially dangerous items in the environment conveys the message that safety is also their responsibility.

Behavioral criteria that indicate safety has been achieved include absence of injury to self and others. Increase in the patient's attention to environmental safety may be evidenced by such things as reduced encounters with objects in the environment, increased neatness in the management of personal space, and the wearing of protective clothing such as coats or boots in cold weather.

Maintenance of physical health

Personal physical needs such as daily hygiene requirements are often neglected by agitated individuals. The nurse's attention to such details is important for maintenance of physical health and serves the added purpose of helping the patient focus on goal-directed tasks that are easily achieved.

The energy expended by the agitated individual drains both physiological and psychological reserves. The constant activity that characterizes especially the late stages of agitation can lead to malnutrition and dehydration. If the patient has a preexisting health problem such as diabetes or a cardiac condition, physiological crises could develop as a result of the hyperactivity and increased metabolic demands.

Patients should be monitored for weight loss and levels of nutritional and fluid intake and output. High-calorie and high-protein foods should be provided. When the patient is so active that sitting long enough to eat is a problem, finger foods, which can be ingested quickly while the person is moving, should be provided. Electrolyte imbalances of sodium and potassium are also a potential risk when the patient is being treated with lithium carbonate,[7] a drug that is often used to control mood swings. At times fluid intake has to be limited to help stabilize the blood levels of this medication. When the patient is taking this drug, electrolyte levels should be monitored daily via blood tests.

Often the patient has much difficulty sleeping, and this lack of sleep, in addition to increased activity, could result in exhaustion. Providing the patient with a quiet environment with soft lighting and opportunities for frequent naps can facilitate the return to a regular sleep pattern.[15]

At times it may be necessary for the patient to expend energy intentionally. If the inability to focus seems to be due to an excess of energy, physical exercise can be used as an avenue of release. Caution must be taken, however, since certain kinds of exercise may be too stimulating. A moderate amount of large-muscle activity can usually provide an effective amount of controlled release.[7] The nurse will need to make a judgment as to what type of exercise (e.g., a brisk walk versus a comfortable stroll) is the most beneficial for a particular patient. Eventually, patients can be asked and encouraged to identify activities that are and are not helpful for them. Exploring the effects of physical activities on the patient's overall sense of well-being helps the individual become aware of physiological and psychological reactions. Such awareness facilitates the patient's ability to identify cues indicative of increased levels of agitation.

Criteria indicative of physical health maintenance relate to the specific need areas. Examples of some appropriate behavioral criteria are increased hours of sleep, increased intake of needed nutrients, increased personal hygiene care, and decreased energy expenditure.

Increase of understanding of current experiences

Agitated patients often need help in understanding the reality of their situation. Although such patients are usually not "out of touch with reality," they are often unable to perceive their situation clearly and may only selectively attend to the environment. What is real to an individual and the way that individual functions psychologically depend on how reality is perceived.[24] To assist in clarifying perceptions, the nurse first needs to understand the agitated patient's perception of events and experiences. Often the agitated patient needs reality-based information from the nurse's perspective. However, the patient often can process only a limited amount of information. An extremely agitated patient will be able to process only short bits of information that are concrete and to the point. Reality must be identified in a direct manner, as in the following illustration. Jerry was disturbing all the other patients on the ward by butting into conversations and telling others how to play their card games, while at the same time he was unable to sit still long enough to finish a game himself. The nurse might structure reality by saying, "Jerry, you are having difficulty finishing a game here with the rest of the patients in the day room. Let's go back to the sun porch where just the two of us can play." In agitation of a lesser extent patients should be included in the structuring of reality so they can begin to make decisions, gain some sense of control over their situation, and have the opportunity to communicate needs and feelings. The next day Jerry was still actively moving about the ward but was apparently in better control of his need to interfere with other patients' activities. At this time the nurse could point out the change, give an interpretation of reality, and attempt to return additional control to the patient by saying, "You seem to be having a better day today but still have a lot of excess energy. Would you like to go back to the sun porch as we did yesterday, or would you like to play cards with some of the other patients out here in the day room?"

Admission to the hospital can be a fearful experience. Keeping the patient as informed as possible concerning routines of the hospital, upcoming procedures or tests, and changes that might occur such as room reassignment helps the patient maintain cognitive control and gain a sense of consistency.

Some situations and experiences in the hospital prove to be particularly stressful and potentially agitation-producing for certain individuals. The nurse should identify what seems to be especially stressful for a particular patient. Eliminating or modifying the effects of certain events can help the patient focus on reality and alleviate the potential for escalation of the patient's agitation, as in the following example. After the last two visits from her physician, Marjorie was increasingly tearful and restless. Although the physician's visit could not be eliminated from the patient's daily routine, its impact could be modified. By spending time with Marjorie before and/or after the physician comes and helping her deal with the feelings that result from the visits, the nurse can decrease the potential for agitated behavior.

Behaviors that indicate increase in the patient's understanding of current experiences include lengthened attention span, ability to make simple decisions without increased agitation, and decreased impulsive, boisterous behavior.

Development of feelings of trust and security

Agitated behavior rarely occurs without warning. Alert health care personnel who notice and respond to the cues presented in the discussions of behavioral definitions can often prevent agitation from escalating. By functioning as a nonjudgmental, neutral, human buffer between agitated individuals and their environment, the nurse can help patients focus on the present, improve concentration, and begin dealing with immediate problems and needs.

Altering the environment to decrease stimuli and minimize distractions can have a soothing effect on agitated patients. The nurse should attempt to remain calm, use a low-pitched voice, and use a firm but kind approach. Shaming or scolding can decrease an agitated person's self-esteem further and increase the potential for escalation of the agitation.

Setting limits is an effective way of conveying to agitated patients that their safety and well-being are important and expected.[22,35] Agitated individuals often need externally imposed controls just as adolescents do. Through the specific guidance of what is and is not expected of them, they can gain a greater sense of security. Limits set by the nurse also help patients believe that they are worthy of the nurse's attention and that the nurse is competent and concerned. The ultimate aim of limit setting is better self-control by the patient and can be communicated in positive expectations by matter of fact statements such as "I will not let you harm yourself"; "I cannot allow you to hit the other patients; you will have to stay in the quiet room until you can refrain from hurting others"; and "You will be able to control yourself; I will help you until you can do it on your own." The security provided by the concern and interest of the nurse enables the patient to more comfortably recognize and deal with the causes and events of behaviors.

Patients can perceive the concern and interest of the nurse through interpretive statements that respond to the tone of the patient's behavior, as explained later in the discussion of increased self-awareness. By showing that it is important to have an accurate understanding of the patient's thoughts and feelings, the nurse can lay the foundation for trust.

As trust continues to develop between the patient and the nurse and as agitation decreases, more opportunities for examining the patient's situation will become available. By asking for concrete explanations of events from the patient's perspective, the nurse can begin to help the patient focus on the patient's reality.[1,13] When the patient knows that the nurse can be counted on to listen and to help sort out what has happened, the patient's anxiety will be reduced. Consistent follow-through by the nurse concerning appointments and commitments is paramount to the building of a trusting relationship. As anxiety decreases, energy conservation results, which in turn facilitates the patient's ability to devote more time and energy to problem solving and self-awareness.

Behaviors indicative of trust development are increased tolerance for the physical presence of the nurse as noted by a reduction in physical activity (e.g., pacing) when the nurse is present. Increased ability to accept delay, tolerate frustration, and take no for an answer without a need for physical energy release are other indicators. Additional cues of trust development are approach behaviors such as seeking the company of the nurse, sitting by the nurse, asking for company on a walk, or asking for time to talk.

Increase of self-awareness and verbalization of feelings

Agitated individuals are adept at shutting out awareness of how they are responding to their experiences. The activities in which they become involved, particularly during the advanced stages of agitation, serve as a means of avoiding feelings. Once agitated patients are able to experience a degree of security and establish some trust in others, they can begin to work on developing a more open and direct awareness of self.

If throughout early contacts with the agitated patient the nurse gradually identifies the individual's responses to what is happening, the patient will become consciously aware of feelings experienced and will become ready to examine them. During nurse-patient interactions attention should be focused on underlying themes, nonverbal gestures, and tone of voice rather than strictly on verbal content.[13] Addressing these factors brings into the open that which is actually occurring. When the nurse focuses on the immediacy of the situation and the message that the patient's behavior is conveying, the patient can begin to make connections between the overt behavior and the underlying affective component.[1,13] For example, the nurse might say, "I can see from your pacing and the expression on your face that something must really be upsetting you." When the patient realizes that the nurse is sensitive to internal reactions as well as external behavior, bonds of understanding and trust develop. As the nurse is able to elicit expressions of immediate and relevant interpersonal themes, the patient becomes more secure in the further exploration of self-awareness. Behavioral responses that are more acceptable than agitation can then be explored, and measures can be initiated to help the patient substitute alternate behavior. For example, the nurse may suggest, "When you feel yourself getting upset, come tell me and I will talk with you. Together we can sort out what is happening."

Conceptualizing the self into the following four parts is helpful in understanding how self-awareness can be promoted for agitated patients:

1. *The public self:* that which is presented by the individual and is evident to others.
2. *The semipublic self:* that which others perceive. The individual may not be aware of this part.
3. *The private self:* that known only to the individual. It is not intended that this be revealed to others.
4. *The inner self:* that which is unconscious. This part is not known to the individual because it is too anxiety laden to be acknowledged in a conscious way.[21]

As a person becomes more cognizant of these various parts of the self, there is an increase in feelings of mastery of one's actions and emotions. The person becomes consciously aware of elements of the self that previously were unavailable to the individual's working knowledge.

Developing an increase in self-awareness comes from interpersonal exchanges involving three steps: (1) listening to oneself, (2) listening to others, and (3) telling others about yourself and letting others listen to you.[16]

Listening to oneself. Listening to oneself means becoming aware of a feeling, identifying that feeling, and then attempting to bring into conscious awareness the cause of the feeling. True introspection of this nature helps the person become knowledgeable about previously unknown areas of the self.

Haber et al.[16] suggest that the following questions are useful in helping patients work through the process of listening to themselves:

1. *How do I feel now?* This first question can usually be answered in general terms (e.g., good, bad, relaxed, tense, anxious).
2. *What is the feeling I am experiencing?* Answering this question involves a more in depth examination and labeling of feelings (e.g., fear, anger, guilt, joy, sadness, frustration).
3. *Why am I feeling this way?* or *What happened to make this feeling arise?*

Since agitated behavior diverts attention from such issues, the agitated individual may find it difficult to answer these last two questions. Explanations offered may be rationalization by the patient or may be attempts to avoid looking at the real motivations behind the behaviors. An agitated patient has probably received little encouragement in the past to examine and explain behaviors and/or feelings. The nurse can help such a patient identify hidden feelings and their meaning by persistently extending the discussion past superficial levels. For example, the patient may say, "I don't know what is wrong; it just seems that I never know what's going to happen next." A response such as "I know what you mean. None of us knows what to expect next around here," would close off further examination of feelings. A better response would be "You don't feel you are being kept well enough informed?" This question encourages the patient to clarify the reason for the feeling.

Listening to others. Listening to others has a twofold benefit for increasing self-awareness. As one listens to what others are saying, awareness of the semipublic self increases. Getting feedback from others allows an individual to identify behaviors and attitudes that should be modified and to receive reinforcement for positive aspects of the self.

The second benefit is increased knowledge about what other individuals experience in given situations and how they respond. Understanding others helps people have a better understanding of themselves.

The way agitated patients can be helped by listening to others depends on the patient's level of agitation. The extremely agitated patient usually is able to process only very simple input. As agitation is reduced, the patient can begin to develop listening skills through two methods. The first approach uses role modeling of the nurse's listening skills. The nurse reflects, restates, and clarifies the patient's statements, showing that the patient has been heard and demonstrating effective communication techniques throughout all interactions with the patient.[6,13,31,32] When the nurse and the patient reach the point at which they can become actively involved in improving listening skills, the nurse can point out the listening techniques that have been used and encourage the patient to practice them.

The second approach involves identifying nonverbal cues such as eye contact, body posture, and intonation of voice that indicate active involvement on the part of the listener.[6] Just bringing these cues out into the open is often enough for patients to become aware of the nonverbal messages they are sending. However, some patients may need more direct nonverbal communication identification.

Telling others about oneself. Self-disclosure is the main process in this step of self-awareness development. Self-disclosure means sharing with another person parts of the self that were heretofore primarily hidden in the private self. As individuals discover and reveal to others their feelings, strengths, weaknesses, and potentials, they become more knowledgeable about these areas. Verbal acknowledgment to others of a particular characteristic requires close scrutiny of oneself.

One way to help a person learn to be open is to identify personal characteristics that are perceived to be the least favored and then to discuss how the person feels about these characteristics, how it feels to discuss them with someone else, and what should be done about these characteristics. Through this process of developing self-awareness and examination of feelings, the person begins to gain a sense of objectivity about self. Decisions to change behavior patterns can follow naturally.

Behavior that indicates that a patient is increasing self-awareness and sharing feelings includes the patient's agreement that certain feelings are being experienced, statements regarding what is being felt, explanations for these current feelings, identification of how others might have responded to a situation, and presentation of possible reasons for others' behavior. Behaviors related to improvement in listening skills include the use of reflecting, restating, and clarifying statements in conversions and the use of nonverbal cues that reinforce verbal messages.

Development of alternative behavior patterns

For many patients the development of self-awareness and exploration of feelings is a major change in their approach to handling experiences. Helping patients proceed step-by-step through the examination and expression of feelings often precipitates changes in behavior patterns.

Changes in behavior patterns will persist only if verbal communication continues to receive reinforcement. For this reason it is important to include family members or significant others in the treatment plan. The patient's action-oriented behavioral responses were not developed in a vacuum, and lasting changes cannot be expected to occur if the interactive mode between a patient and the patient's support group is not modified.

However, changes in the patient's behavior may not be welcomed or wanted by the family. If the person begins to express feelings rather than suppressing them and occasionally using the escape valve of agitated behavior, family members may become uncomfortable. Expression of feelings may force the family members to look at themselves and their interpersonal relationship with the patient. Family members may prefer the occasional upheaval.

Therapy that focuses on the family as a unit provides an avenue to help replace disruptive family relationships with supporting interactions. This approach facilitates the expression of feelings by members of the family as well as by the patient. The four general principles of family therapy are (1) identify the problem as a family one, (2) create a family client rather than an individual one, (3) help the family understand the operation of family triangles, and (4) help each member differentiate a sense of "I."[34]

Assertiveness training can also be used independently or in conjunction with family therapy. The use of assertive techniques by agitated individuals can help them constructively restructure their way of dealing with life situations.[2] Assertive behavior is the identification and expression of the emotions generated by a situation rather than arrest of feeling identification and expression at the level of anxiety.[29] Through assertiveness training individuals can learn how to express their feelings and recognize the difference between nonassertive, assertive, and aggressive behavior. One of the greatest realizations that occurs during the process of learning assertive techniques is that to be assertive does not mean to be hostile.[9]

Once the patient is able to label feelings and recognize interpersonal dynamics, more permanent alternative behavior patterns in response to the environment can begin to be established. The following are indications that these new behaviors have been learned: rather than act out feelings, the agitated individual uses assertiveness, identifies feelings, and acts on them; fear is expressed verbally rather than through hyperactivity; sadness is acknowledged and dealt with directly rather than fought; and frustrations are expressed and worked through rather than bottled up to the point of explosion.

CONCEPT OUTLINE

I. *Conceptual definition:* Agitation is a psychological state of ambivalance wherein an individual uses actions or body language to release energy, communicate needs, and postpone a fight or flight decision.

II. *Antecedent conditions*
   A. Developmental arrest
   B. Environmental uncertainties and inconsistency
   C. Catecholamine levels

III. *Behavioral definition*
   A. Objective data
      1. Motor-behavioral response
         a. Mild agitation
            (1) Restlessness
            (2) Finger tapping
            (3) Foot bobbing
         b. Moderate agitation
            (1) Periodic pacing
            (2) Increased muscle tension

(3) Inability to sit still; sitting on edge of chair
(4) Impulsivity, attention seeking, and limit testing
c. Severe agitation
(1) Constant movement
(2) Negative, argumentative responses
(3) Overreactions to frustration
2. Cognitive response
a. Mild agitation
(1) Heightened cognitive abilities
b. Moderate agitation
(1) Perceptual narrowing
(2) Focus on isolated thoughts
(3) Decreased attention span
(4) Decision-making process quick and changeable
c. Late-moderate to severe agitation
(1) Only fleeting focus on topics
(2) Poor reality testing
B. Subjective data
1. Affective response
a. Emotional lability
b. Verbalization or denial of anxiety
c. Excessive energy

IV. *Intervening variables*
A. Environmental support
1. Social environment
2. Physical environment
B. Current developmental level

V. *Nursing interventions—goals*
A. Provision of safe environment
1. Patient helped to focus on present and to take responsibility for own safety
2. Environment policed for safety hazards
B. Maintenance of physical health
1. Nutrition and sleep needs monitored
2. Electrolyte balance monitored
3. Use of high-calorie, high-protein diet
4. Use of finger foods
5. Provision of balanced activity and rest schedule
C. Increase of understanding of current experiences
1. Patient asked to identify perceptions of situations
2. Provision of reality-based information from nurse's perspective
3. Provision of opportunity for patient to limit own behavior
D. Development of feelings of trust and security
1. Decrease of environmental stimulation
2. Setting of activity and behavior limits
3. Consistent fulfillment of commitments
E. Increase of self-awareness and verbalization of feelings
1. Patient asked to verbalize feelings currently being experienced
2. Patient asked to identify source of feelings
3. Patient helped to develop listening skills
4. Identification of nonverbal communication
5. Discussion of perceptions of personal characteristics
F. Use of alternative behavior patterns
1. Verbal exploration of feelings
2. Initiation of family therapy
3. Use of assertive techniques to accomplish goals

VI. *Evaluation criteria*
A. Absence of injury to self and others
B. Increased attention to environmental safety
C. Wearing of clothing appropriate to environment
D. Increased hours of sleep
E. Increased intake of needed nutrients
F. Increased personal hygiene care
G. Decreased random energy expenditures
H. Lengthened attention span
I. Increased ability to make decisions
J. Decreased impulsive, boisterous behavior
K. Increased tolerance for physical presence of nurse
L. Reduced pacing when nurse is present
M. Seeking company of nurse
N. Identification of present feeling
O. Identification of how others might respond to situation
P. Use of listening skills
Q. Use of assertive techniques
R. Verbal expression of feelings

REFERENCES

1. Ackerhalt, J.: The nurse-client relationship. In Haber, J., Schudy, S. M., Leach, A. M., and Sideleau, B. F., editors: Comprehensive psychiatric nursing, New York, 1978, McGraw-Hill Book Co.
2. Alberti, R. E., and Emmons, M. L.: Your perfect right: a guide to assertive behavior, ed. 3, San Luis Obispo, Calif., 1978, Impact Publishers, Inc.
3. Barber, J. M., Stokes, L. G., and Billings, D. M.: Adult and child care, a client approach to nursing, St. Louis, 1973, The C. V. Mosby Co.
4. Bergmann, M. V.: On the relationship between words and actions: examples of technique from psychoanalytic practice. In Milnar, D., and Goldman, G. D., editors: The neurosis of our times; acting out, Springfield, Ill., 1973, Charles C Thomas, Publisher.
5. Blos, P.: The concept of acting out in relation to the adolescent process. In Rexford, E., editor: A developmental approach to problems of acting out, rev. ed., New York, 1978, International Universities Press, Inc.
6. Brammer, L. M.: The helping relationship: process and skills, Englewood Cliffs, N.J., 1973, Prentice-Hall, Inc.
7. Carter, F. M.: Psychosocial nursing: theory and practice in hospital and community health, New York, 1976, Macmillan Publishing Co., Inc.
8. Clack, J.: Nursing intervention into the aggressive behavior of patients. In Burd, S., and Marshall, M., editors: Some clinical approaches to psychiatric nursing, New York, 1963, Macmillan Publishing Co., Inc.
9. Duke, M. P., and Nowicki, S., Jr.: Abnormal psychology: perspectives on being different, Monterey, Calif., 1979, Brooks/Cole Publishing Co.
10. Eisenberg, L.: A developmental approach to adolescence. In Rogers, D., editor: Issues in adolescent psychology, New York, 1969, Appleton-Century-Crofts.
11. Fenichel, O.: The psychoanlytic theory of neurosis, New York, 1945, W. W. Norton & Co., Inc.
12. Fromm-Reichmann, F: Selected papers of Frieda Fromm-Reichmann. In Bullard, D. M., editor: Psychoanalysis and psychotherapy, Chicago, 1959, The University of Chicago Press.
13. Goodman, G., and Dooley, D.: A framework for help-intended communication, Psychotherapy: Theory, Research, Practice **13**:106, 1976.
14. Greenacre, P.: General problems of acting out, Psychoanal. Q. **19**:455, 1950.
15. Haber, J.: The client who threatens the self concept. In Haber, J., Schudy, S. M., Leach, A. M., and Sideleau, B. F., editors: Comprehensive psychiatric nursing, New York, 1978, McGraw-Hill Book Co.
16. Haber, J., Leach, A. M., Schudy, S. M., and Sideleau, B. F.: Self awareness. In Haber, J., Schudy, S. M., Leach, A. M., and Sideleau, B. F., editors: Comprehensive psychiatric nursing, New York, 1978, McGraw-Hill Book Co.
17. Josselyn, I.: The adolescent today. In Sze, W. C., editor: Human life cycle, New York, 1975, Jason Aronson, Inc.
18. Kalkman, M.: Psychosis. In Kalkman, M., and Davis, A. J., editors: New dimensions in mental health psychiatric nursing, New York, 1974, McGraw-Hill Book Co.
19. Kety, S.: Biochemistry of the major psychoses. In Freedman, A. M., Kaplan, H. I., and Sadock, B. J., editors: Comprehensive textbook of psychiatry, vol. II, ed. 2, Baltimore, 1975, Williams & Wilkins Co.
20. Loomis, M.: Nursing management of acting out behavior, Perspect. Psychiatr. Care **8**:168, 1970.
21. Luft, J., and Ingham, H.: The Johari window, a graphic model of awareness. In Luft, J., editor: Group processes: an introduction to group dynamics, Palo Alto, Calif., 1963, National Press Books.
22. Lyon, G. G.: Limit setting as a therapeutic tool, J. Psychiatr. Nurs. **8**:17, 1970.
23. Maas, J., Fawcett, J., and Dekirmenjian, H.: Catecholamine metabolism, depressive illness and drug response, Arch. Gen. Psychiatry **26**:252, 1972.
24. MacKinnon, R. A., and Michels, R.: The psychiatric interview in clinical practice, Philadelphia, 1971, W. B. Saunders Co.
25. Maslow, A. H.: Motivation and personality, ed. 2, New York, 1970, Harper & Row, Publishers, Inc.

26. Mattheis, R.: Psychodynamics concepts relating to health. In Haber, J., Schudy, S. M., Leach, A. M., and Sideleau, B. F., editors: Comprehensive psychiatric nursing, New York, 1978, McGraw-Hill Book Co.
27. Monea, H.: Developmental reactions in adolescence. In Kalkman, M., and Davis, A. J., editors: New dimensions in mental health–psychiatric nursing, New York, 1974, McGraw-Hill Book Co.
28. Peplau, H. E.: A working definition of anxiety. In Burd, S. F., and Marshall, M. A., editors: Some clinical approaches to psychiatric nursing, New York, 1963, Macmillan Publishing Co., Inc.
29. Price, P. A.: Theoretical models, In Haber, J., Schudy, S. M., Leach, A. M., and Sideleau, B. F., editors: Comprehensive psychiatric nursing, New York, 1978, McGraw-Hill Book Co.
30. Rexford, E. N.: A developmental concept of the problems of acting out. In Rexford, E. N., editor: A developmental approach to problems of acting out, rev. ed., New York, 1978, International Universities Press, Inc.
31. Rogers, C.: Counseling and psychotherapy: newer concepts in practice, Boston, 1942, Houghton Mifflin Co.
32. Rogers, C.: Client-centered therapy: its current practice, implications, and theory, Boston, 1951, Houghton Mifflin Co.
33. Schildkraut, J. J.: Neuropsycho-pharmacology of the affective disorders, Boston, 1970, Little, Brown & Co.
34. Winstead-Fry, P.: Family theory and application. In Haber, J., Schudy, S. M., Leach, A. M., and Sideleau, B. F., editors: Comprehensive psychiatric nursing, New York, 1978, McGraw-Hill Book Co.
35. Wolfe, N. A.: Setting reasonable limits on behavior, Am. J. Nurs. **62**:104, 1962.

ROSE MARIE FRIEDRICH

SONJA I. LIVELY

thick
smothering
choking
creeping conqueror
penetrating
the marrow and soul,
rising
like an iceberg
freezing thought and feeling
commanding constant attention,
life
passes
just out of reach.

PAULETTE R. Di ANGI

Chapter 4

PSYCHOLOGICAL IMMOBILIZATION

CONCEPTUAL DEFINITION

Immobilization is defined as a restriction or limitation of movement, and psychological means of the mind and/or mental processes.[15] The term "psychological immobilization," then, signifies limitation of movement of the mental processes. Key words found in the literature in conjunction with this term include "emotional paralysis," "psychologically overwhelmed," "emotional cripple," and "frozen with fear."[2,11]

Wu[16] and Carnevali and Brueckner[2] relate psychological immobilization to the severe threat that overwhelms the individual. The individual reacts to a situation or loss that is perceived as potentially harmful but uncontrollable. As a consequence, behavior is directed toward dealing with the anxiety arising in response to the personal threat rather than toward meeting the problem. The individual focuses energy inward in an attempt to preserve ego and integrity and to decrease feelings of personal threat.

Psychological immobilization is not an uncommon reaction to loss. It generally occurs when an individual confronts an overwhelming situation. However, the intensity and value of the response vary. Lazarus[6] points out that the individual's belief regarding the ability to deal with a loss is of utmost importance in determining the degree of perceived threat. Psychological immobilization may be a temporary, normal defense that is associated with the avoidance-denial stage of illness.[11] When this response is used as a temporary measure, its adaptive effect is the temporary relief or alleviation of painful anxiety. In addition, immobilization has a restorative function of energy conservation that may facilitate the healing process.[16]

If this reaction is prolonged, it becomes maladaptive. Increasing amounts of psychological energy are directed toward control and repression of negative feelings rather than toward problem-solving behavior. This lowering of adaptive efficiency interferes with achievement and need gratification, affecting every aspect of the person's life. Eventually, the individual may give up and assume a self-imposed cripple role.[11] After the temporary threat such as acute illness passes, the person may fail to reassume role responsibilities, may continue a dependence pattern, and may make no attempt to become self-sufficient.

Psychological immobilization is a psychological condition in which an individual has restricted, decreased, or absent responses to physical, emotional, and/or social stimuli. The sequential dynamics of this condition are that an individual (1) perceives a threat to self that is overpowering, (2) responds to the high anxiety precipitated by the threat by directing psychological energy inward to protect the self from further struggle and pain, and (3) withholds energy expenditures from interaction with external reality. This response may be temporary and adaptive, or it may be prolonged, severe, and maladaptive.

ANTECEDENT CONDITIONS

Stress situations involving the threat of death, injury, or mutilation result in severe emotional disturbance in nearly everyone.[6] In the acute care setting an individual is likely to experience innumerable losses that involve a high level of danger and that impinge on the person's safety and security. These losses may be related to the disease process itself such as loss of body function, body part, or even life itself. Other losses may be related to environmental factors such as exposure to totally unfamiliar surroundings or social role changes in which there is a disruption of social relations and normal life patterns.[6,11]

For psychological immobilization to be precipitated by a specific loss, usually one or more of the following antecedents are also present: (1) meaninglessness or ambiguity of event; (2) unsuccessful resolution of past developmental tasks; (3) inadequate learning; (4) altered levels of neurotransmitters.

Meaninglessness or ambiguity of event

An individual who is admitted to an acute care setting is often unable to perceive the situation realistically because of lack of knowledge or familiarity with the environment. The patient may not ask questions because no one seems interested or perhaps because of fear of unpleasant reports. As a consequence, the bombardment of unfamiliar stimuli is likely to overwhelm the individual. If an agent of harm is ambiguous, threat will be intensified because ambiguity limits the individual's sense of control over the situation.[6] When the perception of an event is distorted, the person may even be unable to see a connection between the event and the feelings of stress.[1] Only the individual who understands this relationship as well as the impact of the illness on the life situation can deal with these changes in an effective, problem-solving manner.

As the individual is bombarded with unfamiliar stimuli, anxiety mounts. This compounds the problem, since perceptual focus narrows and the person becomes increasingly unable to reach out to others for clarification of the situation. As a consequence, the patient is unable to communicate fears and fantasies to others. The individual begins to dwell on the details of the situation, unable to see the link between events and feelings. Questions remain unanswered, and uncertainty and fear become more and more troublesome. In an attempt to create order out of the unknown, the individual withdraws from external reality into a more familiar subjective world.

Unsuccessful resolution of developmental tasks

Individuals who have experienced highly unsatisfactory family relationships in the formative years and whose usual behavioral pattern was that of submission usually use the same response pattern in an illness situation. When the individual becomes ill, this submission is apt to become exaggerated and intensified.

Successful completion of Erikson's task of trust development appears to be particularly critical. Mereness,[9] in the discussion of the dynamics of withdrawal behavior, describes this behavior as evolving from family situations in which it was impossible to develop warm, positive relationships with others. Consequently, individuals from such families direct energy toward themselves rather than risk nonacceptance and rejection from others. Individuals who have seldom been able to count on others to have needs met are more likely to withdraw than to reach out in an illness situation.

The extent to which an individual feels in control is also important in the appraisal of threat and consequent coping. The successful completion of Erikson's second task of development, autonomy, lays the basis for feelings of mastery over the environment. The belief of control over the situation can greatly reduce feelings of helplessness.[6] Conversely, a person who doubts self-adequacy and self-worth is more prone to experience threat than the individual who is confident of abilities. If the person believes the environment is uncomfortable and overpowering, the ability to take independent action against the threat is reduced.

Inadequate learning

Through the process of daily living an individual learns methods of coping with anxiety. An individual confronted with a stressful situation chooses response strategies from an available repertoire of past learning.[4] The demands for coping with situations that arise with acute illness frequently cannot be anticipated, and consequently, often there are no ready-made, previously learned coping mechanisms in the repertoire to help reduce the threat. All the individual's past knowledge and skills may seem totally inadequate and irrelevant, making the individuals helpless to take goal-directed action.

Johnson[4] contends that individuals learn powerlessness through repeated experiences of having events controlled by forces outside themselves. Powerlessness may be learned through negative reinforcement of independent activity. For example, an individual may have been hospitalized in the past and received negative feedback for attempting active involvement in care. The person may have been labeled a bad patient and identified as someone who was interfering with care. To avoid the adverse feedback, the patient responded with the maladaptive behavior of withdrawal and passivity. When confronted with the threat of acute illness again, this patient is apt to use the same maladaptive response and to shun active participation in care.

The pattern of learned powerlessness may also evolve from modeling of undesirable behavior in childhood. A child observes and imitates the behavior of others. The child who is exposed to frequent modeling by parents of a defensive reaction to threat (i.e., not facing and dealing realistically with problems) may assume this method of coping, especially if this behavior is rewarded by approval from the parents. The avoidant life style becomes self-reinforcing because it reduces anxiety. Whenever the individual feels severely threatened, this pattern of impotence and withdrawal is used.

Altered neurotransmitter levels

Research evidence lends support to the hypothesis that depression is associated with a deficiency of the brain neurotransmitter norepinephrine. Elevated dopamine levels in the central nervous system have been associated with schizophrenia. The catecholamine hypothesis is discussed in Chapter 3.

BEHAVIORAL DEFINITION

The gradation of the individual's behavioral response to the perceived threat depends on the balance between the perceived harm-producing situation and the individual's resources to counter harm. Since severe threat cannot be directly observed, it must be inferred from the motor-behavioral response, cognitive response, and specific affective behavior.

Objective data

Motor-behavioral response. The person who is psychologically immobilized does not strike out at the world but withdraws. The overall behavioral pattern is inaction with no demands on the environment. There is a decrease or absence of spontaneous activity. The psychologically immobilized person becomes passive and depends on others for direction.[2,11]

The individual may appear to want to be left alone. When approached, the person may not return a greeting or make eye contact. The patient may have difficulty initiating a conversation, and if a sentence is begun, it may not be completed. Answers to specific questions are apt to be brief, frequently monosyllables such as yes and no. Crying may be present, but even that may be silenced as the individual becomes overwhelmed with feelings, perhaps to the point of becoming mute. Outward behavior is likely to discourage rather than invite interaction. Mr. B. provides an example. He had been admitted to the hospital to confirm a possible diagnosis of cancer of the colon, and he had been informed of this condition. When the nurse entered Mr. B.'s room, she saw that his body was rigid and his eyes were glued to the television. When she said, "You look uncomfortable. How are you feeling?" Mr. B responded, "Fine," and continued staring at the television.

The body posture indicates withdrawal from active involvement in surroundings. There is a minimum of gestures and movements. Rigidity and tension characterize the body musculature; consequently, movements are slow and deliberate, as if the limbs were weighted down. As the withdrawal from external reality increases, posture may become that of flexion, in which the body appears to fold onto itself, and progress to a fetal position. This extreme regression in outward behavior is best exemplified in catatonic schizophrenia. In this condition there may be total absence of spontaneous behavior. The individual's position does not vary unless someone else actively changes it. Even within the general hospital population extreme behaviors occur. Mrs. A. is an example. She had the diagnosis of terminal cancer but had never discussed the illness with any of the professional staff. When a nurse asked, "Have you considered how your illness may affect your plans when you go home?" Mrs. A. turned to her side, drew her knees up to her chest, closed her eyes, and pulled the sheet over her head.

Cognitive response. The severe threat and anxiety that accompany psychological immobilization disrupt cognitive functioning. High degrees of threat are associated with regressive or primitive thought processes, but effective methods of coping require undisturbed cognitive functioning.[6] Generally, as anxiety increases, there is a narrowing or limiting of the perceptual field and the individual becomes less able to consider the situation in its entirety; consequently, only part of the situation is perceived. The perceptual distortion impedes decision making and problem solving because of the reduced ability to relate ideas. Details of a problem may be considered and exaggerated, but the relationships between these details are missed. For example, an individual may spend countless hours ruminating about specific aspects of the misfortunes experienced, but be unable to move past these details to see how the present behavior relates to the problems or to think through behavioral alternatives to handle the threat.[7]

Perceptual narrowing reduces the ability to concentrate on external stimuli. The attention span may be so severely impaired that the person cannot follow what others are saying, especially if the communication is lengthy. The patient is likely to misunderstand or forget when someone attempts to clarify the present situation. Perceptual distortion may become so severe that the individual becomes unaware of the environment. Then the patient may not respond to the presence of others in the room and may seem not to hear. Disorientation to time, place, and person and vulnerability to environmental dangers such as scalding water may appear as receptivity decreases.

Subjective data

Affective response. One problem inherent in the assessment of the emotional status of the psychologically immobilized person is that a combination of emotions can occur simultaneously. Assessment of this state is difficult because the emotions are turned inward and the individual cannot express them. Because of this difficulty with verbal expression, clues to the individual's feelings come primarily from nonverbal behavior.

Anxiety, the inevitable initial response to threat, is prominent, and no clear action is generated.[6] Lack of control over the threatening situation results in feelings of helplessness. The person feels powerless. If the situation continues and no problem-solving behavior is found, the helplessness may progress to hopelessness. Under these circumstances the individual cannot foresee any eventual resolution of the problem, which produces a lack of confidence in future events. Sadness and dejection may be present. The affect associated with such a condition of hopelessness is depression.[6] Depression may be seen in the facial expression of the individual whose eyes look sad or vacant. The following excerpt describes the sadness detected by one nurse who cared for a psychologically immobilized individual:

> I found as I sat with him I became absorbed with his mood. Though in the dayroom with many people around it was as though we were in a room alone somewhere. His mood seems to surround him like a wall that he carries around with him and envelopes anyone who gets near. Listening to him I began to feel more and more sad. His eyes were full of expression. They hold no tears but look as if they were crying. . . . I wanted to cry myself. *

Particularly poignant are the feelings of alienation and isolation. The example cited graphically describes the inability of the person to reach out to others either physically or emotionally. The decreased ability to openly share feelings with another results in an emotional gap in which the person feels alone and misunderstood. There may be a mutual withdrawal as others find it increasingly difficult to approach the affected individual. Significant others may take a detached stance, which only reinforces the patient's belief that no one cares.

The inability to deal with the threat and the withdrawal from meaningful interaction may be accompanied by feelings of worthlessness and self-dislike. Although words may not express "I'm no good," the body posture suggests low self-worth. Lack of spontaneity, absence of eye contact, and muscle rigidity indicate a view of self that perceives personal failure.

INTERVENING VARIABLES

Several variables can influence an individual's response to threat and the precipitated psychological immobilization.

Situational support

A person's significant others (family, friends, and health team) become supportive if they communicate the message, "We know you are sick, but we still see you as a person of value." Supportive family and friends can help the person remain a viable member of the family and social group by sharing events from home, keeping

*From Ioder, M.: Personal communication, 1974.

the person's role in the family as much the same as possible, indicating they want to be with the patient, and offering comfort when it is needed. The support radiates from the communication of the individual's perceived worth. When the message is the reverse, that is, when the person is seen as sick and dependent and therefore not a worthwhile person, social groups become nonsupportive. A nonsupportive message can be communicated by not allowing adequate time to be with the individual, by belittling the patient's fears (e.g., "That's silly; it doesn't hurt when I take your blood pressure"), by not taking the initiative in communication, or by exhibiting disgust for the person's immobile behavior. Another way of belittling the person's worth is to treat him or her as a child by responding or making decisions for the individual or by avoiding discussion of emotions. These attitudes subtly encourage the immobilization. The person is expected to be a quiet, complacent patient who follows instructions and does not bother others.

Social role

Occupational and societal relationship patterns influence society's expectations regarding acceptable behavior in various social roles. When the behavioral norms of a person's social role are not in conflict with the expected behavior during the illness situation, this social role is a supportive variable. However, when they are in conflict, social role becomes a nonsupportive variable. For example, a person engaged in an occupation that rewards action and independence may have a difficult time as a patient, when forced into the dependent sick role. A woman whose husband is the sole decision maker assumes a passive, dependent role in her daily life. For her, being placed in a dependent role during acute illness poses no great change in her method of relating with others; therefore her role is supportive.

The traditional female role in America is a passive one. It is acceptable for the female to be dependent and emotional when she is sick. Because of this, it is often easier for the female to release her emotions through crying and talking. The traditional male role is one of independence accompanied by lack of expressed emotions. The male is expected to "be brave," "don't cry," and "don't discuss feelings." With the advent of women's liberation, acceptable sex role behavior is changing and there is more openness and equality in the show of emotions. The nurse must assess the patient's sex role identity. The traditional female role may be supportive, whereas the traditional male role may be nonsupportive.[5]

Current developmental level

The current stage of development can influence the response to immobilization, especially for children less than 5 years of age. Infants are particularly vulnerable because they are in an almost completely helpless developmental stage. They have no vocabulary to communicate the nature of discomfort to others; crying is their primary means of expressing distress. Feelings of security and relief from distress are achieved through physical contact with a consistent care-taking adult. Later in infancy this consistent care-taking adult is increasingly important in the creation of security because infants respond selectively to this person. When infants are confronted with acute illness, there is an interruption in the method of establishing security and decreasing anxiety. The problem is further compounded because infants lack a repertoire of alternative coping mechanisms. This problem can become so severe as to lead to anaclitic depression or even death.[12,14]

The immobilization of acute illness can be devastating for children less than 2 years of age, whose cognition and interaction with the world are derived from sensation and movement. Mobility provides a means of exploring the environment, which in turn leads to autonomy and control. In addition, mobility is a critical outlet for intense anger and frustration. Although they have growing ability to communicate verbally, toddlers have incomplete comprehension and use of the language. They use gross speech and cannot verbally explain and communicate needs and distress. Concreteness of thinking typifies their thought processes, and they lack the ability to analyze and synthesize new experiences. They often misunderstand explanations of others and may feel threatened and afraid when confronted with strange objects or experiences such as hospitalization.[12] As children mature and begin to expand their social and physical environment, they learn to deal with anxiety through play and fantasy. When children are confined in an acute care setting, their sense of being can be threatened because they no longer have the usual means of interacting with the world.[14]

NURSING INTERVENTIONS—GOALS AND EVALUATION CRITERIA

The primary goal of nursing intervention for the person who is experiencing psychological immobilization is for the person to gain increased control over the experience of acute illness as evidenced by the following behaviors: (1) increased participation in own physical care, (2) use of alternates such as physical activity for expressing feelings, (3) increased verbalization of feelings, (4) seeking of information from others when the situation is unclear, and (5) active participation in problem solving.

The areas of nursing intervention that should be considered with these persons correlate with Maslow's hierarchy of needs. Basic needs must be met before the more sophisticated ones. On the basis of this format, the following goals of nursing intervention will be discussed: (1) maintenance of physical health, (2) provision of safe and secure environment, (3) development of feelings of belonging, and (4) development and support of self-esteem.

Maintenance of physical health

A person who is psychologically immobilized may be unaware of internal clues that signal problems with physiological functioning or may not communicate these clues. The nurse needs to use observational skills to identify signs and symptoms signaling illness and/or injury. Many of these signs and symptoms are considered specifically in Chapter 5.

In addition to these potential risk areas, the nurse must also monitor how the patient is meeting such basic needs as nutrition, elimination, and sleep.[8,10] Often the psychologically immobilized patient is so preoccupied as to have no energy to eat and drink adequately. Records of intake and output should be kept. If the patient has difficulty maintaining adequate intake, it may be necessary to establish a nutrition routine such as frequent small meals or meal supplements. In addition, assistance may be needed during meals. This may entail simply reminding the person to continue to eat or may require verbal directions to put the food onto the fork and into the mouth. If this is not effective, the person may need to be fed, with reminders to chew and swallow. In some cases tube feeding and intravenous therapy are required to provide adequate nourishment.

Constipation is another common problem of the immobilized patient because of decreased intake, slowed physiological functioning, and decreased exercise. The nurse should be aware of the patient's elimination habits. Increased physical activity, fluids, and/or laxatives may be needed to manage this problem.

An immobilized patient may have problems with insomnia. Often the person can fall asleep but awakens within 3 to 4 hours and cannot return to sleep. The nurse should assess the patient's normal routine for inducing sleep. An opportunity to ventilate feelings to the nurse, a quiet environment, a warm bath, a cup of warm milk, or reading may facilitate sleep. In addition, increasing physical activity during the day may assist in releasing enough tension that sleeping during the night can be achieved. If insomnia is present, keeping the patient awake all day usually does not precipitate sleeping through the night. Because the patient sleeps for only short intervals, it is vital to provide periods of uninterrupted rest during the day.

Since personal hygiene activities such as oral care, shampoos, bathing, and nail care may be omitted by the patient, special routines may need to be established. This may simply require the establishment of the routine that these activities are to be done at a certain time, with the reminder to do them at that time. More severely affected persons may require step-by-step assistance through the activity. A kind, directive approach in the performance of activities of daily living may be warranted. For example, telling a severely immobilized patient that it is time to shower will not suffice. Instead, the nurse may have to give step-by-step instructions (e.g., "Mr. Smith, it is time for your shower. Come into the shower room. Remove your clothes and hang them on this hook. Turn on the water. Soap your body . . ."). This patient, because of the decreased level of functioning, needs adequate time to complete tasks. Whether the patient is doing tasks or the nurse is giving direct care, extra time should be allotted.

Behaviors indicative of an increase in the patient's control over maintenance of physical health include increased level of active participation in personal hygiene activities. Other criteria to be used to determine effectiveness of maintenance procedures relate directly to the basic need areas such as achievement of a particular level of protein and/or fluid ingestion or increase in number of night hours slept.

Provision of safe and secure environment

If the patient is so severely regressed as to be in danger during interaction with the environment, close supervision will be necessary. The patient might be unaware of scalding bath water or broken glass on the floor.

The hopelessness that may accompany immobilization also has safety implications. Hopelessness can lead to suicidal ideation and intent; consequently, the nurse should be alert for safety hazards in the environment (e.g., the hoarding of pills). If a suicide decision is reached, the person will have moved out of the state of psychological immobilization. Nursing intervention for the suicidal person is discussed in Chapter 6.

The isolation that is commonly present in the acute care setting can be frightening and can increase the individual's insecurity. A patient in a private room has much time alone with these fears. The mere physical proximity of other patients can increase this person's sense of security. It is often beneficial to place a psychologically immobilized person in a room with a carefully chosen roommate. The roommate should not be one who is also immobilized and withdrawn, since this may only serve to reinforce the withdrawal. On the other hand, an extremely active patient may be too overwhelming, increasing the environmental ambiguity.

Increasing the patient's familiarity with the environment also helps promote security. This may be accomplished by encouraging the patient to bring familiar possessions from home (e.g., pictures of family, books). These personal possessions should be placed where the patient can see and reach them. A familiar environment may also be created through maintenance of the patient's prehospitalization routine in the activities of eating, sleeping, and bathing. A predictable routine that incorporates the individual's preferences helps reduce feelings of helplessness by increasing the familiarity of the setting. This routine may be a specific daily schedule (e.g., 7:00 AM—get up, brush teeth, take shower, get dressed; 7:45—breakfast; etc.). Adherence should be maintained to provide the patient a sense of consistency and familiarity. Knowing what to expect provides a feeling of control over some aspects of the environment.[2]

A third measure useful in increasing security is provision of brief explanations to the patient about the care. This information allows the individual to gain confidence regarding ability to predict and control what is happening. A patient being prepared for treatment should be helped to establish an understandable frame of reference for the event about to be experienced. However, unless the frame of reference has meaning for the patient, it will not serve its purpose. Lengthy, detailed explanations may only upset and confuse the immobilized patient whose perception has narrowed and whose ability to see relationships is constricted.

Evaluative criteria for the effectiveness of provision of a safe and secure environment are absence of injury, adherence to a predetermined routine, and verbalization of understanding regarding aspects of care.

Development of feelings of belonging

Since the nurse has the opportunity for frequent contact with the psychologically immobilized patient, there is potential for developing a trusting nurse-patient relationship. However, it is frequently difficult to initiate this relationship because the patient often does not reciprocate. The nurse may believe that time is being wasted and may decide to leave the patient alone until the patient initiates conversation. This tendency for mutual withdrawal must be recognized and avoided.

To feel comfortable, the patients must believe that the nurse cares about them and will not desert them. The initial contacts lay the groundwork for this belief. When approached, the patients should be addressed by name, thereby giving them recognition as individuals. It is important to speak even to unresponsive patients. Lack of response does not mean the persons cannot hear. Care must be taken regarding what is discussed in the patients' presence. A caring attitude is often conveyed nonverbally by willingness to remain with patients, apparent comfort while with the patients even though they are silent or crying, and assisting or assuming responsibility for tasks the patients are unable to complete.

A common pitfall at the initiation stage of trust development is an overly warm or cheerful approach (e.g., smiling broadly, "Mr. Jones, it's great to see you up. You look so good"). The depressed patient tends to react by withdrawing further. He feels uncomfortable, unworthy, unable to believe the comments, and unable to reciprocate. The nurse should be neutral, pleasant, and matter-of-fact (e.g., "Mr. Jones, it's time for breakfast. I'll walk with you to the cafeteria"). The depressed person uses an "evaluative factor," which reflects the person's own value, in the perception of the world.[13] Because of the evaluative factor, the individual is vulnerable to instances that imply good or bad. It is better for the nurse to refrain from using value-laden words. Instead of saying, "You look so good today," it is more descriptive to say, "It looks as if you have just had your hair washed and set." Similarly, it is more helpful to describe the weather as sunny or rainy rather than good or bad.

Throughout all interactions with the psychologically immobilized patient, it is vital to maintain a hopeful attitude. Verbally, this can be done by conveying both recognition of the person's present feeling and the belief that improvement can occur. For example, it is better to advise a patient to defer an important decision "until you are feeling better" than "because you aren't up to it."[8] The first comment demonstrates that the patient will feel better, whereas the second reinforces the hopelessness of the present situation. Nonverbally, a hopeful attitude is conveyed in a variety of ways. Remaining with the patient conveys respect and that the nurse will stay even though the patient does not talk. Relaxed body language and eye contact convey concern and patience.

Behaviors indicative of the patient developing feelings of belonging include muscle relaxation when with others and an increased eye contact. There may also be indications that the patient has developed a relationship with the nurse (e.g., inquiring where the nurse is and participating in activities when the nurse is present).

Development and support of self-esteem

Self-esteem is concerned with the view of self as a worthwhile person and an awareness of one's individuality.[3] The psychologically immobilized individual has feelings of worthlessness and self-dislike. Although the initiation of a trusting nurse-patient relationship lays the groundwork for personal growth, opportunities must be provided for the individual to interact with the environment and to attain feelings of control and personal satisfaction through self-expression and independent activity. The primary measures used to achieve self-esteem are provision of alternate outlets for expression of feelings, promotion of verbalization of thoughts and feelings, and support of socialization.

Provision of alternate outlets for expression of feelings. When the immobilized patient begins to feel secure with the nurse, increased interaction and verbalization become possible. Providing alternate outlets for expression of feelings can assist the patient in developing feelings of self-esteem by reducing feelings of tension. Physical activity forces the person to interact with the external environment. However, this interaction can be less threatening than verbal interaction. Physical activity does not require as much trust. When psychologically immobilized, the individual uses emotional energy to keep feelings suppressed. Before initiation of an activity plan, it is useful to know the patient's usual activity outlets. However, if the patient is severely withdrawn, it may be necessary to present a suggestion rather than a choice. For example, rather than asking what that patient would like to do, it may be helpful to state, "I need a partner for this game; you be my partner." Activities that are noncompetitive and can be carried out in a dyad, between the nurse and patient, are preferable to competitive group activities, in which failure is possible. Letter writing, looking at books, and doing puzzles are activities in which the individual can set the pace and the extent of participation.

The intense feelings of the psychologically immobilized person may be expressed verbally only with difficulty. If activities are used to facilitate the release of anger and frustration, the nurse should select those appropriate for the patient's developmental level. These activities include such things as pounding designs into leather, tearing paper, using a punching bag, and running.

Promotion of verbalization of thoughts and feelings. Simple verbalization of fears can reduce tension. Feelings and ideas that can be verbalized can be faced more easily than unclear emotional sensations.[13] When the person begins to verbalize, many angry or self-derogatory feelings may be expressed. The patient needs to discuss these emotions with a person who will be supportive. The nurse, through the use of active listening and therapeutic communication skills, can facilitate the patient's exploration of feelings. Reflective statements and validation of perception can help the patient pinpoint feelings.

It is important to listen to the feeling tone so that the nurse can respond to the patient's need and not introject value judgements. A format that facilitates this type of response is "You feel __________ because __________." For example, in response to "I'm so irritated with my wife; she leaves the kids alone all day," the nurse says, "You feel angry because your wife doesn't spend time with the kids." This response is concise and does not introject feelings; it conveys that the nurse understands and is empathetic. A response such as "You feel your wife is an unfit mother," is value laden and could be very threatening to a psychologically immobilized patient who is just beginning to reach out. Once the anger or self-derogatory feelings have been verbalized, the patient may be ready to start evaluating the present situation and identifying how to gain control over it and develop a more positive self-concept. One way to help with this process is to explore the situation that occurred prior to depression with the patient. This may assist in altering the individual's focus from a negative self-image to more positive aspects of life.

In addition to being supportive when the patient verbalizes feelings, the nurse can become a working partner in problem solving. The nurse can identify themes that recur in the patient's discussions of feelings (e.g., feelings of loss relating to spouse's death). After a secure relationship has been established, these themes can be explored (e.g., "Mrs. Jones, you have spoken often of your husband's death. I wonder if that is a concern for you now"). By using therapeutic communication skills, the nurse can help the patient identify problem areas and establish realistic goals and plans.

Support of socialization. The patient's communication with other patients, friends, and especially family members can further assist in increasing self-esteem. This communication can be via visits, phone calls, or letters. The nurse can facilitate as well as support the person's progressive involvement with others by providing a comfortable environment for the patient and family to visit or by engaging in a small, informal group discussion with the person and a few other patients.

Stability and support from family and friends are critical in helping the patient increase self-esteem and reassume social role. However, the effect depends on the message they communicate. Consequently, it is important for the nurse to work with the family to assess their needs in relationship to the patient's needs, to help them understand the changes that have occurred because of the illness, and to help them openly communicate with one another.

Behaviors indicative of increased self-esteem are increased participation in ward activity, self-initiation of physical activity when tension increases, initiation of situation clarification, increased expression of feelings, active participation in decision making, and resumption of social and family roles.

CONCEPT OUTLINE

- I. *Conceptual definition:* Psychological immobilization is a psychological condition in which an individual has restricted, decreased, or absent responses to physical, emotional, and/or social stimuli.
- II. *Antecedent conditions*
  - A. Loss accompanied by meaninglessness or ambiguity of event
  - B. Loss accompanied by unsuccessful resolution of developmental tasks
  - C. Loss accompanied by inadequate learning
  - D. Altered neurotransmitter levels
- III. *Behavioral definition*
  - A. Objective data
    - 1. Motor-behavioral response
      - a. Decreased spontaneous activity
      - b. Lack of eye contact
      - c. Decreased verbalization
      - d. Muscular rigidity
      - e. Minimum of gestures
    - 2. Cognitive response
      - a. Narrowing of perceptual field
      - b. Difficulty in decision making
      - c. Decreased attention span
      - d. Disorientation to time, place, and person
      - e. Unawareness of environmental dangers
  - B. Subjective data
    - 1. Affective response
      - a. Anxiety
      - b. Helplessness
      - c. Hopelessness
      - d. Depression
      - e. Alienation and isolation
      - f. Worthlessness
- IV. *Intervening variables*
  - A. Situational support
  - B. Social role
    - 1. Occupation
    - 2. Societal relationship pattern
  - C. Current developmental level
- V. *Nursing interventions—goals*
  - A. Maintenance of physical health
    - 1. Observation for signs and symptoms of physical illness
    - 2. Nutrition, elimination, and sleep monitored
    - 3. Routine for personal hygiene established
  - B. Provision of safe and secure environment
    - 1. Assessment of safety hazards
    - 2. Avoidance of isolation
    - 3. Increase of familiarity with environment
    - 4. Provision of explanations about care
  - C. Development of feelings of belonging
    - 1. Initiation of nurse-patient relationship
    - 2. Speaking directly to patient
    - 3. Remaining with patient in comfortable silence
    - 4. Avoidance of overly warm or cheerful approach
    - 5. Refraining from use of value-laden words
    - 6. Maintenance of hopeful attitude
  - D. Development and support of self-esteem
    - 1. Provision of alternate outlets for expression of feelings
    - 2. Promotion of verbalization of thoughts and feelings
    - 3. Support of socialization
- VI. *Evaluation criteria*
  - A. Increased participation in own physical care
  - B. Absence of injury
  - C. Adherence to predetermined routine
  - D. Verbalized understanding of care
  - E. Increased eye contact
  - F. Muscle relaxation
  - G. Increased participation in activities
  - H. Use of alternate methods for expressing feelings
  - I. Increased verbalization of feelings
  - J. Seeking of information from others
  - K. Active participation in problem solving

REFERENCES

1. Aguilera, D., and Messick, J.: Crisis intervention: theory and methodology, ed. 3, St. Louis, 1978, The C. V. Mosby Co.
2. Carnevali, D., and Brueckner, S.: Immobilization—reassessment of a concept, Am. J. Nurs. **70**:1502, 1970.
3. Haber, J., Leach, A., Schudy, S., and Sideleau, B.: Comprehensive psychiatric nursing, New York, 1978, McGraw-Hill Book Co.
4. Johnson, D. E.: Powerlessness: a significant determinant in patient behavior? J. Nurs. Educ. **6**:39, 1967.
5. Jourard, S.: The transparent self, New York, 1971, Van Nostrand Reinhold Co.
6. Lazarus, R. S.: Psychological stress and the coping process, New York, 1966, McGraw-Hill Book Co.
7. Luckman, J., and Sorenson, K.: Medical-sur-

gical nursing—a psychophysiologic approach, Philadelphia, 1974, W. B. Saunders Co.
8. Mackinnon, R., and Michels, R.: The psychiatric interview in clinical practice, Philadelphia, 1971, W. B. Saunders Co.
9. Mereness, D.: Essentials of psychiatric nursing, ed. 9, St. Louis, 1978, The C. V. Mosby Co.
10. Risley, J.: Nursing intervention in depression, Perspect. Psychiatr. Care 5:65, 1967.
11. Roberts, S. L.: Behavioral concepts and the critically ill patient, Englewood Cliffs, N. J., 1976, Prentice-Hall, Inc.
12. Scipien, G., Barnard, M. U., Chard, M. A., Howe, J., and Phillips, P. J.: Comprehensive pediatric nursing, New York, 1975, McGraw-Hill Book Co.
13. Stockwell, M.: Depression: an operational definition with themes related to the nurse's role. In Zderad, L., and Belcher, H., editors: Developing behavioral concepts in nursing, Atlanta, 1968, Southern Regional Education Board.
14. Waechter, E., and Blake, F.: Nursing care of children, ed. 9, Philadelphia, 1976, J. B. Lippincott Co.
15. Webster: New twentieth century dictionary, ed. 2, New York, 1968, The World Publishing Co.
16. Wu, R.: Behavior and illness, Englewood Cliffs, N. J., 1973, Prentice-Hall, Inc.

FRANCES K. MILDE

Chapter 5

PHYSIOLOGICAL IMMOBILIZATION

CONCEPTUAL DEFINITION

The ability to move freely and easily without restrictions is a prized physical possession that generally is not fully valued until it is lost or altered. Mobility affords an individual the means to fulfill the requirements of life such as withdrawing from danger, maintaining homeostatic balance, and seeking pleasurable experiences. The body functions best with the changing of positions. Metabolic processes and functions of organs and body systems are directly or indirectly enhanced when the individual is standing. For example, in the kidney all but the lower calices drain when the body is upright; the axes of the bronchioles, except for the middle lobes, are in the vertical plane; and the functioning of joints, muscles, bones, and tendons is dependent on the stress of movement.

Unrestricted mobility is, however, not always possible. In fact, in each individual's life there are multiple occurrences that dictate varying degrees and durations of immobilization. This loss in mobility has social, psychological, and physical implications that result from the unnaturalness of the situation.

Immobilization or decrease in the level of activity has beneficial physiological effects. Rest decreases metabolic needs and oxygen requirements and thus provides a simple and safe means of reducing the work load of the heart. The musculoskeletal system relaxes in a supine position, which may assist in the relief of pain and may decrease tension of injured tissue. In addition, the effects of gravity on the circulation are reduced, which may prevent or assist in the reduction of venous and lymphatic engorgement.

All diseases and states of rehabilitation involve some degree of immobilization. Immobilization interacts with and is inseparable from the majority of concepts associated with acute illness such as hypoxia, ischemia, and fluid and electrolyte imbalance.

Immobilization is present whenever physical movement is restricted, decreased, or absent. This definition, without qualifiers, would include behaviors of "healthy" individuals such as a night's sleep or a period of rest following a vigorous tennis match. The qualifiers of control, duration, and degree provide a reference base both for exclusion of an individual from consideration under the concept of immobilization and for prediction of the effect of the experience for an individual.

Control refers to an individual's ability to determine the quality and quantity of physical movement. The greater the degree of physical immobilization, the greater is the state of physical powerlessness an individual experiences. The individual's physical resources are inadequate to overcome the precipitating event or to meet the demands of the body's systems.

Decreased movement associated with "healthy" individuals would therefore not meet this qualification. When an individual requires a period of rest after vigorous activity, the individual retains the ability to move from danger and to meet the demands of the body systems. The immobilized individual requires assistance from external resources such as people or appliances. The amount and type of assistance required are determined by the extent and duration of immobilization. For example, an individual with segmental immobilization of a body part such as from a splinted finger would need less assistance than an individual with a more involved immobilization problem that requires a total body cast.

Duration is another qualification to the definition of immobilization. Duration does not refer to some arbitrary time value such as a week. Rather, it is relative to the potential for untoward involvement. The transitory decrease in activity that occurs with rest is thus excluded from this definition of immobilization, since the length of the rest is relatively predictable and is not associated with untoward reactions. An individual immobilized with a fractured arm will experience segmental immobilization for approximately 6 to 8 weeks. Involvement will probably be restricted to the area of the mechanical cast restraint. In contrast, an individual immobilized as a result of surgery under general inhalation anesthesia has the potential for much greater involvement. The duration of immobilization may be less, but the potential for untoward effects to the body system is much greater.

The last qualifying factor of immobilization is the degree, extent, or severity of the limitation. Three separate but interactive components determine the degree of involvement. They are physical inactivity, restriction to movement, and constancy of body position in relation to gravity.[163] Physical inactivity refers to the decrease in body movements that results from a lack of energy such as that which occurs in hypoxic individuals. Restriction to movement incorporates all forms of limitation to movement such as motor paralysis and casts. Constancy of body posture occurs when a position is sustained for a time without alteration of the gravitational effect on the body. Since physiological control mechanisms are not required for adjustments to the changes in gravitational forces, there is a decrease in or loss of ability to adjust to posture changes.

The greater the physical inactivity, restriction to movement, and constancy of body posture, the greater the potential for untoward effects. Physiological problems can be precipitated.

The effects of musculoskeletal, respiratory, and cardiovascular deterioration, disturbances of elimination, and integumentary changes will be presented. The focus, however, will be those predictable pathological responses in which nursing activities have the potential to prevent the pathological response.

Musculoskeletal deterioration

Immobilization produces rapid and progressive changes in the musculoskeletal system. The results are losses of muscular strength and endurance, skeletal strength, and joint mobility.

Loss of muscular strength and endurance. Muscular strength is dependent on the tension of frequent contractions of muscle fibers.[101] When no tension is produced within a muscle, a loss of strength and a concommitant loss in muscle mass result.[42,111,125] This loss of strength can range from 0.04% to 5.5%/day, with the greatest decrease occurring during the initial period of immobilization.[42,125] These losses plateau as the period of immobilization lengthens.[125,190] The rate of loss depends primarily on the amount of muscle contractions. Elevated metabolic demands, which accelerate endogenous protein catabolism, such as occur with fever or trauma also increase the loss of muscle mass.[110]

Not all muscles of the body are equally affected by immobilization. Those most affected are the antigravity muscles that facilitate locomotion and the maintenance of an upright position.[21] These muscles are the gastrocnemius-soleus group, quadriceps, glutei, and erector spinae.

As muscle strength and mass decrease, so does endurance.[100] During immobilization the diameter of individual muscle fibers decreases because of the loss of myofilaments.[147] This results in decreased ability of the muscle to sustain activity without fatiguing.[69] If circulation is impaired, muscular endurance is further reduced because the mechanisms for supplying the muscle with nutrients and removing waste products are impeded. With immobilization the muscles' venous pump is less active, which contributes to impaired circulation.[101]

Loss of skeletal strength. Normally the skeletal structure is in a constant state of remodeling with absorption and replacement of bone tissue. This continual remodeling is dependent on mechanical factors such as muscle contraction.[1,75,92,109] Physical stress stimulates deposition of bone. Immobilization disrupts this normal process of bone formation and reabsorption. The result is a net increase in reabsorption of bone.* The cause of this phenomenon is unknown. Intramedullary hypervascularity,[64] circulatory stasis,[104,173] reduced lymphatic flow,[172] and local acidotic response of cellular degradation[26] have been postulated as the cause. These hypotheses are based on the idea that the primary mechanism underlying the bone changes is curtailment of an adequate supply of nutrients to keep pace with increased cellular activity.

The imbalance between bone production and destruction results in a loss of bone tissue and the pathological condition of osteoporosis, which literally means porous bone. Concomitant to the loss of bone matrix is a loss of bone minerals, principally calcium and phosphates. The degree of immobilization and the ability of the body to impose muscular "stress" on the bone affect the extent of loss. The amount of calcium excreted in the urine and feces increases with increased degrees of immobilization.

Not all bones are equally affected by immobilization. Bones with a high turnover rate of calcium are most susceptible to the loss of mechanical stress. The long bones of the lower extremities, the os calcis, and the bodies of the vertebrae are

---

*See references 16, 21, 69, 75, and 141.

most involved.[111] In addition, segmental loss of bone mass occurs with immobilization. The part of the body restricted, as from a cast, will be affected, whereas the remainder of the skeleton will remain essentially unaltered.[26]

The rate of bone mineral loss changes during the period of immobilization. A plateau is reached in extended immobilization.[42,76,149] Excretion of calcium has been found to increase rapidly from the third day to the third week of immobilization and to reach a peak during the fifth or sixth week.[42,46] At this time a new equilibrium in the calcium reabsorption-deposition process appears to be reached, which prevents the skeleton from becoming increasingly porous. Often, however, there are coexisting or preexisting causes of osteoporosis. The total effect to the skeletal system of multiple processes is an extremely fragile skeletal system. Pathological fractures may occur as the bones become so porous that they are unable to support the weight of the body. Such fractures may occur on ambulation without external trauma.

Calcium mobilization, which occurs as a result of bone reabsorption, is most severe in adolescent males.[87,115,149,188] In immobilization, hypercalciuria generally exists without significant hypercalcemia.[42,76] However, immobilization may precipitate hypercalcemia in the adolescent male without evidence of preexisting metabolic or bone disease. Although the cause for this phenomenon is unknown, the anabolic cycle of adolescence with its rapid bone growth is presumed to be a factor in its development.[87,115]

Loss of joint mobility. Motion in joints is maintained by daily movement of body parts through their range of motion. Normally there is a continual turnover of the components of connective tissue by breakdown and replacement. Organization of these components in a functional system is dependent on the type and amount of movement. For example, the collagen fibers of the tendons and ligaments become arranged linearly in the long axis of the body part, whereas the connective tissue between structures such as the joint capsule become arranged in a loose, areolar network.[67,73,101]

Progressive and deleterious changes occur in the joint structure during immobilization. Histological evidence of joint structure changes has been reported as early as the fourth day of immobilization.[89] The ligaments and tendons shorten,[40,140] the composition of connective tissue changes,[2] and intra-articular degeneration occurs.[54,57] The result of these changes is a dense network of connective tissue (fibrosis). The manifestation of these changes is gradual and insidious. Initially, there is less flexibility of the joint. Although movement is possible, the effective range of motion is curtailed. As this process continues and the joint becomes stiffer, range of motion is further restricted. Finally, if the condition is allowed to progress, destructive changes in the joints occur.[54]

Changes in joint structure can be accelerated when immobilization is accompanied by pain, edema, trauma, impaired circulation, spasticity, inflammatory exudate, and/or degenerative changes in the joint. Any interference with delivery of nutrients or removal of waste products will interfere with the normal dynamics of the joint. An individual with multiple processes is especially prone to the development of restriction in the effective range of motion. This individual may assume a flexed position for maximum relief from pain. Contracture of the flexed joint may result.

Although all joints are susceptible to these structural changes, the hip, knee, and ankle are most frequently affected. Factors responsible for the higher risk of these joints include the effects of gravity, the difficulty of their full extension or range of motion when the body is in a supine position, and the strength of the flexor muscles. Only when the individual is standing are the hip and knee in full extension with the glutei muscles holding the hip in extension.[126] When the body is supine, in a lateral recumbent position, or sitting, partial flexion of the hip is always present. Even in the prone position, hip extension is 10 to 20 degrees less than in an upright position.[101] Full extension of the knee while the person is in bed seldom occurs without deliberate effort. The predominant muscles of the knee, the hamstring muscle group, contribute to continued flexion of the knee. Other factors contributing to the development of knee and hip flexion contractions are painful disability such as arthritis, stationary positions such as prolonged sitting, and positions with knees flexed such as when pillows are placed under the knee or the headrest is elevated.

Normally the angle at the ankle is approximately 90 degrees, with repeated dorsiflexion and plantar flexion during walking. When the body is supine, the foot, from the effects of gravity and the predominant plantar flexor muscles (gastrocnemius and soleus), assumes a plantar flexed position. The dorsal flexor muscles attempt to override the action of the plantar flexor muscles. However, gravitational force and the added stress from bedclothes contribute to the fatigue of these muscles. If this position is maintained, a drop-foot deformity results, which makes ambulation difficult or impossible.

Respiratory deterioration

Immobilization per se does not produce deleterious effects on the respiratory system. In studies with normal subjects, changes in the respiratory system were transitory with position and did not produce any regional or systemic effects. The loss of muscular strength and endurance, however, is associated with an increase in the work of breathing. Immobilization in the presence of such factors as decreased level of awareness, illness, and restraint of chest expansion results in the respiratory complications of atelectasis and/or pneumonia. The pathogenesis of these complications resides in three concurrent respiratory phenomena: (1) abnormal patterns of ventilation, (2) retention of secretions, and (3) aspiration.*

*See references 10, 32, 50, 74, and 79.

Abnormal patterns of ventilation. The normal tendency of the alveoli is to collapse because of the surface tension and elastic elements in the tissue. Stability is achieved by the alveolar epithelial secretion of surfactant, which lowers the surface tension.[29,35,156,159] Constant low-volume ventilation for several hours, however, reduces the amount of surfactant production and thus increases the surface tension, which forces the collapse of alveoli.[13,31,35,69] Sedatives, narcotics, thoracic restraint such as from a cast, body position, and pain are factors that interfere with or prohibit periodic hyperinflation.*

A supine position decreases the vital capacity by approximately 4%.[21] Factors responsible are elevation of the diaphragm, change in the shape of the chest, and redistribution of blood from the legs to the chest. When the body is in a supine position, gravity forces the abdominal contents toward the head, thereby forcing the diaphragm to rise approximately 2 to 6 cm. When the body is in a lateral recumbent position, the dependent hemidiaphragm rises even further.[29,180] Gravitational forces and external pressure as from the bed alter the shape of the chest. These changes reduce the maximal inspiratory capacity of the lung by restricting maximal inflation of the alveoli. Diffuse alveolar collapse, atelectasis, may result.

Retention of secretions. The lungs are continuously exposed to pathogenic organisms. Protection from these organisms is afforded by mucus produced by the goblet cells, the action of the ciliated epithelial cells, and the cough reflex.[29]

When the body is supine, the outward traction of the negative intrapleural pressure decreases, blood is redistributed to the thorax, and the diaphragm rises. The net effect is a reduction in the diameter of the bronchus.[21] The result is an increase in the thickness of the layer of mucus surrounding the lining of the bronchus. In addition, gravity draws the mucus toward the dependent portion of the lungs, resulting in a disproportional layer of mucus.[21] The upper surface of the lung has a thin coat of mucus that may easily become dry, thereby decreasing or abolishing the movement of the cilia. In contrast, the dependent surface becomes covered with an overabundance of mucus, which overwhelms the cilia. The result is that the normal cephalad ciliary activity becomes ineffective.[156]

The ability of the cilia to transport mucus is dependent on characteristics of the mucus. Thin, watery secretions are transported more easily than thick, tenacious, viscid secretions. Lack of humidification (either internal or external), dehydration, and secretion-suppressing drugs such as atropine increase the viscosity of secretions.

The cough is a protective reflex or voluntary maneuver to prevent the accumulation of secretions. The phases of a cough are inspiration, compression, and expulsion. During the first phase a large volume of air is inhaled, followed by an inspiratory pause to allow dissipation of air to distal segments of the lung. The compressive phase begins with tight closure of the glottis while the diaphragm and expira-

*See references 12, 29, 35, 49, 69, 128, 147, 156, and 179.

tory intercostal and abdominal muscles contract. A high intrathoracic pressure is achieved. Then the glottis abruptly but slightly opens to allow a rush of air and/or secretions to be expelled.[88,154] The result is a violent, explosive, clearing movement of air from the respiratory system. The effectiveness of the cough depends on the degree of positive pressure achieved and the volume of air inspired prior to the compressive phase.[29,105]

Muscle weakness such as that precipitated by immobilization restricts forceful contractions of muscles. Other variables that may affect the immobilized person's cough effectiveness are abdominal surgery or peritonitis, which limit the ability to contract the abdominal muscles; muscle weakness from neuromuscular disease or electrolyte imbalances (e.g., hypokalemia); and the use of narcotics or anesthetics that depress or abolish the cough reflex.

Any impairment of the protective defenses results in some degree of secretion retention. The greater the impairment, the greater the potential pathological effects. If the impairment is sufficient, the bronchioles become obstructed with mucus, which prevents the ventilation of distal segments of the lung. Absorption of alveolar air distal to the obstruction (absorptive atelectasis) results in alveolar collapse. The alveolar gases are absorbed into the circulating pulmonary blood because of the pressure gradient of the gases between the alveolar air and mixed venous blood. When the person is breathing ambient air, this diffusion process, leading to alveolar collapse, takes several hours because of the small pressure gradient of nitrogen between the alveoli and blood. If 100% oxygen is breathed and a nitrogen washout of the lungs occurs, this diffusion process may be completed in minutes.[29,39,181] The alveolar collapse does not, however, impede the secretory activity of the mucous glands.[156] As a result, stasis of secretions and pneumonia are precipitated.

Aspiration. Aspiration is another cause of respiratory problems for the immobilized individual who has a decreased level of awareness. When the pharyngeal or laryngeal reflexes are obtunded, the body's protection against aspiration is lost. A comatose individual or one who has had general anesthesia or local anesthesia of the pharynx or larynx has a high risk of aspiration.

The aspiration of gastric contents into the lungs results in an inflammatory reaction accompanied by hyperemia, edema and cellular infiltration (pneumonitis), pooling of secretions, atelectasis, and pneumonia. The severity of the response depends on the general status of the individual and the quantity and acidity of the aspirant. The larger the amount of aspirant, the greater the insult to lung tissue. Likewise, the lower the pH, regardless of volume, the greater the damage.[17,156]

Cardiovascular deterioration

Physical immobilization associated with recumbency affects the cardiovascular system by reducing the skeletal muscles' peripheral pumping action and by changing the direction of the gravitational pull on the system. The primary responses are changes in the blood and vessels (thromboembolism) and decreased ability of the body to adjust to postural changes (orthostatic intolerance). In addition, there is the potential for detrimental effects from normal hemodynamic mechanisms: increased work demands on the heart when the body is in a supine position and the use of the Valsalva maneuver in movement.

Thromboembolism. The anatomical arrangement of the muscles and vessels in the lower extremities provides a peripheal pumping action during movement, which assists in the maintenance of venous flow.[4,37,191] The veins empty during contraction and fill during relaxation. When the limbs are inactive, the peripheral pump's action is abolished, decreasing the emptying of vessels, particularly those of the calf.

Gravity augments the stasis produced by the reduction in peripheral pumping action. The anatomical arrangment of the veins most frequently involved in thrombosis, the soleal veins, is such that marked stasis occurs in them when an individual is supine and inactive.[59,96,134] When the leg is horizontal and supine, the valveless soleal veins are dependent, resulting in slow emptying of these vessels.[135] In addition, when the body is in this position, external pressure from the bed is also applied to this region.[15]

Stasis predisposes and facilitates the development of venous thrombosis by preventing the removal of coagulation products by the reticuloendothelial system[162] and liver[43,185] and by promoting endothelial damage via migration of leukocytes to the vessel wall.[167,185] Stasis of blood flow alone, however, is not enough to initiate thrombosis. Hypercoagulability or injury of a vessel must also be present.[183]

Other vessels besides the soleal veins that are frequent sites for thrombosis development, in order of decreasing incidence are peroneal, posterior tibial, popliteal, gastrocnemius, femoral and iliac veins and the inferior vena cava.[65,155] The incidence of thrombosis in these veins, except for the gastrocnemius, follows the ascending anatomical relationships of the vessels. The gastrocnemius generally is not involved except with the femoral vein because of the anatomical arrangement of the vessels. The gastrocnemius bypasses the posterior tibial and peroneal veins to drain directly into the popliteal vein.[65]

In approximately 45% of individuals with thrombosis thrombi originate in the vessels of the calf,* with the majority of these thrombi originating in the soleal veins.[30,133] In another 40% of individuals the calf thrombus extends from the calf vessels to the more proximal veins of the thigh and pelvis.[24,136,167] The proximal popliteal, femoral, and iliac veins have been found to be involved independent of the distal calf veins in approximately 15% of individuals with thrombosis.[24,167]

Thrombi generally have one of three outcomes: organization in the wall of the vein, growth, or dislocation from the attachment site and embolism.[11] The majority (78%) of thrombi organize in the vessel wall and remain localized in the calf[24,95]

*See references 24, 59, 95, 96, 127, 129, 133, 136, and 174.

without further problems, and only 22% extend to the proximal vessles.[95] In 10% to 25% of individuals with thrombosis, fragments dislodge, and pulmonary embolism results. Clinical evidence of embolus generally evolves from proximal vein thrombosis,[11,95] whereas the silent, small pulmonary emboli usually evolve from involvement of the distal calf veins.[24]

Thromboembolism does not affect every individual who is immobilized. The incidence varies depending on individual factors and diagnostic methods used. Estimates from postmortem studies indicate that 23% to 60% of all immobilized individuals develop thrombosis[11,65,83] and that the incidence for the elderly and for trauma victims is 80% to 100%.[155] Young children rarely have been found to be affected by thrombosis.[65,71] Venographic and isotopic studies have identified that high-risk candidates for the development of thrombosis are individuals who are elderly, severely ill, obese, have a malignant disease, or have a history of thromboembolism or varicose veins.*

A direct relationship has been found between the duration of bed rest and the occurrence of venous thrombosis. The longer the period of immobilization, the greater the risk. In a postmortem study of injured and burned patients, thrombosis was found in 19% of those who died within 3 days of injury, in 47% of those who died within 4 to 7 days, and in 75% to 90% of those who died after 7 days.[155]

Isotopic and venographic studies have revealed that calf thrombosis begins almost immediately after the initiation of immobilization. Thrombi have been found during the first week of immobilization in persons who have been paralyzed and in those who were admitted to the hospial for treatment of a medical problem.[77,127,136,182] Thrombi have also been found in patients on their first and third postoperative day.[63,80,94,174] After 2 to 4 weeks of immobilization, there is a high incidence of thrombosis originating in the thigh and pelvis.[65,131,155] This is particularly significant, since the majority of fatal pulmonary emboli originate from the veins of the thigh and pelvis. Up to one-third of the individuals who have thigh or pelvic thrombosis will develop pulmonary emboli, with death resulting in 5% to 25% of these individuals.† Approximately 80% of these deaths occur suddenly.[55]

Orthostatic intolerance. After a period of immobilization cardiovascular deconditioning can result in an altered ability to adjust to postural changes. The usual response when an individual changes from a supine to an upright position is a decrease in arterial pressure and an increase in heart rate. The baroreceptors immediately elicit sympathetic stimulation to produce vasoconstriction and increase the arterial pressure.[69]

After a period of immobilization this normal physiological response to position is less effective. Although the exact mechanism of this orthostatic intolerance is un-

---

*See references 7, 11, 18, 22, 60, 63, 77, 80, 96, and 124.

†See references 23, 95, 127, 152, and 182.

known, the most prevalent theory relates to a failure of normal postural reflexes. This reflex failure results in vasodilation.[21] As a result of the hydrostatic pressure gradient, venous peripheral pooling occurs, resulting in reduced circulating blood volume, decreased venous return, decreased cardiac output, increased pulse rate, and decreased blood pressure.[21,103,142,164] Postural reflexes are altered to some degree within the first hours of recumbency. In a study of healthy subjects mild but significant orthostatic tachycardia was produced after 6 hours of bed rest.[116] More pronounced effects were reported to occur after 1 or more weeks of immobilization. In studies with passive tilting to an upright postion all subjects demonstrated marked increase in pulse rate, ranging from 10 to 40 beats/minute over their immobilization levels, * and an increased incidence of syncope.[42,86,119-121] These changes occurred whether the subject's immobilization position was supine or sitting.[104]

Decreases in muscular strength and blood volume have also been implicated as factors in the development of orthostatic intolerance. Since muscular strength decreases with immobilization, the effectiveness of the peripheral venous pump and the external pressure applied to vessels by the muscles are decreased.[103,114] The result is a lack of external pressure to counterbalance the increased pressure in the veins.

Blood volume decreases during prolonged immobilization. An average 5% to 17% reduction in plasma volume occurs.† The maximum reduction in volume occurs within the second[120,121] to tenth day[120,177] of immobilization. These losses in volume are due to changes in hydrostatic pressure and the redistribution of blood.[110]

Hemodynamic effects. Two normal but potentially detrimental effects on the cardiovascular system of some immobilized individuals result from the Valsalva maneuver and the work demands on the heart. The individual with a compromised cardiovascular system is especially vulnerable if subjected to such stress.

The Valsalva maneuver, by definition, is an increase in intrathoracic pressure by forcible exhalation against a closed glottis.[148] Pushing, pulling, or straining movement such as turning, lifting oneself with the aid of a trapeze, getting on a bedpan, and forceful defecation can result in involuntary production of this maneuver. When the glottis is closed and the chest fixed, such movements are more effectively accomplished.

The Valsalva maneuver produces a series of changes in the cardiovascular system. Normally there are minor fluctuations of intrathoracic pressure that augment venous blood return. When, however, there is a sustained increase in pressure, venous blood flow is greatly inhibited.

With the onset of straining as venous return is reduced, there is an initial de-

*See references 16, 42, 86, 119-121, 166, and 178.

†See references 16, 42, 68, 120, 121, 138, 166, 172, 176, and 178.

crease in pulse rate and a transient increase in systemic blood pressure. Sustained straining increases the pulse from prebaseline levels and decreases blood pressure. The immediate effect of the release of pressure is a further reduction in blood pressure and a responding increase in pulse rate. After about 5 seconds, with the rapid increase in venous return, the blood pressure rises to levels greater than the baseline and the pulse falls.[51,148]

These physiological changes are not deleterious to a normal heart; however, for individuals with compromised cardiovascular system, potential detrimental effect may result. Arrhythmias from hypoxia may result.[36] In addition, when the maneuver obstructs the venous return, dilation of distal veins is produced.[21] This may cause existing thrombi to dislodge and be swept through the heart and into the pulmonary arteries with the rapid influx of blood that occurs when the intrathoracic pressure is released.

The second potentially detrimental hemodynamic effect can be produced from the redistribution of blood in the cardiovascular system. When a supine position is assumed, approximately 11% of the total blood volume is redistributed from the legs. Of this, approximately 80% enters the thoracic region, with the rest entering the systemic circulation of the arms, head, and abdomen.[158] As a result, the heart works harder when the body is in a flat, supine position. Research evidence indicates that in an individual with a normal cardiovascular system the heart works approximately 20% more when the body is in a recumbent position than when it is in a sitting position. This load is doubled in individuals who have cardiovascular disease.[33]

Disturbances of elimination

Immobilization contributes to changes in the gastrointestinal and urinary systems. The primary gastrointestinal tract symptom observed is constipation. Problems of the urinary system occur in relation to drainage of the renal pelvis and bladder.

Constipation. The barrage of radio, television, and magazine advertisements for laxatives suggests that the entire human species is affected with constipation. In reality, most people have well-established patterns and habits of defecation. These patterns, however, are easily interrupted by changes in the environment, diet, or routine. In addition, the physiological effects of immobilizaton (e.g., muscle weakness) and of the therapeutic regimen (e.g., response to opiates and anticholinergic drugs) contribute to the development of constipation.

Defecation in Western culture is a private act. A bedpan, a bedside commode, or a toilet facility at one side of the room provide varying degrees of visual, olfactory, and auditory invasion of privacy. For example, a curtain pulled around a bed can provide only visual, not auditory or olfactory, privacy. The impact of this invasion of privacy depends on the sensitivity of the immobilized individual. A person who is sensitive to the sounds and smells associatd with defecation will suppress the urge to defecate.

The response of the rectum to the retention of feces is relaxation and accommodation. A greater volume of feces is then required to reelicit the urge to defecate.[69] Some of the retained feces returns to the sigmoid or decending colon, where more water is absorbed. The rectum is thought to be impermeable to water.[41,161] As the feces lose water and become hardened, passage becomes more difficult.

Compounding the problem of elimination for an immobilized individual is the change in position used during defecation. Although considered primitive, the ideal position is squatting, which aligns the rectum and sigmoid and increases intra-abdominal pressure.[5] The usual sitting position for defecation approximates the squatting position, especially if the individual leans forward, resting the arms on the thighs. When a person must use a bedpan, the position assumed does not approximate the ideal position. Even when the head of the bed is elevated, the hips are flexed less than 90 degrees. In addition, the legs are extended, not flexed. The result is an increase in the duration and amount of intrathoracic pressure needed to accomplish defecation and inefficiency of the abdominal muscles to increase intra-abdominal pressure.[41,72]

Increased intrathoracic pressure is accomplished by the Valsalva maneuver. The glottis is closed, and the chest muscles are contracted. The detrimental effects noted previously can result from straining to defecate.

A decrease in an individual's level of activity contributes to the development of constipation. Physical activity increases the motor activity of the colon, particularly the propulsive movements after meals.[82] Inactivity, especially that associated with recumbency, removes this effect. In addition, the postural and gravitational effects that aid elimination are removed.[161]

Passage of fecal material is enhanced by relaxation of the ileocecal valve and propulsive contraction of the colon. Entry of food into the upper small intestine initiates a reflex response, the gastroileal reflex, which leads to the movement of fecal material from the ileus into the rectum.[69] Within a few minutes of eating, contraction of the colon markedly increases, particularly in the sigmoid.[82,146] Recumbency alters this effect of meals on the activity of the colon. Although the segmenting pressure activity of the colon increases, the propulsive activity of the bowel remains essentially unchanged.[81,82] Hence the passage of fecal material is delayed, and an increased absorption of water occurs.

The type of food eaten affects the motility and characteristic of the stool. Contents from high-residue diets pass more rapidly through the intestinal tract than those from low-residue diets. Vegetables and bran stimulate intestinal motility by adding bulk.[27] The average weight of the stool is doubled with such a diet because most of the indigestible fiber is excreted.[41,47]

Micturition. Difficulty in micturition frequently occurs in individuals confined to bed. Although the exact mechanism of this difficulty has not been identified, it is thought to be due to the difficulty in achieving relaxation of the perineal muscles and the external sphincter when the body is in a reclining posture.[21,99] Individuals with additional obstruction to urine flow such as hypertrophy of the prostate have even greater micturition difficulties. Bladder distention from retention of urine results.

Renal calculi. Immobilization contributes to the production of renal stones by impairing renal drainage and by altering calcium metabolism and urinary pH. The stones associated with immobilization differ from the usual ambulatory stones, which generally consist of oxalate and urate. The stones of recumbency are predominately composed of calcium phosphate.[34,53,144] Because of the effects of immobilization on the skeletal system, both calcium and phosphates are present in the urine in increased amounts.[42] In addition, immobilization increases the time available for the precipitation and aggregation of these crystalloids, since the supine position impairs drainage from the renal calices.[21]

Normally, urinary pH fluctuates during the day from 4.5 to 7.0, with an "alkaline tide" occurring after meals.[186] With prolonged immobilization the urine becomes more alkaline because of the absence in the urine of acidic metabolites, which are the product of muscle metabolism.[21,52,160] As the urine becomes more alkaline, less calcium is held in solution.[53]

Contributing factors implicated in the development of renal calculi are infection and dehydration.[21,147,169] Urinary tract infection can contribute to stone formation by providing bacterial nuclei around which stones can form.[160] In addition, some bacteria such as *Proteus* species contribute to alkaline urine by their urea-splitting ability.

Dehydration predisposes an individual to the formation of renal stones via two mechanisms: disproportionate ratio of solids to fluid and reduction of washout of particulate matter. Precipitation of crystalloids is facilitated by this stasis and supersaturation.

Integumentary changes

One of the major problems confronting any individual who is immobilized for a prolonged period is ischemic changes of the skin and muscle. Ischemia results from prolonged external pressure that exceeds the tissue capillary pressure.[14,98] A detailed discussion of this phenomenon is included in Chapter 14.

ANTECEDENT CONDITIONS

The major categories of factors that result in immobilization of the body or of its parts include interruption of or interference with the function of the musculoskeletal and neurological systems, altered cellular function, restrictive or suppressive therapeutic regimens, and psychological immobilization.

Decreased musculoskeletal function

The body is dependent on the skeleton for structural stability and on functioning muscle cells for movement. Without a functioning musculoskeletal system, a person's ability to stand upright and to sustain movement on two appendages is altered.

Disorders of the musculoskeletal system may primarily involve the muscles, bones, joints, or a combination of these structures. Atrophy, dystrophy, and injury of muscles; infection, fracture, tumor, osteoporosis, and osteomalacia of bones; and arthritis and tumor of joints will all decrease the functioning of this system. The primary responses to these pathological processes are muscle weakness, increased fatigability, and decreased ability to move body parts as a result of structural changes and associated pain and edema.

Pain is one of the body's protective mechanisms that warns of impending danger. When pain is experienced, an individual restricts movement and activity of the injured part in an attempt to decrease pain. The degree of immobilization that occurs depends on the severity of the injury or the nature of the process that is producing the pain and on the individual's interpretation of the situation.

Muscle movement may be prevented or decreased by an increase in interstitial fluid. Edema may result from a host of factors, among which are inflammation and impeded venous blood return.

Altered neurological function

The nervous system provides the control functions of the body. The rapid activities of the body such as muscular contraction and reflexes are dependent on an intact nervous system. Any interference with sensory reception, impulse propagation, information processing, or motor response will result in some degree of immobilization, from involvement of a single motor unit to the total body. Alterations of neurological function can be produced by such conditions as infections (e.g., encephalitis), tumors, trauma, drugs, vascular diseases (e.g., cerebral infarction), demyelinative diseases (e.g., multiple sclerosis), degenerative diseases (e.g., Parkinson's disease), exposure to toxic products (e.g., carbon monoxide), nutritional disorders, and metabolic disorders (e.g., hypoglycemia).[69]

Responses to such disorders include alteration in level of awareness, loss of strength, loss of muscular coordination, paralysis, and tremors. Paralysis may take the form of spasticity or flaccidity, depending on the underlying pathological mechanism. Although spasticity is often thought of as an increase in motor activity, the result of muscle spasticity is stiffening or rigidity of the body, especially of the extremities.

Altered cellular function

Energy is necessary to provide the fuel for movement and to sustain life. The cells use energy for such activities as synthesis and growth, muscular contraction, active transport of electrolytes and nutrients across cell membranes, and propagation of nerve impulses.[69]

The cells' ability to produce adequate energy is reduced by conditions such as hypoxia, ischemia, malnutrition, toxemia, edema, fluid and electrolyte imbalance, acid-base imbalance, and shock. The common denominator of all such conditions is an alteration in cellular function. When physiological demands on the body or on its parts exceed its ability to respond, rest is necessary to protect the body from damage and exhaustion. The body will attempt to reduce its activity to a level that is within its capacity to meet the energy demands.[99]

Restrictive or suppressive therapeutic regimens

Medical regimens often affect the quantity or quality of an individual's movement. Mechanical factors such as traction and casts facilitate healing by inhibiting movement. Pharmaceutical agents such as sedatives, analgesics, tranquilizers, and anesthetics used to alter a patient's level of awareness also reduce or eliminate movement.

Bed rest can be either a therapeutic, prescriptive factor or the inadvertent result of illness or disability. Rest is often required to reduce body system demands on diseased or injured organs. Rest decreases metabolic needs and oxygen requirements. Also, bed rest is the simplest and safest means of reducing the work load of the heart. Rest decreases blood pressure, heart rate, and cardiac output, which favors healing of a diseased heart. The musculoskeletal system is allowed to relax. Pain is relieved, and excessive irritation of injured tissue is prevented. Rest can overcome the effects of gravity, which is valuable in the prevention and treatment of venous and lymphatic engorgement.

Thus, although rest is often required to reduce demands made on diseased or injured tissues, the hospital environment structured around the bed may promote inactivity when it is not necessary. There are few provisions in the hospital for the ambulatory patient; a decrease in activity is thereby encouraged. One research study found that the greatest increase in time spent in bed by surgical patients occurred immediately after admission to the hospital, not after surgery. When these persons were at home, they spent only 30% of the day in bed. On admission to the hospital these preoperative patients spent approximately 63% of the time in bed. During their first 3 postoperative days they spent approximately 90% of the time in bed. The amount of time spent in bed increased 33% after admission to the hospital, whereas it increased only 27% after the surgical event.[20]

The surgical experience is unique in that the medical regimen enforces immobilization of patients in almost every conceivable avenue. The pharmaceutical agents used not only reduce movement of the musculoskeletal system but also affect the respiratory and cardiovascular systems. Trauma to tissues from cutting and manipulation precipitates both pain and edema. The energy demands placed on the body to clear its system of toxins and to heal its tissue deplete energy reserves.

Mechanical restraints such as casts, splints, bulky dressings, and binders may be used postoperatively to assist in wound healing. In addition, supportive measures used to assist in recovery such as intravenous fluid administration, gastric suctioning, and oxygen administration further restrict movement.

Psychological immobilization

An individual may perceive the situation to be so overwhelming and the self so helpless or powerless as to become psychologically immobilized. If this state persists, varying degrees of physical immobilization can result. The concept of psychological immobilization is addressed in Chapter 4.

BEHAVIORAL DEFINITION

The parameters that identify the severity or potential risk level of an immobilizing event are (1) the duration or length of the event, (2) the degree of restriction to movements, (3) the amount of the body affected by the restrictions, (4) the degree to which an upright position can be assumed, and (5) the individual's control of both the quantity and quality of movements.

The data that indicate that an immobilization event is precipitating pathological or physiological changes reside in the systems of the body being affected. The data will be presented by the categories of effects of immobilization on the body.

Musculoskeletal deterioration

Objective data. Primary indications of the severity of the effects on the musculoskeletal system are decreases in the tone, strength, size, and endurance of the muscles; in the range of joint motion; and in skeletal strength. Data must be compared with baseline information obtained at the onset of the immobilization episode to the useful monitors of these changes.

Reduced tautness of muscles when a body part is relaxed indicates reduction in tone. Decrease in the level of resistance a muscle group can offer indicates decreased strength. Decrease in the circumference of the involved parts indicate reduced muscle size. Reduced muscle endurance can be evidenced by reduction in the time that general activities can be sustained. For example, reduction in the length of time that an individual performs an activity such as hair combing is an indication of reduced muscle endurance. Also, increase in cardiac and respiratory rates during these activities indicate that such activities are becoming more stressful or that the muscles' endurance is decreasing. Decrease in range of motion is evident from a measurement of the degrees of joint movement by the use of a goniometer or from a functional interpretation of movements during normal activities such as the manipulation of a fork to eat.

Evidence of decreases in skeletal strength can be obtained from laboratory and radiological studies when the results of such studies are available. X-ray evidence is a late clinical sign of the development of a fragile skeletal system. The loss of bone minerals, especially calcium, provides diagnostic evidence of changes in the bone. However, it has been estimated that 10% to 50% of the total skeletal calcium must be lost before changes become radiologically apparent.[21,42] Elevations in serum and urine calcium levels occur earlier and are generally more readily available indicators of bone decalcification.

Objective signs of hypercalcemia, which are often initially vague and nonspecific, include vomiting, weight loss, constipation, hypertension, metabolic acidosis, bradycardia, seizure, and coma.[87,115,188,189] The onset of these signs occurs most frequently during the fourth to eighth week after injury.[87,115,188,189] This time frame is consistent with the rates of calcium excretion of normal immobilized men, in whom peak values are reached during the fifth and sixth week of immobilization.[42]

Subjective data. Reduced muscle strength or endurance is often reflected by weakness, fatigue, or muscle heaviness. Stiffness and pain reflect changes in joint mobility. Symptoms of hypercalcemia include anorexia, nausea, lethargy, weakness, headache, and abdominal pain or cramping.

Respiratory deterioration

Objective data. The effect of immobilization on the respiratory system is determined on the basis of clinical data. Elevation in temperature and accompanying or prior increased heart rate are two of the initial signs of respiratory complications. When atelectasis involves a portion of the lungs, physical signs include decreased chest movement, dullness to percussion, and reduced or absent breath sounds and vocal fremitus over the involved area. If the atelectasis is massive, the trachea will deviate to the side of involvement. In pneumonia the physical signs vary with the degree of involvement. Decreased movement of the chest cage, dullness to percussion, bronchovesicular to bronchial breath sounds over the affected area, a midline position of the trachea, egophony, and whispered pectoriloquy indicate lobar involvement. Rales, predominately during the last phase of inspiration, are frequently present over the area of involvement.[29] Other evidence can be obtained from arterial blood gas analyses and chest radiography. The degree of hypoxemia depends on the level of involvement. Consolidation and mediastinal shift are evident from radiological studies.

Subjective data. Vague and nonspecific subjective data accompany the effect of immobilization on the respiratory system. Dyspnea may be present, especially with massive atelectasis and pneumonia.

Cardiovascular deterioration

Objective data. The cardiovascular system does not provide direct or conclusive evidence of the development of vascular complications. Clinical signs and symptoms are unreliable for the detection of thromboembolism. Isotopic and radiological studies have indicated that thrombosis was present in 20% to 50% of the individuals without any clinical evidence of thrombosis.* Likewise, when clinical signs such as erythema, edema, tenderness, and Homans' sign were present, no radiological or isotopic evidence of thrombus could be found in approximately 50% of the individuals.[56,70] When clinical signs indicated thrombophlebitis and objective parameters indicated thrombosis, the proximal thigh and pelvic veins were involved in approximately 69% of the individuals, and the distal calf veins in approximately 10% of individuals.[3] Of individuals with both positive clinical signs and positive radiological or isotopic signs, pain or calf tenderness was present in approximately 60%, ankle or calf edema in approximatly 40%, and positive Homans' sign in approximately 10%.[59,70,96]

The first evidence of massive embolic occlusion of the main pulmonary arteries may be shock and death. For smaller embolic episodes there are few clinical signs.[93] Arterial blood gas levels provide evidence of hypoxemia. The magnitude of the oxygen deficit depends on the degree of pulmonary vascular occlusion. Chest radiography, electrocardiography, lung scanning, and pulmonary angiography can provide definitive evidence to support a diagnosis of pulmonary embolus.

An increase in pulse rate after assumption of an upright position is an early indication of orthostatic intolerance. Other signs of inadequate cerebral blood flow or orthostatic intolerance are pallor, tremor of the hands, sweating, difficulty following commands, syncope, and decreased blood pressure.[164]

Subjective data. Pain or calf tenderness is present in approximately 60% of persons with thrombosis. Orthostatic intolerance is often accompanied by dizziness, nausea, and blurred vision. Dyspnea is the symptom reported most frequently by individuals with pulmonary embolism; it is present in approximately three fourths of these patients.[93]

Disturbances of elimination

Objective data. Evidence indicative of constipation includes the passage of hard, dry stools and of stools of insufficient quantity or frequency.[5,41] Deviations from an individual's usual pattern determine changes in frequency and characteristics of the stool. Other data that indicate the development of constipation include distended abdomen, especially the lower quadrants, and a palpable mass in the descending colon.

Objective evidence of difficulties with micturition result from the retention of urine. Physical signs include distention of the lower abdomen between the symphysis pubis and umbilicus, a line of demarcation to percussion between the bladder and the air-containing intestines, and palpable bladder margin. In addition,

---

*See references 23, 95, 96, 127, 129 and 174.

the urine output is decreased or absent. Small, frequent voidings may be noted.

Often the only objective evidence of renal calculi is hematuria, either gross or microscopic, and positive radiological reports.[28] Nonspecific signs such as restlessness and frequency of urination may be present.

Subjective data. Subjective sensations of constipation include lower abdominal discomfort, sense of fullness, pressure on or incomplete emptying of the rectum, anorexia, nausea, restlessness, malaise, mental depression, irritability, weakness, and headache.[5,41] Statements such as "I can't go on the bedpan," and, "I have to be alone," may be indications of this problem.

Symptoms of micturition difficulties include inability to void, pressure in the lower abdomen, pain, and discomfort.

The passage of a renal stone into the ureter causes renal colic. Typically the onset occurs after a position change.[28,144] Characteristically this pain is located in the flanks or radiates to the lower abdomen. Restlessness and frequency of urination may accompany this pain.

Integumentary changes

Signs of integumentary changes are discussed in Chapter 14.

INTERVENING VARIABLES

Each individual enters a period of immobilization with resources and liabilities. These physiological and psychological variables affect the duration, extent, and sequela of an immobilization episode. The immobilized individual will not develop all the complications that immobilization can produce. The major categories of interactive intervening variables affecting the severity of or the level of risk produced by immobilization relate to (1) the characteristics of the immobilizing event, (2) the physiological reserve of the immobilized individual, and (3) the individual's perception of the threat evolving from the immobilization.

Event characteristics

The degree and duration of immobilization are the major interactive characteristics that define the level of risk. The degree refers both to the extent and the severity of the limitations. Dimensions of degree include the amount of bodily involvement, the extent of imposed restriction to movement, and the extent of limitation to the assumption of an upright position. Duration refers to the length of time of the immobilization event. The interactive effect of these characteristics is exemplified by the difference in the risk from a broken arm and from surgery. The segmental immobilization of a fractured arm for 6 to 8 weeks carries a lower complication risk than a 3-hour period of total immobilization caused by the effects of general anesthesia. Although duration does influence the results, the greater impact evolves from degree.

Physiological reserve

Immobilization has the potential of affecting directly or indirectly all systems of the body. Together with the event characteristics, the health status of the body when immobilization is initiated determines the potential effects of immobilization. For example, two individuals with the same antecedent conditions (e.g., fractured leg from identical impact injuries) may be affected differently. If one of these individuals is a young, healthy, active person without any known physical limitations, the impact would be minimal for the total body system. If the second individual has multiple body systems involvement such as seen in cardiac and pulmonary disease, the impact could be catastrophic.

The normal aging process as well as concomitant diseases reduce the body's ability to adjust to lowered levels of mobility. The more directly mobility supports normal functioning of a system, the greater the risk to that system when factors that compromise the system are present. For example, alertness and responsiveness depend on the individual's contact with changing environmental stimuli as well as the ability to receive those stimuli. If a person who is hard of hearing or has impaired vision becomes physically immobilized, most of the avenues for interaction with the environment become impaired. This individual's risk of becoming confused and psychologically immobilized is much greater than that of an individual with no additional sensory impairment.

Anyone who is subjected to the immobilization of a surgical event and also has a reduction in the compliance of the respiratory system has a much greater risk of developing the complications of atelectasis and/or pneumonia. The ability to take a deep breath can be considerably decreased by such respiratory problems as pulmonary fibrosis. Pulmonary complication occurs three to five times more frequently in surgical patients with preexisting pulmonary diseases than in those without them.[165,187]

Threat perception

The restriction of one's ability to move from physical danger is a threat to one's safety. The importance that society attaches to mobility accentuates the threat of immobilizing events. Self-esteem, body image, success in role activities, and one's very identity are related to the control over mobility. When it appears to an individual that an immobilizing event will interfere with goal achievements that support the person's identity, the chances are greater that the individual will feel the helplessness of loss of control. The interactive cycles of psychological and physiological immobility are discussed in Chapter 4.

NURSING INTERVENTIONS—GOALS AND EVALUATION CRITERIA

The primary approach to the neutralization of the effects of immobilization is maximizing mobility within the limits of the individual's condition. The ultimate goals under the concept of immobilization are maintenance of the preimmobilization abilities and functions and prevention of impairment. These goals direct the selection of interventions designed to prevent body positions and conditions that predispose body systems to deterioration. Preventive interventions should be initiated at the beginning of the immobilization episode.

Essential factors to consider when selecting goals and interventions are the pathological process causing the immobilization event (antecedent condition), the limits imposed by medical therapy, the preimmobilization status, and the intervening variables. Without this knowledge, inappropriate or potentially detrimental nursing care can be prescribed.

The initial step in the selection of goals and interventions for a specific patient is assessment of the individual's preimmobilization health status and of the individual's resources and potentials. The behaviors to be used in the evaluation of the attainment of goals are derived from these assessment data. For example, changes in muscle size, strength, and tone evidence success of interventions in the maintenance of muscle strength and endurance.

No specific activity or exercise program will be outlined in this chapter because the type and amount of exercise and activity depend on the particular patient's capability, physical status, and medical limitations. If a potential exists for detrimental effects (e.g., from an exercise regimen), medical consultation should be obtained prior to initiation of the activity.

The following subgoals of intervention for physiological immobilization relate to supporting the normal functioning of the body systems that are most affected by the immobility: (1) maintenance of strength, flexibility, and endurance of the musculoskeletal system, (2) maintenance of normal ventilation, (3) maintenance of adequate venous circulation, (4) maintenance of vascular tone (5) neutralization of normal circulatory hemodynamic effects, (6) maintenance of normal bowel and bladder function, and (7) maintenance of normal renal function.

Maintenance of strength, flexibility, and endurance of the musculoskeletal system

The prevention of deterioration of the musculoskeletal system from the effects of immobilization must include three major areas. The maintenance of muscle strength and endurance involves a daily conditioning exercise program. Exercises include both isometric, or "setting," and isotonic, or "resistive," contraction. In addition, deep breathing and coughing exercise the abdominal muscles.[97] Interventions for maintenance of skeletal strength depend on mechanical stress on the bone. Forces applied to bone by contracting muscles are the most effective means of preventing loss of bone mass. Ambulation and resistive exercise provide the necessary stress. Ambulation that involves active participation by the individual is the ideal measure. This approach, because of the very nature of the problem of physical immobilization, is not always feasible. Exercise, except for the individual with flaccid paralysis, has proven beneficial to decrease the loss of calcium from bone.[112] Other interventions such as provision of diet with adequate calcium levels and active range of motion (ROM) exercises also help reduce skeletal mineral loss. The maintenance of flexibility or joint mobility can be assisted by ROM exercises, proper positioning, and activities of daily living.

If muscle mass is lost, the return of muscle strength and circumference to preimmobilization status is a slow process. When there is no planned exercise program, recovery of muscle strength will take a few days after a short period of immobilization and from 4 to 6 weeks after a 6-week period of inactivity.[21,42,168] Muscle endurance can be increased only by increasing muscle strength and improving circulation.

Isometric muscle contraction. An isometric muscle contraction is one in which muscle tension increases but the length of the total muscle does not change.[40] No joint movement is involved. These contractions "tighten" a muscle, but they do not produce work or movement. Isometric exercises are used to maintain strength of particular muscle groups. They are especially useful in maintaining the strength of the antigravity muscles (the quadriceps, abdominal, and gluteal muscles).

If an exercise program is used during immobilization, loss of strength can be reduced or prevented.[168,189] In normal subjects muscle strength has been demonstrated to increase with a daily schedule of five maximal isometric contractions for 6 seconds each with a 2-minute rest period between contractions.[125] It has been found that one contraction at half-maximal strength per day is enough to prevent a decrease in strength.[125]

Isometric muscle contractions are also used when an increased cardiovascular load or energy expenditure from dynamic isotonic muscle contractions must be avoided.[125] Isometric contractions, however, do place some increased demands on the cardiovascular system. Sustained contraction causes elevation of both systolic and diastolic blood pressures.[8,137] These changes persist only during the exercise period and are of no consequence for people with a normal cardiovascular system. Further stress to the cardiovascular system can result from the inadvertent use of the Valsalva maneuver during exercise. This effect can be prevented by having the patient breathe through an open mouth. If a compromised cardiovascular state exists, as with congestive heart failure, medical consultation must be sought to determine work load tolerance before such exercises are initiated.

Isometric muscle contractions are performed by alternately tightening, or contracting, the muscle as hard as possible and then relaxing it. The stronger the muscle contraction, the greater the total benefit. On the basis of research by Muller,[125] it is recommended that five daily maximal contractions of 6 seconds each be performed at intervals of 2 minutes. To maximize contraction effort, the exercise period should be scheduled at a time of peak physical ability (after a rest period or during the early morning hours for most people).

Isotonic muscle contraction. An isotonic muscle contraction is one in which the length of a muscle changes but muscle tension remains unaltered.[40] Muscles shorten and lengthen. These contractions produce movement and do work. Isotonic, or resistive, exercises are performed by pushing or pulling against a stationary object. Examples of resistive exercises for bedfast, immobilized individuals include (1) pushing the feet against a foot board, (2) lifting oneself with the aid of a trapeze bar, (3) pulling oneself to a sitting position with the aid of a rope attached to the foot of the bed, (4) pushing oneself up from a prone position, and (5) pushing against the bed with the arms while in a sitting position.

Isotonic exercises produce changes in blood pressure, primarily in the systolic level.[40] For a patient with a compromised cardiovascular status, the changes produced by the dynamic work of isotonic exercise may be contraindicated. These effects can be compounded by the use of the Valsalva maneuver during the exercise.

The use of isotonic exercises to increase the strength of a muscle is most beneficial to individuals with segmental immobilization or who are recovering from an acute illness. Normal movements can be maximized for select muscle groups. For example, if the lower legs are in skeletal traction and cannot be moved, movement of the upper body and arms can be encouraged. The use of the trapeze bar over the bed not only allows the patient independence in movement in bed, but also provides active resistive and ROM exercise for the shoulders and arms. If such activities do not provide for full range of motion, supplemental exercise should be performed. Occupational therapists can often help identify other activities patients may use to retain maximal function and range of motion.

Diet. To prevent skeletal changes, the diet should contain the recommended daily dietary intake of calcium (800 mg for adults). Research on healthy individuals has demonstrated that calcium ingested at this level or higher is associated with the least loss of bone mass.[112] Caution, however, should be exercised; consistent high intake of calcium may contribute to elevated calcium levels in the blood or urine.

Positioning. Good body alignment is essential regardless of the position assumed—sitting, lying on side, prone, or supine. "Proper" alignment in bed strives to meet the same postural dynamics as when the body is in an upright position. The spine should be kept straight, with the head and extremities in the normal relationship to the trunk of the body; the normal curves of the body should be maintained, by support if needed; and the bed should be kept flat, or as flat as possible based on the patient's individual requirements.[38]

A firm mattress, possibly with a bed board, is needed to provide the support required for correct body alignment. A sagging mattress increases the risk of hip flexion contractures.

Special care must be taken to prevent flexion contractures of the hip and knees and plantar flexion contractures of the ankles. If possible, a person confined to bed should assume a prone position at least once daily to provide maximal in-bed extension of the hip joint. Flexing the knees by using pillows or raising the gatch of the bed should only be done intermittently. The predominant position of the hips and knees should be that of extension. Elevation of the head should likewise only occur intermittently so that the extension offered by a flat supine position can occur.

The feet require firm support to prevent plantar flexion contracture of the ankle. A foot board perpendicular to the long axis of the leg can be used to approximate the neutral upright posture position. Foot boards are especially critical for patients who are weak and unable to sustain dorsiflexion or who have paralysis of the lower extremities. Bedclothes should be positioned over the foot board in such a fashion that their weight is not supported by the feet. A foot board serves the multiple purpose of preventing foot-drop by maintaining the foot at approximately a 90-degree angle, preventing excessive pressure on the foot from bedclothes and providing a firm surface for exercising lower extremities against resistance.

Evaluation criteria. Areas to be evaluated to determine the success of exercise programs and body position maintenance include tone, strength, and size of muscles; endurance; range of motion; and skeletal strength. Maintenance of preimmobilization functioning levels indicates success. Muscle tone can be evaluated by observing muscle groups with the individual in a relaxed, comfortable position. The degree of tautness indicates tone. The strength may be assessed with an ergometer, if available, or by subjective assessment. To increase the accuracy of subjective assessment, the same examiner should do the evaluating at least once a week.

Circumferential measurements of each appendage should be used to determine size maintenance. A prominent landmark such as the patella should be selected, from which the distance to the measurement point can be identified repeatedly and accurately.

Endurance can be evaluated by means of normal activities such as personal hygiene care. The individual's subjective response of fatigue or weakness as well as objective responses of pulse and respiratory rate can be used to assess endurance maintenance. The patient's verbal indication of being tired, cessation of performance of the activity earlier than usual, and/or increase in heart and respiratory rates during the activity reflects decreased endurance.

The evaluation of the range of joint motion involves a functional interpretation and a measurement of the degrees of joint movement. The functional range of motion can be determined from an individual's ability to conduct activities of daily living such as manipulation of a fork to eat.

The accuracy of measuring the degree of movement is increased by the use of a goniometer. Often, however, subjective interpretation of joint movement must be made without the use of specialized equipment. To increase the accuracy of such evaluation, the same examiner should do the weekly assessment. Limitations to movement from both resistance and pain are indicative of joint changes.

Skeletal strength can be assessed from indirect studies when they are available. X-ray films can evidence a loss in bone minerals. Earlier and generally more readily available indicators are serum and urine calcium levels. For individuals who have a greater risk for the development of hypercalcemia (e.g., adolescent males and individuals with metastatic bone cancer), the Sulkowitch test may be used to screen for excessive urinary excretion of calcium. This test is simple and easy; it can be performed by a nurse on a random urine specimen. An early morning specimen should be used because of the diurnal variation in calcium excretion.[186]

Maintenance of normal ventilation

To prevent respiratory deterioration in the immobilized individual, normal ventilation must be maintained. Measures include periodic hyperinflation (deep breathing and exercise) and mobilization and removal of secretions (coughing, humidification, turning, positioning, chest physical therapy, and adequate fluid intake). In addition, positioning is used to help prevent aspiration of gastric contents.

Hyperinflation. To inflate a maximal number of alveoli, deep breathing should be performed with muscles relaxed and with movement of the thoracic structure and diaphragm unimpeded. Sitting is the ideal position for this exercise. In this position the abdominal muscles relax, the liver and abdominal structure fall downward, vascular engorgement of the thorax decreases, and diaphragmatic movement is unimpeded, allowing for maximal lung capacity. In this position the feet should be supported to stabilize the body and provide support for the abdominal muscles. When the body is supine, relaxation of abdominal muscles and minimal restriction to the thorax can be accomplished with positioning. The head of the bed should be elevated slightly; the knees should be flexed with either a pillow or elevation of the knee gatch of the bed; and the arms should be at the side of the trunk. Each inspiration should be slow and deliberate. Quick, sudden movements are ineffective, and in the abdominal surgical patient they may produce pain. There should be a pause between inspiration and expiration to allow maximal dispersion of air and inflation of the alveoli. A yawn, which has a long, deep inspiration, pause, and slow expiration, is an ideal maneuver to maximally inflate the alveoli.[9] Deep breathing should be interspersed with normal (tidal volume) breaths. Repeated hyperinflation can result in excessive elimination of carbon dioxide.

If an individual cannot breathe deeply, hyperinflation can be accomplished via a mask and ventilation bag. Prior to the use of this maneuver, the physician should be consulted. Individual hazards and precautions should be clearly defined. Voluntary cooperation of the patient is required to accomplish this maneuver. The patient is instructed to take a slow, deliberate breath through an open mouth to maintain the glottis in an open position. At the same time manual hyperinflation is provided via a mask and bag. If the individual has an endotracheal or tracheostomy tube, hyperinflation can be provided via these artificial airways with a bag.

Hyperinflation should be performed periodically, at least every 2 hours. If the patient is receiving oxygen or has an altered level of awareness, the deep breathing exercises should be more frequent. When the individual is receiving narcotics, deep breathing should be performed 30 to 60 minutes after intramuscular injection of the narcotic, that is, during the peak of the medication's respiratory depressant effects.[66] In one study on morphine and its effect on breathing, the major effect noted after intravenous administration of morphine was the lack of sighs for approximately 1 hour.[49]

When an individual cannot initiate voluntary breathing exercises, involuntary, or reflexive, hyperventilation can be produced. Movement of the limbs increases the rate of breathing.[35,159] To elicit this reflex, joint movement must occur because the mechanoreceptors do not respond to muscle contraction without joint movements.

Mobilization and removal of secretions. When an individual has the ability to deep breathe, coughing can be accomplished. The individual who is in pain or is fearful that coughing will produce pain may be unable or reluctant to cough. Positioning, pain medication, and external support may be needed to reduce or control the pain that coughing may produce.

The ideal position for the cough maneuver is sitting with shoulders rotated inward, head and spine slightly flexed, and forearm relaxed. The individual should take a deep breath, hold it for several seconds, and then forcibly cough. As the individual forcibly coughs, leaning forward increases intrathoracic pressure. If the individual lacks abdominal muscle strength or has had surgery, splinting the abdominal muscles or the incision area will increase the strength and effectiveness of the cough. If an individual cannot assume an upright position, the supine deep breathing position can be used. External abdominal supports are also helpful in this position.

For those individuals who cannot cough, mechanical stimulation of the cough reflex may be needed. Coughing can be stimulated by such measures as direct external stimulation of the trachea, instillation of a small amount of solution into the trachea via a subcutaneous catheter, and endotracheal stimulation by a catheter.[78,175] Measures that may be used to remove secretions (rather than prevent their occurrence) are postural drainage[61] with or without clapping, vibrating and tapping maneuvers of the chest,[102] and endotracheal suctioning.[90,91,139]

The lack of humidification leads to drying of mucus and predisposes to retention of secretions. Increased moisture may be added to a room by a room humidifier or vaporizors. Devices for individual use include nebulizers and humidifiers. The main difference between these two types of devices is that the nebulizer delivers a maximum number of water particles to the respiratory tract, whereas the humidifier delivers a maximum amount of water vapor with a minimum of particulate water.[48] Use of a nebulizer increases the risk of bacterial contamination[48,143] because bacteria can attach themselves to the particulate water for direct transport to the lower respiratory tract. Room humidifiers and vaporizors share this contamination disadvantage because their output also contains large water particles.

Humidified air should be provided for the individual who must mouth-breathe for any extended period of time as well as for anyone with a new tracheostomy or endotracheal tube. Normally, inspired ambient air is 80% to 90% humidified at the carina of the trachea. If this air is inhaled via an open mouth, it is 60% humidified in the oropharynx and 100% at the tracheal carina.[108,153] If the air is inhaled via a tracheostomy or endotracheal tube, humidification occurs in the tracheobronchial tree. Lack of air humidification leads to the use of water from the mucosa and mucous blanket of the tracheobronchial tree.[156] When oxygen, which is a dry gas, is administered, it should be humidified to prevent the drying of mucus and of mucous membranes. Mucus with decreased water content becomes dry, thick, and crusted.

Adequate body hydration is important to support moist mucus production. Abnormal loss of body water from the skin, lungs, gastrointestinal tract, and kidneys or inadequate fluid intake[147] will result in less available water for mucous composition. Secretions would then become inspissated. For an adult, a fluid intake of approximately 30 to 40 ml/kg of body weight/day should prevent the formation of thick, tenacious secretions.[29]

To prevent pooling of secretions in the dependent lung, the patient's position should be changed frequently. Lateral, prone, supine, and upright positions should be used and varied in effors to mobilize secretions and promote maximal inflation of lung areas. The position should be changed at least every 2 hours. Patients with a high risk of respiratory complications should have the position changed every hour to prevent extensive atelectasis of the dependent lung. Ray et al.[145] found that movement every hour was associated with restoration of ventilation and lower levels of deterioration.

Prevention of aspiration. Persons who have lost or have minimal pharyngeal or laryngeal reflexes should be positioned so that gravity will keep fluids from entering the airway. Lateral recumbent and Trendelenburg's positions promote gravity drainage.

Evaluation criteria. The primary indicators that normal ventilation is being maintained are normal breathing patterns, temperature and arterial blood gas levels; the presence of moist nonviscous mucus; and the absence of adventitious lung sounds.

Maintenance of adequate venous circulation

The primary emphasis for this area of intervention is prevention of thrombosis and emboli. Mechanical, anatomical, and pharmacological methods can be employed to prevent stasis and hypercoagulation of the blood.

Mechanical methods. To prevent stasis of blood in the lower extremities, various mechanical methods have been employed, including electrical stimulation,[25,44,45] intermittent pneumatic compression of the lower leg,[30,80,106,151] and passive exercise by a motorized foot mover.[151] Of these methods, intermittent compression of the lower leg is proving to be the most versatile and useful, since it provides the normal physiological dynamics of walking. This compression provides for cyclic emptying and refilling of the veins of the legs. The use of pneumatic compression devices is contraindicated for patients with acute thrombophlebitis or suspected thrombosis.[106]

Anatomical methods. Anatomical methods include elastic compression, elevation of the legs, exercise, and prevention of the Valsalva maneuver. Elastic compression can be provided by elastic stockings or wraps; however, the use of these devices for prevention of thrombosis is being critically evaluated. Research has presented conflicting evidence as to their effectiveness in preventing thrombosis, with the majority of the reports indicating marginal effectiveness[107,150] and potentially detrimental effects. Compressive pressure can cause constriction, with the stocking acting as a tourniquet.[85,107]

Elastic compression, in theory, produces its effect by establishing a pressure gradient. The externally applied circumferential pressure produces graduate pressure, with the highest pressure exerted distally at the foot. The pressure is transmitted to all tissues, compressing the veins and enhancing venous return.[84,113,170] Elastic compression stockings have been found to speed the clearance of a dye from the tibial veins but to delay clearance in the femoral and soleal veins,* the site of the greatest incidence of thrombosis development. The most notable assistance from elastic compression stockings has been seen in patients with varicose veins.[84]

When elastic compression devices are used, they should be removed at least once daily for inspection and care of the skin of the legs and feet. Removal should be more frequent if the pressure gradient effect is not present or if bunching of the stocking occurs, which can result in a tourniquet effect. Since the increased flow velocity produced by compression tends to persist for only 30 minutes after the compression is released,[157] it is recommended that the stocking be reapplied within 30 minutes of their removal.

Elevation of the legs is another method used to prevent venous stasis. Passive drainage of the vessels of the lower leg can be promoted by elevating the lower

---

*See references 84, 107, 130, 132, and 157.

legs. A 15- to 20-degree elevation of the legs in a Trendelenburg position increases the velocity of blood flow from the major vessels of the lower legs.[107,117,118] The clearance of these vessels is six times slower when the legs are horizontal rather than elevated.[117,118]

Elevation of the leg with hip flexion promotes venous return from only the lower legs. Elevation of the entire leg without hip flexion increases the emptying of the thigh vessels. If the legs are elevated when the trunk of the body is horizontal, the emptying of proximal thigh veins is delayed. This may be a result of extraluminal compression from the hip flexion.[107] Venous stasis of the smaller dependent vessels, most notably the soleal veins, is not as greatly affected by leg elevation because of the posterior position of these vessels.[170]

Turning the patient from side to side and to the prone position prevents external pressure on and promotes gravity drainage of the soleal veins, the site of origin of most venous thromboses. All positioning and turning must be accomplished in such a manner that venous return is unimpeded. Extraluminal pressure, which alters venous blood flow, could result from such activities as flexion of the hip with elevation of the head, flexion of the knee from pillows, lateral recumbent position without support for the upper leg, and leg compression from the bed. Another source of extraluminal pressure that can result in turbulence and dislodged emboli is massage of the leg. Since no research has yet indicated that massage does not produce turbulence, this activity should not be conducted until studies delineate its impact. Abdominal distention as from ascites or pregnancy can also cause extraluminal compression and reduced venous flow.

Venous return can also be impeded by positions in which the legs are dependent. A normal chair-sitting position with the legs dependent causes retarded venous return and, potentially, edema and thrombosis. A patient at high risk for thrombosis formation should be positioned with minimal leg dependency and compression of the veins. Elevation of the legs on a footstool or hassock will prevent blood pooling in the lower extremities.

Exercise minimizes venous stasis via the muscle-pumping action. The most effective exercise to promote venous flow is plantar flexion of the foot against resistance repeated two times.[132] This maneuver empties the soleal and tibial veins equally. Plantar flexion of the foot once every 4 seconds is also effective in promoting clearance of the soleal vein, but without resistance it is not as effective in emptying the tibial veins.[132,135] Another exercise that could be beneficial, but for which there is presently no experimental evidence as to its effectiveness, is active flexion and extension of the hip and knee. Deep breathing also helps promote venous return through changes in abdominal and intrathoracic pressure.

To be effective in preventing venous stasis, exercises should be repeated at least every hour. Studies on blood flow have revealed that activity has no lasting effect.[19,84] Within 1 hour after exercise the blood returns to its resting flow rate.

Individuals with a high risk of thrombotic development should exercise, turn, and move with the glottis open to prevent the Valsalva maneuver from dislodging an embolus.

Pharmacological methods. Pharmaceutical agents such as low-molecular-weight dextran, aspirin, and heparin may be used to reduce the blood's coagulability. A detailed discussion of this type of intervention and the nurse's responsibility associated with it can be found in Chapter 14.

Fluids. Sufficient fluids should be ingested to prevent a reduction in blood volume from dehydration. The amount of fluid loss and the function of the kidney and cardiovascular system are indicators of the level of fluids required, as well as of tolerance levels.

Evaluation criteria. Data evidencing maintenance of adequate venous circulation include absence of redness, of increased size of extremities, of edema, and of increased warmth of the lower extremities. Palpation of the extremities should reveal full pulses, absence of calf tenderness, and inability to elicit Homans' sign.

Maintenance of vascular tone

Prevention of orthostatic intolerance has been difficult to achieve. Exercise during immobilization has demonstrated little effect on orthostatic tolerance.[121,171] Exercise, however, has some effectiveness in preventing a reduction in blood volume.[62,171] Supportive measures to maintain vascular tone include changing of body position in relation to gravity, elastic compression, and adequate fluid intake. Sufficient fluids should be ingested to prevent dehydrating reductions in blood volume.

Altering the body's position in relation to gravity is helpful in preventing orthostatic intolerance by periodic stimulation of the postural neural reflex. Measures include periodic elevation of the head of the bed, having the patient sit on the side of the bed or in a chair, and ambulation by the patient. It is important to maximize the individual's participation in position changes, since active movement promotes venous return via the peripheral venous pump.

Elastic compression provides external pressure to the legs to prevent venous dilation and blood volume changes. Quiet standing for 10 minutes has been reported to produce an 11% decrease in plasma volume.[138] This reduction is theorized to result from a shift of body fluids from the venous beds to the interstitial spaces as a result of the hydrostatic pressure gradient.[42,138]

Evaluation criteria. The lack of dizziness, nausea, blurred vision, tremors of the hand, increased pulse rate, decreased blood pressure, pallor, and sweating on ambulation indicates that the body can respond supportively to posture changes. The pulse should be monitored before, during, and after ambulation, since an increasing pulse is an early indicator of orthostatic intolerance.

Neutralization of normal circulatory hemodynamic effects

Measures to prevent untoward effects from normal physiological mechanisms include positioning and elimination of the Valsalva maneuver. In addition, when a patient is receiving supplemental oxygen, its administration should be continued during all movements.

Positioning. To decrease the work load on the heart, positioning is a key intervention. Elevation of the head to a modified Fowler position and chair rest prevent increased return of blood from the legs. This prevents the increased work load on the heart that the supine position precipitates.

Elimination of Valsalva maneuver. The Valsalva maneuver can be eliminated during lifting and straining activities if the patient breathes through an open mouth. It is anatomically impossible to fixate the glottis while actively exhaling, and a conscious effort is required to fix the glottis when the mouth is open. Since straining with defecation produces an involuntary Valsalva maneuver, constipation should be avoided.

Evaluation criteria. A criterion indicative of neutralization of the potentially detrimental hemodynamic effects is maintenance of the preimmobilization cardiac function level as evidenced by minor variations in rate and rhythm patterns.

Maintenance of normal bowel and bladder function

Interventions directed to the maintenance of normal bowel function include environmental preparation, approximation of normal elimination position, maintenance of normal defecation routine, and use of diet, exercise, and drugs. Normal bladder function may be supported by position, privacy, and diet.

Environmental preparation. The immediate environment of an immobilized person should provide auditory, olfactory, and visual privacy. This can be accomplished by removing other people from the patient's immediate environment and by the use of devices to remove or mask odors. The individual should be consulted to help determine what might help minimize the social constraints in the situation.

Position. The usual position for elimination, or as close an approximation as possible, contributes to maintenance of normal function. When an in-bed position is used, the head of the bed should be elevated as far as possible with the patient's knees flexed. Weakened abdominal muscles, which would prohibit increases in intra-abdominal pressure, can be supported by the application of external compression of the abdomen with the hands.

Routine. An individual's usual defecation routine (e.g., time of day) should be followed. For most people defecation occurs approximately 50 to 60 minutes after breakfast, when the spontaneous propulsive motility of the colon is at its peak.[5]

Diet. Natural products such as bran and prunes combined with bulk and roughage such as lettuce will augment and promote a normal elimination pattern. In addition, sufficient fluids should be ingested to prevent excessive dryness of stool.

Exercise. Physical activity should be incorporated in the daily schedule to facilitate motor activity of the colon. Abdominal strengthening exercises are used to prevent muscle weakness and the resultant inability to increase intra-abdominal pressure.

Drugs. Laxatives, which may assist in controlling constipation, are of two classes: bulk formers and emollients. Bulk formers such as methylcellulose and psyllium hydrophilic mucilloid (Metamucil) produce their effects via the polysaccharide or cellulose material they contain, which dissolves and swells in water. An emollient gel or viscous solution is formed, which helps maintain soft, hydrated feces. The surface-acting emollient laxatives such as dioctyl sodium sulfosuccinate (Colace) produce their effect by altering the surface tension, allowing water and fats to penetrate fecal material.[66] To control constipation, the use of these drugs should be initiated before the problem occurs. The effect of bulk formers is usually not apparent for 12 to 24 hours; of emollients, 24 to 48 hours.

Evaluation criteria. The effectiveness of interventions directed to maintenance of bowel function can be noted by the quantity and softness of stools produced, absence of straining with defecation, and a flat, soft abdomen without palpable masses. Indications of effective bladder function include ability to micturate without difficulty, a nonpalpable bladder margin, and adequate urine output.

Maintenance of normal renal function

The maintenance of normal renal function is enhanced by positioning, diet (including adequate fluid intake), and infection control.

Positioning. Change in position is required for facilitation of drainage of the renal pelvis. The intervention of position change has been found to contribute to a marked reduction in the incidence of renal calculi in individuals who are immobilized. In 1936 Armstrong[6] published a report of a 2-year study of the incidence of renal calculi in immobilized patients. Patients who were turned from the supine position as infrequently as every 4 to 10 hours during a 2-week period did not have evidence of renal calculi.

Diet. The diet of an immobilized individual should meet the basic dietary requirements while maintaining normal urinary pH, calcium balance, and urinary excretion. Large quantities of fluid should be included to prevent supersaturation of the urine. Wide variations in intake and output are to be avoided to prevent a wide fluctuation of urinary concentration. Hence fluids should be consumed over a 24-hour period, with increased amounts during the peak hours of calcium excretion and the first 3 hours after meals. Calcium excretion in immobilized individuals is not uniformly distributed over a 24-hour period; rather, 60% to 80% of the calcium excretion, which is increased in response to immobilization, occurs in a few hours in the middle of the day, between 9 AM and 3 PM.[122,123] In addition, the first 3 hours after meals are the peak periods for urine supersaturation.[58]

All types of fluid are allowed; however, inclusion of large amounts of fruit juices and milk or milk products must be evaluated for each patient. Fruit juices, except cranberry, produce an alkaline ash; and alkaline urine compounds the urinary pH effect of immobilization. Milk and milk products may augment the hypercalciuria resulting from the skeletal changes of the immobilized patient. Restriction of dietary calcium and phosphorus to the normal recommended intake values (800 mg for adults) is recommended.[169]

To help prevent urinary pH changes and the precipitation of calcium phosphate, the diet should contain foods that produce an acidic urine. Such foods include meat, fish, and cereal. No rigorous dietary modification, for the most part, is recommended to prevent calcium phosphate renal stones.[58] Rather, the control of dietary intake should be directed to the prevention of alkaline urine.

Infection control. Control of urinary tract infections helps decrease the incidence of stones by preventing changes in pH from urea-splitting organisms and by preventing the bacteria from serving as nuclei for stone formation. When the patient has a catheter, sterile technique is mandatory to prevent the introduction of bacteria into the urinary system.

Evaluation criteria. Primary indicators that normal renal function is being maintained are the absence of flank pain and hematuria and a negative radiological report.

CONCEPT OUTLINE

I. *Conceptual definition:* Physiological immobilization is present when physical movement is restricted, decreased, or absent and the individual has lost the power to determine the quality, duration, and/or degree of physical movement.

II. *Antecedent conditions*
  A. Decreased musculoskeletal function
    1. Atrophy, dystrophy, and injury of muscles
    2. Infection, fracture, tumor, and osteoporosis of bone
    3. Arthritis and tumor of joints
    4. Pain
    5. Edema
  B. Altered neurological function
    1. Altered level of awareness
    2. Loss of coordination
    3. Decrease or loss of muscular function
  C. Altered cellular function
  D. Restrictive or suppressive therapeutic regimens
    1. Mechanical factors
    2. Pharmaceutical agents
    3. Bed rest
    4. Surgical experience
  E. Psychological immobilization

III. *Behavioral definition*
  A. Musculoskeletal deterioration
    1. Objective data
      a. Decreased tone and size of muscles
      b. Decreased endurance
      c. Decreased range of joint motion
      d. Decreased skeletal strength
        (1) Hypercalciuria
        (2) Hypercalcemia
        (3) Decreased density of bone
    2. Subjective data
      a. Decreased muscle strength or endurance
        (1) Weakness or muscle heaviness
        (2) Fatigue
      b. Decreased joint mobility
        (1) Stiffness
        (2) Pain
      c. Changes associated with hypercalcemia
        (1) Anorexia
        (2) Nausea
        (3) Weakness
        (4) Headache
        (5) Abdominal pain

B. Respiratory deterioration
   1. Objective data
      a. Tachycardia
      b. Abrupt elevation in temperature
      c. Abnormal or adventitious breath sounds
      d. Change of percussion from resonant to dull
      e. Reduced arterial oxygen level
   2. Subjective data
      a. Dyspnea
      b. Vague, nonspecific restless feelings
C. Cardiovascular deterioration
   1. Objective data
      a. Thromboembolism
         (1) Positive isotopic, venographic, or radiological studies
         (2) Erythema
         (3) Edema
         (4) Homans' sign
      b. Orthostatic intolerance
         (1) Tachycardia
         (2) Decreased blood pressure
         (3) Pallor
         (4) Sweating
         (5) Syncope
   2. Subjective data
      a. Thromboembolism
         (1) Pain or calf tenderness
         (2) Dyspnea with pulmonary embolus
      b. Orthostatic intolerance
         (1) Difficulty following commands
         (2) Dizziness
         (3) Nausea
         (4) Blurred vision
D. Disturbances of elimination
   1. Objective data
      a. Constipation
         (1) Hard, dry feces
         (2) Stools of insufficient quantity
         (3) Distended abdomen
         (4) Palpable fecal mass
      b. Urinary retention
         (1) Distended lower abdomen
         (2) Changes in percussion sounds
      c. Renal calculi
         (1) Hematuria
         (2) Positive radiological evidence
   2. Subjective data
      a. Constipation
         (1) Lower abdominal discomfort
         (2) Pressure in or incomplete emptying of rectum
         (3) Anorexia
         (4) Nausea
         (5) Restlessness
         (6) Malaise
         (7) Depression
         (8) Irritability
         (9) Headache
      b. Urinary retention
         (1) Inability to void
         (2) Pressure in lower abdomen
      c. Renal calculi
         (1) Renal colic
         (2) Restlessness
         (3) Frequency of urination

IV. *Intervening variables*
   A. Event characteristics
      1. Degree
      2. Duration
   B. Physiological reserve
      1. Aging process
      2. Entry level health status
   C. Threat perception

V. *Nursing interventions—goals*
   A. Maintenance of strength, flexibility, and endurance of musculoskeletal system
      1. Muscle strength and endurance
         a. Isometric exercise
         b. Isotonic exercise
         c. Deep breathing and coughing
      2. Skeletal strength
         a. Ambulation
         b. Resistive exercise
         c. Adequate calcium diet
         d. ROM exercise
      3. Flexibility or joint mobility
         a. ROM exercise
         b. Positioning
         c. Activities of daily living
   B. Maintenance of normal ventilation
      1. Hyperinflation
         a. Deep breathing
         b. Augmented or mechanical ventilation
      2. Mobilization and removal of secretions
         a. Coughing
         b. Humidification
         c. Turning
         d. Positioning
         e. Chest physical therapy
         f. Adequate fluid intake

3. Prevention of aspiration
    a. Positioning
    b. Suctioning

C. Maintenance of adequate venous circulation
1. Mechanical methods
    a. Electrical stimulation
    b. Intermittent pneumatic compression
    c. Passive exercise via motorized devices
2. Anatomical methods
    a. Elastic compression
    b. Exercise
    c. Elevation of legs
    d. Prevention of Valsalva maneuver
    e. Adequate fluid intake
3. Pharmacological methods
    a. Low-molecular-weight dextran
    b. Aspirin
    c. Heparin

D. Maintenance of vascular tone
1. Exercise
2. Positioning
3. Elastic compression
4. Adequate fluid intake

E. Neutralization of normal circulatory hemodynamic effects
1. Positioning
2. Elevation of head
3. Prevention of Valsalva maneuver

F. Maintenance of normal bowel and bladder function
1. Environmental preparation
2. Maintenance of usual defecation routine
3. Approximation of normal elimination position
4. Diet that includes roughage and fluids
5. Exercise
6. Laxatives

G. Maintenance of normal renal function
1. Change in position
2. Adequate fluid intake
3. Diet to promote acidic urine
4. Aseptic management of urinary drainage systems

VI. *Evaluation criteria*

A. Muscle and joint criteria
1. Return to preimmobilization functioning levels of muscles and joints
    a. Tone
    b. Strength
    c. Size of muscle
    d. Endurance ability
    e. Range of motion

B. Skeletal criteria
1. Normal urine and serum calcium levels
2. No osteoporosis evident on radiological studies
3. Absence of nausea, weakness, headache, anorexia, and abdominal pain

C. Respiratory criteria
1. Normal breathing patterns
2. Normal temperature
3. Arterial oxygen, pH, and carbon dioxide levels in normal limits
4. Presence of moist, nonviscous mucus
5. Absence of abnormal and adventitious breath sounds

D. Circulatory criteria
1. Absence of redness and edema of lower extremities
2. Size of lower extremities equal to each other and to preimmobilization circumference
3. Full bilaterally equal pulses of lower extremities
4. Absence of Homans' sign
5. Lack of dizziness, nausea, and pallor with position change
6. Minor fluctuation in pulse rate and blood pressure during ambulation
7. Normal variation in heart rate
8. Absence of arrhythmias

E. Bowel and bladder function criteria
1. Sufficient quantity and softness of stools
2. Absence of straining with defecation
3. Flat, soft abdomen without palpable masses
4. Micturition without difficulty
5. Adequate urine output

F. Renal function criteria
1. Absence of flank pain
2. Absence of hematuria
3. Negative radiological report

REFERENCES

1. Abramson, A. S., and Delagi, E. F.: Influence of weight-bearing on muscle contraction on disuse osteoporosis, Arch. Phys. Med. Rehabil. **42**:147, 1961.
2. Akeson, W. H., Woo, S. L. Y., Amiel, D.,

and Matthews, J. V.: Biomechanical and biochemical changes in the periarticular connective tissue during contracture development in the immobilized rabbit knee, Connect. Tissue Res. **2**:315, 1974.
3. Alexander, R. H., Folse, R., Pizzorno, J., and Conn, R.: Thrombophlebitis and thromboembolism: results of a prospective study, Ann. Surg. **180**:883, 1974.
4. Almen, T., and Nylander, G.: Serial phlebography of the normal leg during muscular contraction and relaxation, Acta Radiol. **57**:264, 1962.
5. Almy, T. P.: Constipation. In Sleisenger, M. H., and Fordtran, J. S., editors: Gastrointestinal disease: pathophysiology, diagnosis, management, Philadelphia, 1973, W. B. Saunders Co.
6. Armstrong, A. C.: Urinary tract complications in prolonged immobilization, Br. Med. J. **1**:1274, 1936.
7. Ballard, R. M., Bradley-Watson, P. J., Johnstone, F. D., Kenney, A., McCarthy, T. G., Campbell, S., and Weston, J.: Low doses of subcutaneous heparin in the prevention of deep vein thrombosis after gynaecological surgery, J. Obstet. Gynaecol. Br. Commonw. **80**:469, 1973.
8. Bartels, R. L., Fox, E. L., Bowers, R. W., and Hiatt, E. P.: Effects of isometric work on heart rate, blood pressure, and net oxygen cost, Res. Q. Am. Assoc. Health Phys. Educ. **39**:437, 1968.
9. Bartlett, R. H., Gazzaniga, A. B., Geraghty, T. R.: Respiratory maneuvers to prevent postoperative pulmonary complications, a critical review, J.A.M.A. **224**:1017, 1973.
10. Becker, A., Barak, S., Braun, E., and Meyers, M. P.: The treatment of post-operative pulmonary atelectasis with intermittent positive pressure breathing, Surg. Gynecol. Obstet. **111**:517, 1960.
11. Beckering, R. E., Jr., and Titus, J. L.: Femoral-popliteal venous thrombosis and pulmonary embolism, Am. J. Clin. Pathol. **52**:530, 1969.
12. Bendixen, H. H., Egbert, L. D., Hedley-Whyte, J., Laver, M. B., and Pontoppidan, H.: Respiratory care, St. Louis, 1965, The C. V. Mosby Co.
13. Bendixen, H. H., Hedley-Whyte, M. B., Chir, B., and Laver, M. B.: Impaired oxygenation in surgical patients during general anesthesia with controlled ventilation, N. Engl. J. Med. **269**:991, 1963.
14. Berecek, K. H.: Etiology of decubitus ulcer, Nurs. Clin. North Am. **10**:157, 1975.
15. Berman, B.: A stocking to help reduce leg phlebothrombosis in bed patients, Pa. Med. **74**:68, 1971.
16. Bohnn, B. J., Hyatt, K. H., Kamenetsky, L. G., Calder, B. E., and Smith, W. M.: Prevention of bedrest induced orthostatism by 9-alpha-fluorohydrocortisone, Aerosp. Med. **41**:495, 1970.
17. Bosomworth, P., Coyer, B. S., and Bryant, L. R.: Aspiration of gastric juice—physiologic alterations, Anesthesiology **26**:241, 1965.
18. Breneman, J. C.: A formula for predicting and a device for preventing postoperative thromboembolic disease, Angiology **14**:437, 1963.
19. Browse, N. L.: Effect of bed rest on resting calf blood flow of healthy adult males, Br. Med. J. **1**:1721, 1962.
20. Browse, N. L.: Observations on the activity of surgical patients, Br. Med. J. **1**:669, 1964.
21. Browse, N. L.: The physiology and pathology of bed rest, Springfield, Ill., 1965, Charles C Thomas, Publisher.
22. Browse, N. L., Gray, L., and Morland, M.: Changes in the blood fibrinolytic activity after surgery (the effect of deep vein thrombosis and malignant disease), Br. J. Surg. **64**:23, 1977.
23. Browse, N. L., Jackson, B. T., Mayo, M. E., and Negus, D.: The value of mechanical methods of preventing postoperative calf vein thrombosis, Br. J. Surg. **61**:219, 1974.
24. Browse, N. L., and Thomas, M. L.: Sources of non-lethal pulmonary emboli, Lancet **1**:258, 1974.
25. Browse, N. L., and Negus, D.: Prevention of postoperative leg vein thrombosis by electrical muscle stimulation: an evaluation with ^{125}I-labelled fibrinogen, Br. Med. J. **3**:615, 1970.
26. Burkhart, J. M., and Jowsey, J.: Parathyroid and thyroid hormones in the development of immobilization osteoporosis, Endocrinology **81**:1053, 1967.
27. Burkitt, D. P., Walker, A. R. P., and Painter, N. S.: Effect of dietary fibre on stools and transit-times, and its role in the causation of disease, Lancet **2**:1408, 1972.
28. Carlson, H. E., and Ockerblad, N. F.:

Stones of recumbency, South. Med. J. **33**:582, 1940.
29. Cherniack, R. M., Cherniack, L., and Naimark, A.: Respiration in health and disease, ed. 2, Philadelphia, 1972, W. B. Saunders Co.
30. Clark, W. B., Prescott, R. J., MacGregor, A. B., and Ruckley, C. V.: Pneumatic compression of the calf and postoperative deep-vein thrombosis, Lancet **2**:5, 1974.
31. Clements, J. A.: Surface tension of lung extracts, Proc. Soc. Exp. Biol. Med. **95**:170, 1957.
32. Codd, J. E.: Postoperative pulmonary complications: a review, Mo. Med. **72**:286, 1975.
33. Coe, W. S.: Cardiac work and the chair treatment of acute coronary thrombosis, Ann. Intern. Med. **40**:42, 1954.
34. Comarr, A. E., Kawaichi, G. K., and Bors, E.: Renal calculosis of patients with traumatic cord lesions, J. Urol. **87**:647, 1962.
35. Comroe, J. H.: Physiology of respiration: an introductory text, ed. 2, Chicago, 1974, Year Book Medical Publishers, Inc.
36. Conrad, L.: The Valsalva maneuver: a clinical inquiry, Am. J. Nurs. **71**:553, 1971.
37. Cotton, L. T., and Clark, C.: Anatomical localization of venous thrombosis, Ann. R. Coll. Surg. Engl. **36**:214, 1965.
38. Covalt, N. K.: Bed exercises for convalescent patients, Springfield, Ill., 1968, Charles C Thomas, Publisher.
39. Dale, W. A., and Rahn, H.: Rate of gas absorption during atelectasis, Am. J. Physiol. **170**:606, 1952.
40. Darling, R. C.: Exercise. In Downey, J. A., and Darling, R. C., editors: Physiological basis of rehabilitation medicine, Philadelphia, 1971, W. B. Saunders Co.
41. Davenport, H. W.: Physiology of the digestive tract: an introductory text, ed. 4, Chicago, 1977, Year Book Medical Publishers, Inc.
42. Deitrick, J. E., Whedon, G. D., and Shorr, E.: Effects of immobilization upon various metabolic and physiologic functions of normal men, Am. J. Med. **4**:3, 1948.
43. Deykin, D.: The role of the liver in serum-induced hypercoagulability, J. Clin. Invest. **45**:256, 1966.
44. Doran, F. S. A., Drury, M., and Sivyer, A.: A simple way to combat the venous stasis which occurs in the lower limbs during surgical operations, Br. J. Surg. **51**:486, 1964.
45. Doran, F. S. A., and White, H. M.: A demonstration that the risk of postoperative deep venous thrombosis is reduced by stimulating the calf muscles electrically during the operation, Br. J. Surg. **54**:686, 1967.
46. Dunning, M. F., and Plum, M.: Hypercalciuria following poliomyelitis: its relationship to site and degree of paralysis, Arch. Intern. Med. **99**:716, 1957.
47. Editorial: bran reduces cholesterol saturation of bile, J.A.M.A. **241**:1088, 1979.
48. Egan, D. F.: Fundamentals of respiratory therapy, ed. 3, St. Louis, 1977, The C. V. Mosby Co.
49. Egbert, L. D., and Bendixen, H. H.: Effect of morphine on breathing pattern, a possible factor in atelectasis, J.A.M.A. **188**:485, 1964.
50. Egbert, L. D., Laver, M. B., and Bendixen, H. H.: The effect of site of operation and type of anesthesia upon the ability to cough in the postoperative period, Surg. Gynecol. Obstet. **115**:295, 1962.
51. Elisberg, E. I.: Heart rate response to the Valsalva maneuver as a test of circulatory integrity, J.A.M.A. **186**:200, 1963.
52. Elliot, J. S., and Todd, H. E.: Calculous disease in patients with poliomyelitis, J. Urol. **86**:484, 1961.
53. Elliot, J. S., Todd, H. E., and Lewis, L.: Some aspects of calcium phosphate solubility, J. Urol. **85**:428, 1961.
54. Enneking, W. F., and Horowitz, M.: The intra-articular effects of immobilization on the human knee, J. Bone Joint Surg. (Am.) **54A**:973, 1972.
55. Evans, D. S.: The early diagnosis of thromboembolism by ultrasound, Ann. R. Coll. Surg. Engl. **49**:225, 1971.
56. Evans, D. S., and Cockett, F. B.: Diagnosis of deep vein thrombosis with an ultrasonic Doppler technique, Br. Med. J. **2**:802, 1969.
57. Evans, E. B., Eggers, G. W. N., Butler, J. K., and Blumel, J.: Experimental immobilization and remobilization of rat knee joints, J. Bone Joint Surg. (Am.) **42A**:737, 1960.
58. Finlayson, B.: Calcium stones: some physical and clinical aspects. In David, D. S., editor: Calcium metabolism in renal failure and nephrolithiasis, New York, 1977, John Wiley & Sons, Inc.
59. Flanc, C., Kakkar, V. V., and Clarke, M. B.: The detection of venous thrombosis in the

legs using ^{125}I-labelled fibrinogen, Br. J. Surg. **55**:742, 1968.
60. Flanc, C., Kakkar, V. V., and Clarke, M. B.: Postoperative deep-vein thrombosis effect of intensive prophylaxis, Lancet **1**:477, 1969.
61. Foss, G.: Postural drainage, Am. J. Nurs. **73**:666, 1973.
62. Fuller, J. H., Bernauer, E. M., and Adams, W. C.: Renal function, water and electrolyte exchange during bedrest with daily exercise, Aerosp. Med. **41**:60, 1970.
63. Gallus, A. S., Hirsh, J., and Gent, M.: Relevance of preoperative and postoperative blood tests to postoperative leg-vein thrombosis, Lancet **2**:805, 1973.
64. Geiser, M., and Trueta, J.: Muscle action, bone rarefaction and bone formation: an experimental study, J. Bone Joint Surg. (Br.) **40B**:282, 1958.
65. Gibbs, N. M.: Venous thrombosis of the lower limbs with particular reference to bedrest, Br. J. Surg. **45**:209, 1957.
66. Goodman, L. S., and Gilman, A., editors: The pharmacological basis of therapeutics, ed. 5, New York, 1975, Macmillan Publishing Co., Inc.
67. Goss, C. M., editor: Gray's anatomy of the human body, ed. 29, Philadelphia, 1973, Lea & Febiger.
68. Greenleaf, J. E., Bernauer, E. M., Young, H. L., Morse, J. T., Staley, R. W., Juhos, L. T., and van Beaumont, W.: Fluid and electrolyte shifts during bed rest with isometric and isotonic exercise, J. Appl. Physiol. **42**:59, 1977.
69. Guyton, A. C.: Textbook of medical physiology, ed. 5, Philadelphia, 1976, W. B. Saunders Co.
70. Haeger, K.: Problems of acute deep venous thrombosis. I. The interpretation of signs and symptoms, Angiology **20**:219, 1969.
71. Haller, J. A., Jr.: Deep thrombophlebitis: pathophysiology and treatment, vol. 7, Philadelphia, 1967, W. B. Saunders Co.
72. Halpern, A., Shaftel, N., Selman, D., Shaftel, H. E., Kuhn, P. H., Samuels, S. S., and Birch, H. G: The cardiopulmonary dynamics of bowel function, Angiology **11**:448, 1960.
73. Ham, A. W.: Histology, ed. 7, Philadelphia, 1974, J. B. Lippincott Co.
74. Hamilton, W. K.: Atelectasis, pneumothorax and aspiration as postoperative complications, Anesthesiology **22**:708, 1961.
75. Heaney, R. P.: Radiocalcium metabolism in disuse osteoporosis in man, Am. J. Med. **33**:188, 1962.
76. Heath, H., Earll, J. M., Schaaf, M., Piechocki, J. T., and Li, T.: Serum ionized calcium during bedrest in fracture patients and normal men, Metabolism **21**:633, 1972.
77. Heatley, R. V., Hughes, L. E., Morgan, A., and Okwonga, W.: Preoperative or postoperative deep-vein thrombosis, Lancet **1**:437, 1976.
78. Hedges, J. E., and Bridges, C. J.: Stimulation of the cough reflex, Am. J. Nurs. **68**:347, 1968.
79. Hewlett, A. M., and Branthwaite, M. A.: Postoperative pulmonary function, Br. J. Anaesth. **47**:102, 1975.
80. Hills, N. H., Pflug, J. J., Jeyasingh, K., Boardman, L., and Calnan, J. S.: Prevention of deep vein thrombosis by intermittent pneumatic compression of calf, Br. Med. J. **1**:131, 1972.
81. Holdstock, D. J., and Misiewicz, J. J.: Factors controlling colonic motility: colonic pressures and transit after meals in patients with total gastrectomy, pernicious anaemia or duodenal ulcer, Gut **11**:100, 1970.
82. Holdstock, D. J., Misiewicz, J. J., Smith, T., and Rowlands, E. N.: Propulsion (mass movements) in the human colon and its relationship to meals and somatic activity, Gut **11**:91, 1970.
83. Hunter, W. C., Krygier, J. J., Kennedy, J. C., and Sneeden, V. D.: Etiology and prevention of thrombosis of the deep leg veins, surgery **17**:178, 1945.
84. Husni, E. A., Ximenes, J. O. C., and Goyette, E. M.: Elastic support of the lower limbs in hospital patients, J.A.M.A. **214**:1456, 1970.
85. Husni, E. A., Ximenes, J. O. C., and Hamilton, F. G.: Pressure bandaging of the lower extremity, use and abuse, J.A.M.A. **206**:2715, 1968.
86. Hyatt, K. H., Kamenetsky, L. G., and Smith, W. M.: Extravascular dehydrationas an etiologic factor in post-recumbency orthostatism, Aerosp. Med. **40**:644, 1969.
87. Hyman, L. R., Boner, G., Thomas, J. C., and Segar, W. E. Immobilization hypercalcemia, Am. J. Dis. Child. **124**:723, 1972.
88. Irwin, R. S., Rosen, M. J., Braman, S. S.: Cough: a comprehensive review, Arch. Intern. Med. **137**:1186, 1977.

89. Jackson, D. S., Flickinger, D. B., Dunphy, J. E.: Biochemical studies of connective tissue repair, Ann. N.Y. Acad. Sci. **86**:943, 1960.
90. Jacquette G.: To reduce hazards of tracheal suctioning, Am. J. Nurs. **71**:362, 1971.
91. Jeffis, L., and Baker, C.: Nasopharyngeal and tracheal suctioning: a clinical study, Am. J. Nurs. **67**:2361, 1967.
92. Jenkins, D. P., and Cochran, T. H.: Osteoporosis: the dramatic effect of disuse of an extremity, Clin. Orthop. **64**:128, 1969.
93. Jones, R. H., and Sabiston, D. C.: Pulmonary embolism, Surg. Clin. North Am. **56**:891, 1976.
94. Kakkar, V. V.: Review of present status of prophylaxis of venous thromboembolism, Proc. R. Soc. Med. **67**:706, 1974.
95. Kakkar, V. V, Howe, C. T., Flanc, C., and Clarke, M. B.: Natural history of postoperative deep-vein thrombosis, Lancet **2**:230, 1969.
96. Kakkar, V. V., Howe, C. T., Nicolaides, A. N., Renney, J. T. G., and Clarke, M. B.: Deep vein thrombosis of the leg—is there a "high risk" group ? Am. J. Surg. **120**:527, 1970.
97. Kelly, M. M.: Exercises for bedfast patients, Am. J. Nurs. **66**:2209, 1966.
98. Kosiak, M.: Etiology and pathology of ischemic ulcers, Arch. Phys. Med. Rehabil. **40**:62, 1959.
99. Kottke, F. J.: Deterioration of the bedfast patient, causes and effects, Public Health Rep. **80**:437, 1965.
100. Kottke, F. J.: The effects of limitation of activity upon the human body, J.A.M.A. **196**:825, 1966.
101. Kottke, F. J.: Therapeutic exercise. In Krusen, F. H., Kottke, F. J., and Ellwood, P. M., editors: Handbook of physical medicine and rehabilitation, ed. 2, Philadelphia, 1971, W. B. Saunders Co.
102. Kurihara, M.: Postural drainage, clapping, and vibrating, Am. J. Nurs. **65**:76, 1965.
103. Lamb, L. E.: An assessment of the circulatory problem of weightlessness in prolonged space flight, Aerosp. Med. **35**:413, 1964
104. Lamb, L. E., Johnson, R. L., and Stevens, P. M.: Cardiovascular deconditioning during chair rest, Aerosp. Med. **35**:646,1964.
105. Langlands, J.: The dynamics of cough in health and in chronic bronchitis, Thorax **22**:88, 1967.
106. Lee, B. Y., Trainor, F. S., Kavner, D., Madden, J. L., Dratz, H. M., and Ejercito, E. M.: Noninvasive prevention of thrombosis of deep veins of the thigh using intermittent pneumatic compression, Surg. Gynecol. Obstet. **142**:705, 1976.
107. Lewis, C. E., Mueller, C., and Edwards, W. S.: Venous stasis on the operating table, Am. J. Surg. **124**:780, 1972.
108. Liese, W., Joshi, R., and Cumming, G.: Humidification of respired gas by nasal mucosa, Ann. Otol. **82**:330, 1973.
109. Little, K.: Bone reabsorption and osteoporosis, Lancet **2**:752, 1963.
110. Long, C. L., and Bonilla, L. E.: Metabolic effects of inactivity and injury. In Downey, J. A., and Darling, R. C., editors: Physiological basis of rehabilitation medicine, Philadelphia, 1971, W. B. Saunders Co.
111. Lynch, T. N., Jensen, R. L., Stevens, P. M., Johnson, R. L., and Lamb, L. E.: Metabolic effects of prolonged bedrest: their modification by simulated altitude, Aerosp. Med. **38**:10, 1967.
112. Mack, P. B., and LaChance, P. L.: Effects of recumbency and space flight on bone density, Am. J. Clin. Nutr. **20**:1194, 1967.
113. Makin, G. S., Mayes, F. B., and Holroyd, A. M.: Studies on the effect of "Tubigrip" on the flow in the deep veins of the calf, Br. J. Surg. **56**:369, 1969.
114. Mayerson, H. S., and Burch, G. E.: Relationship of tissue (subcutaneous and intramuscular) and venous pressures to syncope induced in man by gravity, Am. J. Physiol. **128**:258, 1940.
115. Maynard, F. M., and Imai, K.: Immobilization hypercalcemia in spinal cord injury, Arch. Phys. Med. Rehabil. **58**:16, 1977.
116. McCally, M., Piemme, T. E., and Murray, R. H.: Tilt table responses of human subjects following application of lower body negative pressure, Aerosp. Med. **7**:1247, 1966.
117. McLachlin, A. D., McLachlin, J. A., Jory, T. A., and Rawling, E. G.: Venous stasis in the lower extremities, Ann. Surg. **152**:678, 1960.
118. McLachlin, A. D., Stavraky, W. K., and Sweeney, J. P.: Venous stasis in the lithotomy Trendelenburg position, Can. J. Surg. **10**:414, 1967
119. Miller, P. B., Hartman, B. O., Johnson, R. L., and Lamb, L. E.: Modification of the effects of two weeks of bed rest upon circu-

latory function in man, Aerosp. Med. **35**:931, 1964.

120. Miller, P. B., Johnson, R. L., and Lamb, L. E.: Effects of four weeks of absolute bed rest on circulatory functions in man, Aerosp. Med. **35**:1194, 1964.
121. Miller, P. B., Johnson, R. L., and Lamb, L. E.: Effects of moderate physical exercise during four weeks of bed rest on circulatory functions in man, Aerosp. Med. **36**:1077, 1965.
122. Moore Ede, M. C., and Burr, R. G.: Circadian rhythm of urinary calcium excretion during immobilization, Aerosp. Med. **44**:495, 1973.
123. Moore Ede, M. C., Faulkner, M. H., and Tredre, B. E.: An intrinsic rhythm of urinary calcium excretion and the specific effect of bedrest on the excretory pattern, Clin. Sci. **42**:433, 1972.
124. Morrell, M. T.: Acute illness—an important cause of venous thrombosis and pulmonary embolism, Br. J. Surg. **63**:162, 1976.
125. Muller, E. A.: Influence of training and of inactivity on muscle strength, Arch. Phys. Med. Rehabil. **51**:449, 1970.
126. Mundale, M. O., Hislop, H. J., Rabideau, R. J., and Kottke, F. J.: Evaluation of extension of the hip, Arch. Phys. Med. Rehabil. **37**:75, 1956.
127. Murray, T. S., Lorimer, A. K., Cox, F. C., and Lawrie, T. D. V.: Leg vein thrombosis following myocardial infarction, Lancet **2**:792, 1972.
128. Naimark, A., and Cherniak, R. M.: Compliance of the respiratory system and its components in health and obesity, J. Appl. Physiol. **15**:377, 1960.
129. Negus, D., Pinto, D. J., LeQuesne, L. P., Brown, N., and Chapman, M.: ^{125}I-labelled fibrinogen in the diagnosis of deep-vein thrombosis and its correlation with phlebography, Br. J. Surg. **55**:835, 1968.
130. Nicolaides, A. N.: Venous stasis in the lower limb. In Nicolaides, A. N., editor: Thromboembolism: etiology, advances in prevention and management, Baltimore, 1975, University Park Press.
131. Nicolaides, A. N., and Irving, D.: Clinical factors and the risk of deep venous thrombosis. In Nicolaides, A. N., editor: Thromboembolism: etiology, advances in prevention and management, Baltimore, 1975, University Park Press.
132. Nicolaides, A. N., Kakkar, V. V., Field, E. S., and Fish, P.: Venous stasis and deep-vein thrombosis, Br. J. Surg. **59**:713, 1972.
133. Nicolaides, A. N., Kakkar, V. V., Field, E. S., and Renney, J. T. G.: The origin of deep-vein thrombosis: a venographic study, Br. J. Radiol. **44**:653, 1971.
134. Nicolaides, A. N., Kakkar, V. V., and Renney, J. T. G.: The soleal sinuses: origin of deep-vein thrombosis, Br. J. Surg. **57**:860, 1970.
135. Nicolaides, A. N., Kakkar, V. V., and Renney, J. T. G.: The soleal sinuses and stasis, Br. J. Surg. **58**:307, 1971.
136. Nicolaides, A. N., and O'Connell, J. D.: Origin and distribution of thrombi in patients presenting with clinical deep venous thrombosis. In Nicolaides, A. N., editor: Thromboembolism: etiology, advances in prevention and management, Baltimore, 1975, University Park Press.
137. Nutter, D. O., Schlant, R. C., and Hurst, J. W.: Isometric exercise and the cardiovascular system, Mod. Concepts Cardiovasc. Dis. **41**:11, 1972.
138. Oberfield, R. A., Ebaugh, F. G., Jr., O'Hanlon, E. P., and Schoaf, M.: Blood volume studies during and after immobilization in human subjects as measured by sodium radiochromate (chromium 51) technique, Aerosp. Med. **39**:10, 1968.
139. Ochsner, J. L., and Keller, C. A.: Removing bronchial secretions: intratracheal suction and related measures, Nurs. Clin. North Am. **2**:521, 1967.
140. Peacock, E. E.: Some biochemical and biophysical aspects of joint stiffness: role of collagen synthesis as opposed to altered molecular bonding, Ann. Surg. **164**:1, 1966.
141. Pennock, J. M., Kalu, D. N., Clark, M. B., Foster, G. V., and Doyle, F. H.: Hypoplasia of bone induced by immobilization, Br. J. Radiol. **45**:641, 1972.
142. Pentecost, B. L., Irving, D. W., and Shillingford, J. P.: The effects of posture on the blood flow in the inferior vena cava, Clin. Sci. **24**:149, 1963.
143. Pierce, A. K., and Sanford, J. P.: Bacterial contamination of aerosols, Arch. Intern. Med. **131**:156, 1973.
144. Pulvertaft, R. G.: Nephrolithiasis occurring in recumbency, J. Bone Joint Surg. (Am.) **21**:559, 1939.
145. Ray, J. F., III, Yost, L., Moallem, S., San-

oudos, G. M., Villamena, P., Paredes, R. M., and Clauss, R. H.: Immobility, hypoxemia, and pulmonary arteriovenous shunting, Arch. Surg. **109**:537, 1974.

146. Ritchie, J. A.: Colonic motor activity and bowel function. 1. Normal movement of contents, Gut **9**:442, 1968.
147. Robbins, S. L.: Pathologic basis of disease, ed. 2, Philadelphia, 1979, W. B. Saunders Co.
148. Robertson, D., Stevens, R. M., Friesinger, G. C., and Oates, J. A.: The effect of the Valsalva maneuver on echocardiographic dimensions in man, Circulation **55**:596, 1977.
149. Rose, G. A.: Immobilization osteoporosis, Br. J. Surg. **53**:769, 1966.
150. Rosengarten, D. S., Laird, J., Jeyasingh, K., and Martin, P.: The failure of compression stockings (Tubigrip) to prevent deep venous thrombosis after operation, Br. J. Surg. **57**:296, 1970.
151. Sabri, S., Roberts, V. C., and Cotton, L. T.: Prevention of early postoperative deep vein thrombosis by intermittent compression of the leg during surgery, Br. Med. J. **4**:394, 1971.
152. Sagar, S., Massey, J., and Sanderson, J. M.: Low-dose heparin prophylaxis against fatal pulmonary embolism, Br. Med. J **4**:257, 1975.
153. Sara, C., and Currie, T.: Humidification by nebulization, Med. J. Aust. **1**:174, 1965.
154. Seaton, A.: The management of cough in clinical practice, Scott. Med. J. **22**:99, 1977.
155. Sevitt, S., and Gallagher, N.: Venous thrombosis and pulmonary embolism: a clinicopathological study in injured and burned patients, Br. J. Surg. **48**: 475, 1961.
156. Shapiro, B. A., Harrison, R. A., and Trout, C. A.: Clinical application of respiratory care, ed. 2, Chicago, 1979, Year Book Medical Publishers, Inc.
157. Sigel, B., Edelstein, A. L., Felix, W. R., Jr., and Memhardt, C. R.: Compression of the deep venous system of the lower leg during inactive recumbency, Arch. Surg. **106**:38, 1973.
158. Sjostrand, T.: The regulation of the blood distribution in man, Acta Physiol. Scand. **26**:312, 1952.
159. Slonim, N. B., and Hamilton, L. H.: Respiratory physiology, ed. 3, St. Louis, 1976, The C. V. Mosby Co.
160. Smith, P. H., and Robertson, W. G.: Stone formation in the immobilized patient. In Hodgkinson, A., and Nordin, B. E. C., editors: Proceedings of the renal stone research symposium, London, 1968, J. & A. Churchill, Ltd.
161. Sodeman, W. A., Jr., and Watson, D. W.: The large intestine. In Sodeman, W. A., Jr., and Sodeman, W. A., editors: Pathologic physiology: mechanism of disease, ed. 5, Philadelphia, 1974, W. B. Saunders Co.
162. Spaet, T. H., Horowitz, H. I., Zucker-Franklin, D., Cintron, J., and Bienzenski, J. J.: Reticuloendothelial clearance of blood thromboplastin by rats, Blood **17**:196, 1961.
163. Spencer, W. A., Vallbone, C., and Carter, R. E., Jr.: Physiologic concepts of immobilization, Arch. Phys. Med. Rehabil. **46**:89, 1965.
164. Stead, E. A., and Ebert, R. V.: Postural hypotension: a disease of the sympathetic nervous system, Arch. Intern. Med. **67**:546, 1941.
165. Stein, M., Koota, G. M., Simon, M., and Frank, H. A.: Pulmonary evaluation of surgical patients, J.A.M.A. **181**:765, 1962.
166. Stevens, P. M., Miller, P. B., Gilbert, C. A., Lynch, T. N., Johnson, R. L., and Lamb, L. E.: Influences of long-term lower body negative pressure on the circulatory function of man during prolonged bedrest, Aerosp. Med. **37**:357, 1966.
167. Stewart, G. J.: The role of the vessel wall in deep venous thrombosis. In Nicolaides, A. N., editor: Thromboembolism: etiology, advances in prevention and management, Baltimore, 1975, University Park Press.
168. Stillwell, D. M., McLarren, G. L., and Gersten, J. W.: Atrophy of quadriceps muscle due to immobilization of the lower extremity, Arch. Phys. Med. Rehabil. **48**:289, 1967.
169. Straffon, R. A., and Higgins, C. C.: Urinary lithiasis and foreign bodies. In Campbell, M. F., and Harrison, J. H., editors: Urology, ed. 3, vol. 1, Philadelphia, 1970, W. B. Saunders Co.
170. Strandness, D. E., Jr., Ward, K., and Krugmire, R.: The present status of acute deep venous thrombosis, Surg. Gynecol. Obstet. **14**:433, 1977.
171. Stremel, R. W., Convertino, V. A., Bernauer, E. M., and Greenleaf, J. E.: Cardiorespiratory deconditioning with static and

dynamic leg exercise during bed rest, J. Appl. Physiol. **41**:905, 1976.

172. Taylor, H. L., Erickson, L., Henschel, A., and Keys, A.: The effect of bed rest on the blood volume of normal young men, Am. J. Physiol. **144**:227, 1945.
173. Trueta, J.: The role of the vessels in osteogenesis, J. Bone Joint Surg. (Br.) **45B**:402, 1963.
174. Tsapogas, M. J., Goussous, H., Peabody, R. A., Karmody, A. M., and Eckert, C.: Postoperative venous thrombosis and the effectiveness of prophylactic measures, Arch. Surg. **103**:561, 1971.
175. Ungvarski, P.: Mechanical stimulation of coughing, Am. J. Nurs. **71**:2358, 1971.
176. Vogt, F. B.: Tilt table and plasma volume changes with short term deconditioning experiments, Aerosp. Med. **38**:564, 1967.
177. Vogt, F. B., Mack, P. B., and Johnson, P. C.: Tilt table response and blood volume changes associated with thirty days of recumbency, Aerosp. Med. **37**:771, 1966.
178. Vogt, F. B., Mack, P. C., Johnson, P. C., and Wade, L., Jr.: Tilt table response and blood volume changes associated with fourteen days of recumbency, Aerosp. Med. **38**:43, 1967.
179. Wade, J. F.: Respiratory nursing care: physiology and technique, ed. 2, St. Louis, 1977, The C. V. Mosby Co.
180. Wade, O. L., and Gilson, J. C.: The effect of posture on diaphragmatic movement and vital capacity in normal subjects with a note on spirometry as an aid in determining radiological chest volumes, Thorax **6**:103, 1951.
181. Ward, R. J., Danziger, F., Bonica, J. J., Allen, G. D., and Bowes, J.: An evaluation of postoperative respiratory maneuvers, Surg. Gynecol. Obstet. **123**:51, 1966.
182. Warlow, C., Ogston, D., and Douglas, A. S.: Venous thrombosis following strokes, Lancet **1**:130, 1972.
183. Wessler, S.: Thrombosis in the presence of vascular stasis, Am. J. Med. **33**:648, 1962.
184. Wessler, S.: Factors in the initiation of deep venous thrombosis. In Nicolaides, A. N., editor: Thromboembolism: etiology, advances in prevention and management, Baltimore, 1975, University Park Press.
185. Wessler, S., Yin, E. T., Gaston, L. W., and Nicol, I.: A distinction between the role of precursor and activated forms of clotting factors in the genesis of stasis thrombi, Thromb. Diath. Haemorrh. **18**:12, 1967.
186. Widmann, F. K.: Goodale's clinical interpretation of laboratory tests, ed. 7, Philadelphia, 1973, F. A. Davis Co.
187. Wightman, J. A. K.: A prospective survey of the incidence of postoperative pulmonary complications, Br. J. Surg. **55**:85, 1968.
188. Winters, J. L., Kleinschmidt, A. G., Jr., Frensilli, J. J., and Sutton, M.: Hypercalcemia complicating immobilization in the treatment of fractures, J. Bone Joint Surg. (Am.) **48A**:1182, 1966.
189. Wolf, A. W., Chuinard, R. G., Riggins, R. S., Walter, R. M., and Depner, T.: Immobilization hypercalcemia: a case report and review of the literature, Clin. Orthop. **118**:124, 1976.
190. Wolf, E., Magora, A., and Gonen, B.: Disuse atrophy of the quadriceps muscle, Electromyography **11**:479, 1971.
191. Wright, H. P., Osborn, S. B., and Hayden, M.: Venous velocity in bedridden medical patients, Lancet **2**:699, 1952.

SONJA I. LIVELY
ROSE MARIE FRIEDRICH

Chapter 6

DESTRUCTIVE BEHAVIOR

Some kennelled
denizen of the deep
crevices of dread
leaps the full
length of its chain
then falls back

Shadow-boxing
with feelings
of inadequacy
this monster
bays at the rising fear

The struggle continues
the pattern repeats
until soul
body
and
breath
are consumed
with wild desperation

Control
slipping-sliding
nearly gone

The chain snaps
with the final leap
the beast lunges

PAULETTE R. Di ANGI

CONCEPTUAL DEFINITION

The word "destructive" refers to acts that are detrimental or that tear down or injure. The term "destructive behavior" refers to behavior, either verbal or physical, that results in injury, damage, or other noxious consequences to oneself, others, or the environment. Although the primary intent, or goal, of the behavior may not be to harm or injure, the results are in fact injurious. Descriptive words frequently used interchangeably with destructive behavior include hostile aggression, attack behavior, and violent behavior.[5,18,24]

When persons engage in destructive behavior modes, they are responding to goal blockage or interference with need fulfillment by using the approach of fight rather than flight. Assertive behavior, an approach behavior, is self-enhancing and uses an honest expression of feelings to achieve goals. The person consciously makes a decision regarding how to act. Since the person chooses how to act, a good feeling typically accompanies this type of response, even if the specific goals are not achieved. This occurs because feelings are released in nondestructive, logical ways. The intent of assertive behavior is to express feelings directly and to show respect for others in the situation. A person using this mode of behavior is often perceived as confident, honest, and respectful.[1]

Aggressive behavior is an accelerated fight response that, if it accomplishes goals, usually does so at the expense of others. Aggressive behavior often injures others by not allowing them to make a deliberate choice and by minimizing their worth. The intent in this response is to dominate and "win." The other person's rights are denied, and the recipient of this behavior feels hurt, defensive, and humiliated. Generally, aggressive behavior is self-enhancing at the expense of others.[1]

Escalation of aggressive behavior can result in destructive behavior. During episodes of such behavior the intensity of the person's emotions clouds the need or problem that is being responded to, and irrational thinking predominates. Consideration is not given to future consequences of behavior. Any behavior that will allow the person to feel better for the moment and maintain a feeling of power is called on. The behavior that occurs is impulsive and lacks cognitive control. The destructive person is often desperate enough to do anything to gain control over the situation. Extremes of destructive behavior interfere with the person's ability to function productively. At this level the individual is totally consumed by the destructive response.

Destructive behavior is manifested in varying levels of severity and directions. The potential end points are suicide and homicide. The person who is a threat to self may commit an isolated act such as suicide or may engage in habitual self-inflicted, life-threatening behavior over an extended period. Less immediate forms of self-destructive behavior include drug addiction and abuse, alcoholism, smoking, and other forms of health risk–taking behavior such as overeating and medical noncompliance. Persons who engage in such gradual self-destructive behavior tend to deny the relationship of this behavior to their own eventual death, believing, perhaps, that they can assume control at any time. This fantasy of being able to control the situation perpetuates the problem.[11,30] One example often noted in the literature is patients being treated with hemodialysis. Their noncompliance with the medical regimen is often labeled as suicidal behavior. At the same time, research has shown that massive denial helps these patients cope with their illness situation.[26]

The individual who is a threat to others may display a variety of behaviors having a wide range of intensity and potential for destruction, from subtle behaviors such as gossiping, which affects the reputation of another, to the more physically violent acts of rape and child abuse. Although such attacks may result in physical harm to the recipients, the psychological damage accompanying these attacks may be more devastating, damaging the person for life. Homicide is the ultimate form of destruction to others.

Moderate forms of destructive behavior commonly occur in the acute care setting. As the acutely ill patient progresses from the initial shock and denial phase of illness to the awareness phase, the impact of the loss threat is reexperienced. Anger and hostility accompany this realization. The uncooperative, acting out, or unreasonable behavior exhibited by some patients is often an attempt to maintain dignity in what is perceived to be a highly institutionalized, impersonal setting. Expressions of hostility and anger may be employed to obtain relief from the perceived threat to self-image.[17,25] A survey of 218 student nurses revealed that they often encountered verbal abuse and attempts to inflict physical violence on them by patients in the general hospital.[29]

Although destructive behavior occurs in situations in which goals are blocked, it is not the events themselves but the individual's interperetation of the meaning of events that causes the distress. Destructive behavior is often a result of faulty beliefs or irrational thinking about the situation and is commonly associated with unrealistic expectations. Initially, the feeling of powerlessness may predominate when the person perceives a severe threat to ego integrity. The individual senses failure in the attempt to exert control over self, situation, or others in the immediate environment. The powerless feelings are quickly short-circuited and taken over by the arousal of anger. Hostility and anger serve as a protective reaction to vulnerability and allow placement of blame for the situation outside the person. This emotional response generates a false sense of temporary control.[10,23,25] The intensity of the anger response reflects the degree of perceived danger. The anger may range from mild arrogance to intense fury and rage.[14] As anger increases, a point is reached at which the emotions can no longer be contained and energy must be released. This emotional energy may be directed against self, others, or the environment in attempts to eradicate the perceived unpleasantness. The anger and hostility will be directed outward toward others or the environment if the person believes that it is possible to overcome the harmful circumstance. However, if the individual perceives the situation as completely unmanageable and believes that attacking others or the environment would create additional stress, outward expression of anger will be inhibited. Under these circumstances hopelessness predominates, and the resultant hostility and anger are turned against the self.[18]

Hopelessness accompanies the feelings of worthlessness and powerlessness in the self-destructive individual. There is a high correlation between hopelessness and suicidal impulses.[3] The person feels caught in a trap from which there is no escape. In this situation the drive for power is no longer foremost because the individual is unable to identify resources to deal with the personal threats being experienced. As a result, the person judges that the situation is unbearable and that the loss of power and self-esteem can be dealt with only by leaving life.

The basic process that may lead to destructive behavior is (1) obstruction to goal or unfulfilled need, (2) initial perception of severe threat to integrity, (3) predominant feelings of powerlessness, (4) arousal of anger, (5) possible reassignment of blame, (6) perception regarding the balance of power, and (7) destructive behavior.

The process of the development of outward-directed destructive behavior can be exemplified in the case of a child-abusing father. When the father interacts with his infant, he has an expectation that the child should respond to his commands in a way that bolsters his self-esteem. When the infant cries or fails to respond in accordance with parental expectations, there is interference with the father's need fulfillment. The father interprets the child's crying as evidence that he is a bad parent. He cannot control the infant's behavior and consequently perceives himself as a failure. The resultant powerlessness and helplessness become overwhelming. In response to these feelings, a shift in the perception of the problem occurs. The condition is blamed on the child so that the father can cognitively process, "There is nothing wrong with me; there is something wrong with you." With the outward shift in the conflict, anger mounts as the father convinces himself that the child is at fault. His emotional energy is directed outward, and attack of the child occurs.[13]

Attack behavior provokes aggression in both the attacker and the subject of the attack. There is abundant evidence that ventilating hostility aggressively makes the individual more likely to go on to further hurtful behavior. A study of violence among married couples clearly demonstrated that verbal violence and physical violence are directly associated. Couples who engaged in little verbal aggression had little or no physical violence. In contrast, 83.3% of the most verbally violent couples were also involved in one or more physical fights during the same period.[28] Acting out anger aggressively against another person leads to heightened aggression rather than resolution. In an attempt to exert control the individual actually loses control because the behavior demonstrates to self and others an inability to deal effectively with life's problems. Consequently, self-doubt, powerlessness, and anger intensify, leading to a recycling of the destructive behavior pattern.

Many people regularly engage in some form of destructive activity. However, those who select destructive behavior as the primary mode of adapting to stress frequently become incapacitated in almost every aspect of life.

ANTECEDENT CONDITIONS

Destructive behavior evolves from developmental and physiological factors. Such factors predispose, encourage, or reward an individual's use of aggression or destructive behavior as a coping strategy. However, the precipitation of the progression from aggressive to destructive behavior often requires a triggering event.

Developmental factors

Between the ages of 18 months and 3 years the child is at the developmental stage of autonomy versus shame and doubt.[30] It is during this period that the child begins to learn mastery over the environment. Aggressive behavior is often a natural part of an infant's exploration of the environment.[16] When learning perceptual coordination and manipulative mastery, the child moves about vigorously, sometimes in a potentially destructive manner.[5] With maturation the child's behavior becomes more goal directed as the child begins determining the relationships between environment and self. At this stage the child first experiences conflicts with authority figures, usually parents. Accompanying these conflicts are the ambivalent feelings of love and hate. These ambivalent feelings are the major factors responsible for modifying primitive destructive wishes and actions. To maintain parental love, the child learns that destructive or aggressive feelings must be controlled, and anger channeled into acceptable outlets.[5]

The development at this stage is crucial to the choice of using destructive behavior as a coping mode in later life. Until the age of 3 the child is primarily concerned with meeting immediate needs. Naturally imbedded in such narcissism is the mode of destruction. The number of behavioral alternatives available to respond to stress increases as the child's capability for thinking expands. However, between the ages of 4 and 7 the child still frequently manifests destructive behavior in attempts to gain power and control over the environment.

Destructive behavior can occur in young children for a variety of reasons. In some instances the goal of such behavior relates only to the cognitive power of inquiry. Neither malice nor anger is present, even though the behavior can harm others or destroy property. However, destructive behavior can also evolve from anger, in which case the child strikes out to accomplish control goals.

Between the ages of 6 and 14 the child's cognitive understanding expands from the concrete to the abstract. As the child learns to reason and develops a beginning value system, tools for displacing anger are acquired. As self-control increases, behavioral alternatives become enlarged. The child learns through the approval of adults that self-control over instinctual emotional responses is a positive attribute. The child learns to tolerate delay of need gratification. As a young child experiments with various behaviors, response patterns that achieve desired goals are reinforced. If a behavior is successful in achieving a desired goal, the child continues to use it. An example is the 3-year-old at the store. When the child's request for a treat is denied, a screaming, kicking tantrum occurs. To quiet the outburst, the mother yields to the demand. Thus the child has the foundation of learning that disruptive outbursts achieve results. If such behavior continues to be rewarded in other situations, it becomes firmly integrated as a viable coping tool.[30]

Destructive behavior can also be learned through modeling. In the formative years of life the child's role models are primarily limited to parents or immediate care givers. The child observes these persons responding to frustration and learns how they deal with stress successfully, or in a way that appears successful in the child's eye. For example, the parent who uses drugs to deal with life communicates to the inexperienced child that drug abuse is an appropriate behavior. Research has found a high correlation between parental drug abuse and subsequent abuse patterns of their children.[15]

The child, being a direct target of parental behavior, frequently observes the role model for parenting. The parent who is loving and supportive teaches the child that this is the acceptable way to be a parent. Likewise, the parent who is abusive teaches the child that this is the way to act. Substantial research shows that parents who abuse children were almost always abused as children.[15,28]

Physiological factors

A variety of physiological factors have been related to the precipitation of anger and aggression, with resulting destructive behavior. The release of norepinephrine by the adrenal medulla has been found to correlate with aggressive behavior. Chemical and/or endocrine disorders such as hypoglycemia and some types of allergies also predispose persons to irritation and aggression. Blood levels of male sex hormones, especially testosterone, directly correlate with levels of aggressive behavior. Also, the premenstrual decline of progesterone levels predisposes women to irritability and increased hostility. The symptoms of nervousness, restlessness, and irritability, which are part of the premenstrual tension syndrome, have been related to psychotic or suicidal behavior in some women.[8,20,32]

The physiological effects on the central nervous system of some drugs (e.g., hallucinogens) and organic diseases (e.g., organic brain syndromes) also have been found to precipitate destructive behavior. In these conditions the physiology required for logical thinking is impaired, which can lead to impulsive behavior. Misinterpretation of reality further increases the risk that destructive behavior will accompany these physiological changes. The individual's logical thinking ability is also severely reduced during alcohol and drug withdrawal. It is not uncommon for an individual with delirium tremens to become destructive while experiencing hallucinations, delirium, and/or severe agitation.

An individual who is withdrawing from mind-altering drugs often experiences periods of central nervous system instability, which can precipitate psychomotor hyperactivity.[6] Such individuals commonly experience hallucinations and/or paranoid feelings, which may initiate harmful behavior. The danger of self-inflicted injury or injury to others becomes prominent during withdrawal experiences.

Triggering events

When an individual has a predisposition to respond to stress destructively or aggressively, specific situations may automatically trigger that behavior. Characteristics common to triggering events are the person's perception that there is an urgency to respond and experience of an overwhelming immediate frustration that demands reflex action to protect the self. Logical, rational thinking is bypassed.

A wide variety of situations can provide the type of fuel that will ignite destructive behavior. The destructive-prone person encountering a threatening confrontation almost automatically responds by fighting back. As the person fights to protect the threatened self-esteem, the initiator of the attack may escalate efforts, which in turn escalates the recipient's aggression. An example of such a destructive cycle is an encounter between two men at a bar. Both have ingested alcohol, which lowers their inhibitions. One man accidently bumps the other while passing by his chair. This initates a verbal challenge, which receives a like response with the addition of an uncomplimentary description of ancestry. This exchange is answered by a physical threat, which escalates to a punch being thrown. Then a knife appears, and one or both of the participants are injured or killed.

The predisposing elements in this situation are the basic coping behaviors used by both men, aggression or destruction, and the ingestion of alcohol, which reduced inhibitions. The trigger insult, the bar encounter, provided an environment in which such exchanges might be more tolerated than in some other settings, and one man happened to be carrying a tool for violence, the knife.

A similar reaction might occur in a hospital ward when a destructive-prone person whose inhibitions have been lowered by medications has activity limitations enforced by a nurse. The patient may counter such a challenge by striking the nurse. Given that the nurse is not a destructive-prone person, the escalation cycle would probably be broken at this point when the nurse did not retaliate.

Mind-altering drugs, in particular amphetamines, tend to make a person fearful and even paranoid about the actions of others.[6] The nurse who quietly enters the room of a patient who abuses amphetamines, calls the patient's name, and lightly touches the patient's shoulder can trigger a violent attack response.

Another type of triggering event relates to the simple availability of a tool of violence that can be used impulsively. In the amphetamine situation just described the availability of scissors on the patient's night stand might result in the death of the nurse. A person with suicidal ideation may impulsively use a razor blade found in a drawer. The availability of the knife in the previously described bar fight could allow the fight to escalate to homicide. Police statistics have shown that many domestic quarrels that end in homicide do so not because of premeditation but because of impulsive use of an available tool of violence. The most frequently used tools are knives and guns. Additional aversive stimuli that may elicit aggressive behavior include environmental factors such as overcrowding, heat, and noise.[4]

Crowd or group expectations may also provide a triggering event when individuals no longer think for themselves but act as a group. Mobs can turn violent and destructive on an impulsive response to a suggestion. Behavior norms of some groups or gangs may include violence as a usual mode of behavior. The group's leader needs only to give the order to attack, and impulsively the members do so.[30]

A loss may be the trigger to the "suicidal gun." Significant types of losses are (1) loss of a significant person by death—either a recent loss or an anniversary of the loss, (2) divorce or separation, (3) loss of job and the accompanying prestige and status, (4) loss of health—whether a serious acute illness or a chronic one, and (5) threat of prosecution.[2,4,7]

The suicide risk following such crises is higher in those who do not have stable support systems. The risk is higher for divorced or single people compared to those who are married. The more stable the person's life has been, the lower is the chance for suicide during a crisis situation. Approximately 75% of the persons who kill themselves had made previous attempts. If a person has selected this coping mechanism in the past, another suicide threat should be given great credance.

BEHAVIORAL DEFINITION

Objective data

Physiological response. The body prepares for fight through the arousal of the sympathetic nervous system. The degree of physiological response is directly related to the intensity of the emotional response. Blood flow is diverted from the viscera to the skeletal muscles and the brain. As this occurs, muscle tension increases and sensory alertness accompanies a heightened level of mental activity. An overall increase in the activity of the heart results in increased heart rate and elevated blood pressure. Gastrointestinal tract responses include dryness of mouth and decreased gastric peristalsis. The decrease in peristalsis and tone of the gastrointestinal tract may lead to constipation. As the sympathetic stimulation intensifies, the basal metabolic rate may increase up to 150%. The respiratory rate rises in proportion to the body's increased need for oxygen.[12]

Motor-behavioral response. The increased tension associated with hostility is often visible in the skeletal muscles and body posture. Facial expression often appears intense, with the musculature around the eyes and mouth tightly drawn. Eye contact is direct, glaring, intrusive, and piercing. Emphatic, threatening gestures such as an upraised hand or shaking fist may be directed toward the recipient of the destructive behavior. Standing or towering above the recipient is an attempt to emphasize the individual's power in the situation. Such a posture not only inhibits interaction but also conveys a message of disrespect and power. This position of power may be further emphasized by invasion of the other's personal space.[30]

The angry feelings may be displaced or sublimated. For example, the displacement of intense feelings may result in the banging a table, stamping the feet, or hitting pillows or other objects. Participation in aggressive, physical contact sports such as football is viewed as a healthy method of sublimating aggressive tendencies to constructive channels. Smoking and overeating, although in and of themselves destructive behaviors, are also ways to repress hostile feelings.

Direct physical attack may occur against self or others. The destructive contact could include hitting, shaking, yanking, choking, or rape. Overt signs of self-destruction range from scratching or skin abuse to more severe suicidal gestures such as slashing of wrists, ingestion of an overdose of pills, or self-inflicted gunshot wounds.

The suicidal person manifests many of the motor-behavioral symptoms of psychological immobilization. (See Chapter 4.) However, suicide does not occur when immobilization is present. Most attempts occur between 3 days and 3 months after the depression lifts. At that time the person still has the destructive feelings, and the energy to carry out the destruction is present.

Changes in activity patterns. A person may prepare for suicide by giving away prized possessions, making a will, or dramatically changing patterns of activity. An example is going on long walks when unable to sleep at night. A person who has been a steady worker may stop going to work. Meaningful interactions with family, friends, and peers decrease. The quality of most relationships deteriorates because the individual either antagonizes others or purposely becomes isolated.

Subjective data

Verbal patterns. It is unusual for persons exhibiting destructive behavior to be able to identify their emotions verbally and openly. They may not even be aware of anger and hostility. These hidden emotions must often be inferred from the behaviors described in the previous discussion of objective data.

The destructive individual is often unable to verbalize inner turmoil. This lack of direct expression of feelings covers up a great potential for violence. If the perceived threat is overwhelming and anxiety is extremely high, verbalization may become nonexistent. For example, cessation of communication, expecially with family and significant others, is a particularly ominous sign in the suicidal individual. Likewise, those who physically attack others are often unable to verbalize their rage. The only cues to the intensity of the emotional state may be nonverbal behavior. The indirect verbalization of anger may be so subtle that the message may be missed. For example, the suicidal individual may offer indirect statements such as "There isn't any point in going on," or "Take this jewelry; I won't be needing it anymore." Sarcasm is another mode of verbalization that is often used to express anger or rage indirectly. The message may be so subtle that it may appear that the individual is concerned, interested, and sympathetic. For example, the patient may say to the nurse, "You're such a nice nurse, much better than I expected." Although the statement may be interpreted as supportive, the underlying hostile message is "Nurses are such losers." Often the pattern of delivery conveys the true meaning more accurately than the content. Rapid speech with an angry tone delivered through clenched teeth leaves no doubt about the aggressive message.

More direct statements that refer to underlying needs and feelings may occur, especially in the presence of an empathetic listener. For example, statements of self-harm such as "I'm going to kill myself," should always be taken seriously and not be passed off as manipulation. Fear of losing control may be evidenced by statements such as "I'm going to blow up," or "I'm afraid I'm going to hurt someone." Overt expressions of hostility toward others can include angry statements or shouts that are inflammatory and derogatory. Threats of various forms of physical assault, including threats of hitting or of using tools of violence such as knives or guns, commonly occur as an individual approaches an episode of direct attack. The individual may ultimately state directly, "I'm going to kill you."

INTERVENING VARIABLES

The two categories of intervening variables that most markedly affect destructive behavior are culture and environment.

Sociocultural patterns

Each culture's predetermined norms govern the acceptable use of aggression by its members. Some cultures such as the aborigines of New Guinea deliberately foster fear and aggression in their members.[33] Some primitive societies view cutting a person with the intent of healing as destructive, whereas other cultures view this as the legitimate role of a surgeon.

Laws are often formalized to govern the acceptable use of destructive behavior. For example, destructive behavior is encouraged, honored, and rewarded when it is used to defend one's country against a declared enemy during war. Mass killing and hand-to-hand combat are viewed as positive behaviors when they are initiated under the authorization of the government. However, when a person individually manifests similar behavior, society views that person as a criminal. The major religions of a culture are a primary influence on the value system of its members. In

American society the Judeo-Christian ethic encourages "turning the other cheek" and discourages direct expression of anger. Many Oriental religions encourage quiet contemplation and passivity. The greater society often accepts and allows for religious variations in expression of aggression if the variation supports greater passivity. For example, conscientious objectors are legally permitted to abstain from aggressive acts in the military service.

Culturally determined sex roles also affect aggression norms. In the lower socioeconomic American culture the man is expected to be the authority figure responsible for the decision making of his family. It is relatively acceptable that he exert control in a physically aggressive manner. He is expected to "fight back" and not to let himself or his family get "pushed around." In higher socioeconomic levels more controls are placed on a man's destructive behavior. He is expected to rely on his intellectual ability and not his physical prowess. However, it is acceptable to use sarcastic humor or a demeaning attitude to exhibit aggression, control, or power.

Women in the American culture are expected to be much less physically destructive than men, regardless of socioeconomic level. Women are expected not to become involved in aggressive physical contact, even in sports. They are to exhibit anger by crying or verbalization, not by physical aggression.

Women are more likely to attempt suicide than men, but men are more likely to be successful in their attempts. This seems to be because men tend to use more lethal methods than women.

Environment

The control over one's personal territory is important for maintaining a comfortable, stress-free environment in which to live. Crowding, whether it be in an urban ghetto, a sibling's bedroom, or a hospital ward, is a nonsupportive intervening variable in destructive behavior. As crowding increases, the person whose territory is being invaded experiences a lack of control. The individual is placed in a nonpowerful situation, which increases the probability of an aggressive and potentially destructive response.[30]

NURSING INTERVENTIONS—GOALS AND EVALUATION CRITERIA

The nurse who is faced with care of a patient exhibiting destructive behavior may be hindered by judgmental attitudes that must be overcome to intervene effectively. By becoming aware of the patient's pain and lack of control, the nurse may be better able to deal objectively and sensitively with the destructive patient.[27]

As discussed earlier, destructive behavior runs the gamut from suicide to homicide, with many levels of destructive behavior in between. The most common types of destructive behavior that bring patients to an acute care setting are suicide, hostile aggression, and drug or alcohol withdrawal.

The primary goals of the nursing care of patients manifesting destructive behavior are (1) maintenance of physiological equilibrium, (2) maintenance of safety, (3) identification of personal strengths, and (4) use of alternate methods of expressing feelings.

Maintenance of physiological equilibrium

The person who is potentially destructive to others often gives no attention to basic personal care because of anxiety. The management of this type of patient is discussed in Chapter 3.

Helping the drug or alcohol abuser to regain physiological equilibrium presents a complexity of problem areas, including malnutrition, vitamin deficiencies, dental caries, loss of teeth, respiratory infections, skin abscesses, cellulitis, hepatitis, bacterial endocarditis, constipation, amenorrhea, impotence, and seizures.[34] The patient should be carefully assessed to determine whether such physical problems are present. Medical treatment for the conditions present should be instigated.

Behaviors indicative of the maintenance of physiological equilibrium include the absence of physical illness. Other criteria relate directly to specific need areas such as adequate intake and output.

Maintenance of safety

Limit setting. The destructive individual who is very frightened or angry often requires external control. Although destructive behavior can erupt unexpectedly, usually there are adequate warning signs. The nurse must be alert to changes in behavior that signal possible destructive intent. For example, the suicidal patient may suddenly become sociable and assure everyone that "I'm OK" and "no longer depressed." The activity of the outwardly destructive person may become more agitated, and threatening gestures and remarks may increase, signaling increased loss of control.

Limit setting can be judiciously applied to the person who is potentially destructive.[19] The need for the limit setting must be validated. This intervention should not be used just to increase the comfort of the staff; rather, it must meet the needs of the patient. After these needs have been validated, the expected behavior should be communicated to the patient, for example, "It is time to take your medicine." If communicating the expected behavior does not precipitate compliance, the patient is then informed that the behavior is unacceptable, and a limit is imposed. The limit should not be advanced as a punishment but as a statement of fact. If the nurse decides that explanation of the consequences of noncompliance with the limit is in the patient's best interest, the explanation should be clear and objective, for example, "If you kick the television, you will have to stay out of the television room for 12 hours." After the patient is told what the unacceptable behavior is, it is helpful to offer a substitute, acceptable behavior, for example, "You cannot kick the television when you are angry. You can tell me when you're angry or hit the punching bag." The limit should be clear-cut and total. For instance, if the patient is told, "You can raise your voice when you're angry, but don't yell," the patient is uncertain as to exact expectations.

After the limit is explained, the patient must be helped to understand it. The amount of explanation must vary according to the patient's ability to understand. The limit must be consistently enforced. It must be realistic and possible to be enforced, for example, "If you kick the television, you will not be allowed to go to the occupational therapy department today." If the limit is not followed, the reciprocal action by the staff must be done quickly without lengthy explanation. However, the patient should have the opportunity to ventilate feelings about the limit.

Contracts can be valuable limit-setting tools in working with the destructive person. The nurse asks the patient to make a contract, usually verbal, although it may be written. In order for the patient to agree, a trusting relationship must have been established. For instance, the nurse asks the suicidal patient to make a contract (or a promise) not to attempt to inflict harm during the night. A short-term contract is often more realistic then a long-term goal for the actively destructive person. A helpful type of contract asks the patient to agree to talk with the nurse whenever the person feels destructive.

Constant monitoring may be needed to maintain the safety of the patient. When a patient has indicated that attempts will be made to die, a nurse needs to remain with the patient at all times. The nurse conveys concern verbally by telling the patient, "You have told me you want to die. I know you're feeling hopeless now. I am staying with you to make sure you do not harm yourself." The relationship between the nurse and the patient should not be like that between a guard and a prisoner; rather, the nurse should be available to talk or to remain quiet and comforting.

Provision of environmental safety. Since it is impossible to remove all potentially harmful objects from the environment, common sense should be used in removing the most potentially dangerous objects such as razor blades, nail files, glass objects, belts, drugs, and matches.[11]

The self-destructive patient should not be assigned living quarters that allow the patient to become isolated. A double room close to the nurses' station increases the possibility of persons being in the patient's environment most of the time.

Use of seclusion and restraint. In intervention with a person who is out of control, both the nurse's feelings and the patient's need for external control are important.[22] Verbal intervention should be tried first, for example, "You're upset. Come with me to your room." Such statements should be made calmly and with authority. When such controls are instigated, the nurse must carry through with the commands. If follow-through does not occur, the patient can become more frightened, realizing that nobody will provide the desperately needed control.

If it appears that the patient requires physical restraint, staff members should remove breakable objects such as eyeglasses and jewelry before approaching the patient. The staff should quickly and clearly coordinate the approach prior to coming in contact with the patient. This is best accomplished by designating one leader to coordinate efforts and deciding who will restrain the person's left leg, left arm, etc. The patient should be held securely at the knee and elbow joints for the safest approach. Staff should remain away from the patient's mouth to avoid being bitten. It is important to maintain stride when taking the patient to seclusion so that control of the patient's body is not lost.[22] If the person is walked backward, the individual will be off balance and unable to strike out.

A unified effort is also necessary to release the person in a seclusion room and leave the room without injury to the staff. However, after being placed in seclusion, the person should not be ignored. When a nurse enters the patient's room, another staff member should be present. The nurse's intentions should be explained to the patient, for example, "Mr. Smith, here is your dinner tray." The patient's condition should be frequently assessed to determine when enough control has been regained for the patient to be released from seclusion.

Some patients ask to go to the seclusion room when they are aware of the approaching loss of control. This request should be honored and followed with constant monitoring to provide support.

Use of medications. Medications are useful tools in decreasing destructive behavior. Antidepressant drugs (e.g., amitriptyline hydrochloride [Elavil] are frequently used for the depressed, suicidal person. However, the nurse must be alert to the possibility of medications being kept to be used later in a suicide attempt. It is therefore vital to be certain the medication has been swallowed. A mouth check may be done, but a better alternative would be to use liquid medication.

Medications are also used for the outwardly destructive patient. Often an antipsychotic agent prescribed on an as-needed basis can be used to decrease potentially violent behavior.

Behaviors indicative of the maintenance of safety include the absence or reduction of destructive behavior directed toward the self or others.

Identification of personal strengths

The destructive person has extremely low self-esteem.[30] The person is acting in the only way known to regain control, however misdirected. The base line in intervening with this person is to treat the patient with the respect and concern that communicate that the person is deserving of attention. Through the presence of the nurse the patient learns that the nurse will remain and attempt to help.

Communication and listening skills provide the road to an increase in comfort level and the opportunity for patient verbalization of destructive feelings.[9] The nurse can facilitate the patient's expression of feelings by helping the person realize that it is normal to feel angry, hostile, or hopeless, thus making these feelings more acceptable to the person. To facilitate the expression of feelings, the nurse must communicate that the patient's emotions are acceptable. The destructive behavior can then be discussed in terms of normalcy, and some of the guilt feelings can begin to be alleviated.[25]

Positive attributes should be recognized and praised realistically.[30] However, the nurse should be careful to avoid excessive generalized praise such as "You do such a fantastic job in occupational therapy." This type of interaction is usually not believed or well received. As progress is made, the patient should be helped to identify feelings, particularly positive ones. This is more helpful than the nurse identifying them. For example, the nurse could ask, "How did you feel when you gave the wallet you made to your husband?"

As the nurse gets to know the patient better, the nurse can build on the patient's strengths and provide the patient with positive experiences.[30] This area of intervention is of high priority in helping the person to modify a negative self-image.

If the person has family or friends who are viewed as supportive, they should be integrated in the overall plan of care. These supportive people need to discuss their many feelings about the patient's behavior before they can help the patient. Support groups can then be directly involved in making future plans with the patient. These people are an important part of the patient's personal strengths. By their love and active concern, they show the destructive person that the individual is perceived as a person of worth.[30]

Behaviors indicative of the identification and use of personal strengths are verbalization of destructive feelings, identification of positive attributes, participation in activities viewed as positive, and understanding that family and friends perceive the individual to be of worth.

Use of alternate methods of expressing feelings

After the destructive patient feels comfortable and is able to identify personal areas of strength, the person is ready to begin to learn alternate methods of expressing feelings. At this point in treatment the destructive person is ready to learn how to internally control behavioral expression of feelings.

It is often helpful to explore with the patient the factors that led to the episodes of destructive behavior. By understanding situations and how feelings get out of control, the patient is better able to explore alternative responses for future use.[30] The patient can be helped to compile a list of problems in their order of stressfulness. These can then be dealt with in their order of priority. The pros and cons to various solutions of the priority problem should be considered by asking the patient questions such as "What is the best you could hope for with this solution?" or "What is the worst you could expect?" By carefully exploring various solutions, plans can be made to deal with this stressful problem. After the behavior has been attempted, its effectiveness should be evaluated. The patient may be asked "How did it work when you explained why you were irritated?"[21]

Cognitive restructuring gives the person a different, realistic perception of feelings and reactions. Threats and feelings of lack of control are reduced by clarifying misperceptions.[17] For the self-destructive person the feeling of hopelessness is explored to clarify misconceptions associated with it. The person can then begin to realize that there are viable options for dealing with problems.

A useful therapeutic technique in the identification of alternate methods of expression of feelings is role playing. It is a learning experience in which the nurse and patient act out a situation (past or future) that is stressful for the patient. It gives the patient an opportunity to practice various behaviors. After acting through the situation, the nurse and patient can switch roles, thereby giving the patient an opportunity to better understand the other person's perspective.[31] such role playing should be followed by a discussion about the feelings that occurred and the ability to use new behavior patterns.

Assertiveness theorists believe that each individual has the right to behave in a way that meets the person's needs as long as the behavior does not impinge on the rights of others.[30] One alternative behavior for the destructive person to learn to use is assertiveness.

The destructive patient who is preparing to return to the community should be familiarized with available support groups. These groups provide an important avenue in dealing constructively with feelings. Two examples of such groups are Parents Anonymous, organized for abusive or potentially abusive parents, and Alcoholics Anonymous, a support group to help alcoholics abstain from drinking.

Behaviors indicative of use of alternate methods of expressing feelings include listing stressful problems and various behavioral solutions, identifying misperceptions about thoughts and feelings, identifying and using assertiveness techniques, and joining community support groups.

CONCEPT OUTLINE

I. *Conceptual definition:* Destructive behavior is verbal or physical behavior that results in injury, damage, or other noxious consequences to oneself, others, or the environment.

II. *Antecedent conditions*
   - A. Developmental factors
   - B. Physiological factors
   - C. Triggering events

III. *Behavioral definition*
   - A. Objective data
     1. Physiological response
        - a. Increased muscular tension
        - b. Increased sensory alertness
        - c. Increased heart rate
        - d. Elevated blood pressure
        - e. Dry mouth
        - f. Constipation
        - g. Increased respiratory rate
     2. Motor-behavioral response
        - a. Changes in skeletal muscles and body posture
          - (1) Tightness in facial muscle
          - (2) Glaring eye contact
          - (3) Threatening gestures
          - (4) Body stance of power
          - (5) Invasion of other's personal space

b. Displacement or sublimation of anger
   (1) Hitting objects
   (2) Participation in sports
   (3) Smoking
   (4) Overeating
c. Direct physical attack
   (1) Against others—hitting, yanking, choking
   (2) Against self—scratching to suicidal gestures

3. Changes in activity patterns
   a. Giving away possessions
   b. Making a will
   c. Decreased work involvement
   d. Deterioration in relationships

B. Subjective data
   1. Difficulty identifying and verbalizing emotions
   2. Cessation of communication
   3. Indirect statements of anger
   4. Sarcasm
   5. Statements of self-harm
   6. Communication of impending attack on others

IV. Intervening variables
   A. Sociocultural patterns
   B. Environment

V. Nursing interventions—goals
   A. Maintenance of physiological equilibrium
      1. Monitoring of basic personal care
      2. Medical care of physical problems
   B. Maintenance of safety
      1. Limit setting
      2. Provision of environmental safety
         a. Removal of dangerous objects from environment
         b. Assignment of patient to shared living quarters
      3. Use of seclusion and restraint
      4. Use of medications
   C. Identification of personal strengths
      1. Communication that conveys respect
      2. Encouragement of identification and expression of feelings
      3. Discussion of normalcy of feelings
      4. Identification of patient's positive attributes
      5. Provision of opportunities for satisfying, positive experiences
      6. Identification of supportive significant others
      7. Use of support groups to reinforce perception of person's worth
   D. Use of alternate methods of expressing feelings
      1. Identification of stressful problems
      2. Identification of triggering events
      3. Identification of alternative approach to use in solving problems
      4. Identification of pros and cons of solutions to priority problems
      5. Teaching of assertiveness techniques
      6. Use of role playing to practice alternative behavior
      7. Evaluation of success of techniques attempted, with exploration of feelings and reactions
      8. Development of association with community support groups

VI. *Evaluation criteria*
   A. Absence of injury or physical illness
   B. Verbalization of feelings
   C. Identification of positive attributes
   D. Identification of support structure
   E. Identification of alternative options for problem solution
   F. Use of assertiveness techniques
   G. Identification of misperceptions regarding thoughts and feelings
   H. Participation in community support groups
   I. Reduction or absence of destructive events

REFERENCES

1. Alberti, R., and Emanons, M.: Your perfect right, San Luis Obispo, Calif., 1978, Impact Publishers, Inc.
2. Aguilera, D. C., and Messick, J. M.: Crisis intervention: theory and methodology, ed. 3, St. Louis, 1978, The C. V. Mosby Co.
3. Beck, A., Kovacs, M., and Weissman, A.: Hopelessness and suicidal behavior, J.A.M.A. 234:1146, 1975.
4. Beck, J. C., and Worthen, K.: Precipitating stress, crisis theory, and hospitalization in schizophrenia and depression, Arch. Gen. Psychiatry **26**:123, 1972.
5. Bolman, W.: Aggression and violence in children, Curr. Probl. Pediatr. **4**:3, 1974.
6. Burkhalter, P: Nursing care of the alcholic and drug abuser, New York, 1975, McGraw-Hill Book Co.
7. Caplan, G.: Principles of preventive psychiatry, New York, 1964, Basic Books, Inc., Publishers.
8. Dalton, K.: The premenstrual syndrome,

Springfield, Ill., 1964, Charles C Thomas, Publisher.
9. Egan, G.: The skilled helper, Monterey, Calif., 1975, Brooks/Cole Publishing Co.
10. Foreyt, J., and Rathjen, D.: Cognitive behavior therapy: research and application, New York, 1978, Plenum Press.
11. Frederick, C.: The role of the nurse in crisis intervention and suicide prevention, J. Psychiatr. Nurs. **11**:27, 1973.
12. Guyton, A. C.: Textbook of medical physiology, ed. 5, Philadelphia, 1976, W. B. Saunders Co.
13. Helfer, R., and Kempe, C.: The battered child, Chicago, 1968, The University of Chicago Press.
14. Jasmin, S., and Trygstad, L. N.: Behavioral concepts and the nursing process, St. Louis, 1979, The C. V. Mosby Co.
15. Kemp, W.: Drug abuse: current concepts and research, Springfield, Ill., 1972, Charles C Thomas, Publisher.
16. Kessler, J. W.: Psychopathology of childhood, Englewood Cliffs, N.J., 1966, Prentice-Hall, Inc.
17. Kiening, M.: Hostility. In Carlson, C., and Blackwell, B., editors: Behavioral concepts and nursing intervention, ed. 2, Philadelphia, 1978, J. B. Lippincott Co.
18. Lazarus, R. S.: Psychological stress and the coping process, New York, 1966, McGraw-Hill Book Co.
19. Lyon, G. G.: Limit setting as a therapeutic tool, J. Psychiatr. Nurs. **8**:17, 1970.
20. MacKinnon, I. L., MacKinnon, P. C. B., and Thomson, A. D.: Lethal hazards of the luteal phase of the menstrual cycle, Br. Med. J. **1**:1015, 1959.
21. McClean, L. J.: The client who generates guilt and rejecting behavior. In Haber, J., Leach, A. M., Schudy, S. M., and Sideleau, B. F., editors: Comprehensive psychiatric nursing, New York, 1978, McGraw-Hill Book Co.
22. Nissley, B. H., and Townes, N.: Guidelines for intervention in aggressive behavior. In Backer, B. A., Dubbert, P. M., and Eisenmon, E. J. P., editors: Psychiatric/mental health nursing: contemporary readings, New York, 1978, D. Van Nostrand Co., Inc.
23. Novaco, R.: The functions and regulations of the arousal of anger, Am. J. Psychiatry **133**:1124, 1976.
24. Olweus, D.: Personality and aggression, Nebr. Symp. Motiv. **20**:26, 1972.
25. Roberts, S. L.: Behavioral concepts and the critically ill patient, Englewood Cliffs, N.J., 1976, Prentice-Hall, Inc.
26. Short, M. J., and Wilson, W. P.: Roles of denial in chronic hemodialysis, Arch. Gen. Psychiatry **20**:433, 1969.
27. Stafford, L.: Depression and self-destructive behavior, J. Psychiatr. Nurs. **14**:37, 1976.
28. Straus, M. A., Gelles, R. J., and Steinmetz, S. K.: Behind closed doors: violence in the American family, New York, 1980, Anchor Press.
29. Strong, P.: Aggression in the general hospital, Nurs. Times **69**:21, 1973.
30. Stuart, G., and Sundeen, S.: Principles and practice of psychiatric nursing, St. Louis, 1979, The C. V. Mosby Co.
31. Underwood, P. R.: Communication through role playing, Am. J. Nurs. **71**:1184, 1971.
32. Wetzel, R. D., McClure, J. N., Jr., and Reich, T.: Premenstrual symptoms in self-referrals to a suicide prevention service, Br. J. Psychiatry **119**:525, 1971.
33. Wittkower, E. D., and Dubreuil, G.: Psychocultural stress in relation to mental illness, Soc. Sci. Med. **7**:691, 1973.
34. Zamora, L. C.: The client who generates anger. In Haber, J., Leach, A. M., Schudy, S. M., and Sideleau, B. F., editors: Comprehensive psychiatric nursing, New York, 1978, McGraw-Hill Book Co.

PAULETTE R. Di ANGI

Chapter 7

BIZARRE BEHAVIOR

Bizzare behavior
is
the helpless
distorted
cry for help,
an individual
driven
beyond reasonable limits
of toleration
who has chosen
the most dramatic form possibl
to communicate to others
about the desperate state
in which he finds himself.

PAULETTE R. Di ANGI

CONCEPTUAL DEFINITION

Bizarre behavior is a pattern of behavior that, although meaningful to the person exhibiting the behavior, does not have a recognizable meaning to persons observing it. The behavior is seen as extreme, incongruous, or unorthodox compared to social norms. The behavior pattern does not match that which society has identified as a reasonable, correct, or understandable response to a given situation. A society may allow a great number of behavior options as adaptive responses. However, when an individual rejects all those options and exhibits an entirely different set of responses, that behavior is judged to be bizarre. The behavior appears maladaptive and without purpose or meaning to the observer. The individual exhibiting the behavior is experiencing an alteration in meaningful interaction with reality. Changing the meaning of interaction allows the person to create and respond to a self-chosen reality. This reality is one in which the person constructs the rules that govern interactions. That which is occurring in the person's reality is incongruous with what is actually happening. In some instances bizarre behavior patterns are based on a complete substitution of a false reality. In other instances the restructured reality may relate to only one area of functioning or to only one false idea.

This change in reality's structure affects the person's ability to perceive and process cues from the environment. The person's ability to solve problems, or even to recognize problems, is diminished, if not lost, as the individual becomes more focused on the substituted reality.

Since the person's adaptive responses are dominated by an internal restructuring of reality, the individual's behavior can be influenced by perceptual disturbances of two types: illusions and hallucinations. Illusions are misinterpretations of sensory data received from the environment. The person exhibiting bizarre behavior no longer participates in reality testing and thus believes that these misinterpretations are true. Hallucinations are sensory perceptions without an external stimulus. The person experiences something via the senses, but the stimulus for the sensation is not based in external reality. These visual, auditory, olfactory, or tactile sensations are perceived as real and influence, if not direct, the person's behavior. Others cannot interact with this altered reality because it does not exist for them. Neither can they understand the meaning of the person's behavior patterns. The socially formed self of the hallucinating individual has disintegrated, and society perceives the individual to be experiencing a mental disorder.

Usually, bizarre behavior is episodic rather than a consistent way of life. The behavior occurs when the individual attempts to cope with something that is perceived as an overwhelming threat. Bizarre behavior involves the person's ability to solve problems in a stressful situation. When the coping methods the individual knows do not help to maintain the individual's relationship with the environment, bizarre behavior can occur.

To exist and grow, a personality is in constant process of change and problem solving in response to the environment. When a person is confronted with a problem or crisis that precipitates uncertainty or disequilibrium, the individual will attempt to categorize the problems by making judgments about them. Knowledge of past problems is used for reference. The individual can then project possible solutions either by logical conclusion or by vicarious learning from significant others.

After making a judgment regarding a problem, the person chooses a course of action, tries it, and, if successful, stores the information for further use. When the action is not successful, disequilibrium continues and anxiety increases. If the person tries another approach to the problem which is successful, this information is stored for future reference. If the person is unsuccessful in problem solving and a period of trial and error behavior occurs without relieving the anxiety or disequilibrium, the person becomes more and more immersed in the problem. The person eventually uses up all primary alternatives to problem solution. As frustration continues and anxiety increases, the individual may begin to use internal and external resources not included in the past behavior repertoire. It is at this point that bizarre behavior may begin. It is also at this point that judgment, the ability to see the real problem and to decide on a course of action, is lost.

With the increase of anxiety and frustration and the decrease in ability to deal with reality, personality disorganization may result. The person loses the ability to perceive part or all of reality. In addition, the person is often flooded with painful or unacceptable memories. This situation demands emergency coping measures to reduce the anxiety. If the present reality is overwhelming, the person may choose to escape or to cope by creating a different, less painful reality. The person's response to that reality is seen by an observer as bizarre behavior.[9,21]

ANTECEDENT CONDITIONS

Behavior does not exist in isolation but evolves from relationships to the environment. An individual's life consists of a series of relationships. An individual must learn to manage involvement in many different relationships, yet keep them in some meaningful, coherent order. One's place in situations encountered must be identified by the individual, as must the place of others in the same situations. The feedback evolving out of social interactions provides cues to the appropriateness of behavior and the acceptance of the person by the group.[21]

An individual's behavior can be understood only in relation to the behaviors accepted by the social group to which the individual belongs. At each stage of growth there are social tasks that the child, adolescent, or adult is expected to accomplish. Growth experiences develop behaviors that foster more growth. Relationships with others provide the conditions for the patterning of self. The interactions that occur during an individual's formative years with those persons perceived by the child as being significant have important consequences. These experiences help in the formation of self and the development of identity and control. The child uses the information or cues received from the environment to interpret the world and its expectations. The individual gradually learns to adjust behavior so that it is appropriate to a given time and place. This does not imply conscious planning, but rather a continuous process of sorting the cues and feedback received and then responding.[30]

The child expands the self-concept with "good me," "bad me," and "not me" feedback experiences. At first the family is the primary source of feedback, but as the child matures, other groups such as schoolmates, peers, church groups, and the community supplement self-concept formation experiences.[42] Successful behavior depends on the child's ability to infer the required behavior for a situation and the role of the others in the situation. Since at each stage of growth the individual exists in relationship to others, the definition of self hinges on the individual's ability to read the available cues.

Social interaction precedes the self-concept and provides the building materials for it. The child becomes aware of others before developing a clear image of self. The self is formed and sustained by ongoing interactions with others. Self-concept is composed of learned perceptions, expectations, and hypotheses that are formed through interactions with significant others.[28]

There are endless combinations of possible reasons why an individual would construct an alternative reality. However, all the hypothesized reasons appear to focus on two major sources: interpersonal and biochemical factors. The interpersonal factors are based on inadequate learning of appropriate interaction behavior. The lack of learning opportunity or the receipt of inconsistent or nonunderstandable messages during learning opportunities can prevent the individiual from learning appropriate behavior. The biochemical factors relate to the interruption or alteration of stimuli transmission and neural perception.

Lack of learning opportunity

Parental rejection. Children who receive rejecting cues from significant others perceive themselves as unappreciated, scorned, or deceived. Parents who view the child as unwanted and troublesome precipitate pervasive feelings in the child of isolation in a hostile world. Without basic supports and security in the home, the child lacks confidence to try new things and to venture forth into the world outside. As a result of parental rejection, the child may anticipate rejection by others. The child often learns to avoid others as a defense against further emotional pain. This child may exhibit apathy and indifference as a protective cover to minimize the expected rejection.

Rejection is not the only parental attitude that may precipitate this reaction in the child. Exploitation, seduction, and deception can destroy the trust the child needs to test the outside world. If the child fails to meet parental demands and consistently experiences punishment, an expectation of punishment from all relationships can develop. This expectation can result in hopelessness and discouragement and can cause the person to withdraw and avoid social encounters.[27,35] A sense of being unwanted, however, seems to have the most shattering effect. A child who perceives that significant others are loving and supportive can tolerate a great deal of punishment from the environment.[35,37]

Parental overprotection. Some parents narrowly restrict the child's experiences so that the child fails to learn the basic components of autonomous behavior. Overprotective parents, fearing that their children are too frail or are unable to care for themselves, deny the child opportunities to grow normally. This may foster feelings of inadequacy in the child. The child may be trained to be dependent, deficient, and progressively fearful of leaving the protection of the parent.[10,19,34]

Parental overindulgence. Parents who are overly permissive and undisciplined allow their child's behavior to go unchecked. Their model of undisciplined living reinforces the child's irresponsibility. These children often grow up to be inconsiderate with tyrannical personalities and tend to be aggressively antisocial.[35]

Absence of role models. The lack of significant adults in the family may rob the child of the opportunity to acquire, through imitation, some of the complex patterns of behavior used in adulthood. The most serious deficit is the unavailability of a model of the child's sex. This model does not have to be a parent, but someone who can fill the role of model and be close to the child. This loss can occur either by the absence of a person to fill the role of a sex model or by the lack of the individual's attention to this modeling role when the child is present. This problem may be present, for example, in families in which parents have vocational preoccupations and are frequently absent from the home.[5,8,10,13]

Inconsistent feedback

Conflicting communication. Families have their own style of communication, and the child assimilates these patterns of listening, attending, and conveying thoughts to others. When this pattern is not rational or reciprocal, the child is ill-equipped to function in an effective way.[17] One confusing pattern of communication, called a double-bind, transmits ambivalence.[2] The messages given are erratic with a loss of focus, conveying contradictory meanings through verbal and nonverbal messages. An example is the mother who repeatedly implores her child in a distinctly hostile tone, "Come to Mommy; Mommy wants to hug you, squeeze you, hug you, squeeze you."* The conflicting nature of such verbal and nonverbal messages can immobilize the child. The recipient of the message cannot respond without running head-on into conflict with one or the other aspect of the message. It is

*See references 2, 31, 32, 35, and 40.

a "damned if you do, damned if you don't" situation. Exposure to this type of communication makes it difficult to establish a foundation in reality.

Children exposed to constant bickering are influenced by a lack of consistent models of behavior. When dissension is constantly present in the home, the child is exposed to mistrust, suspiciousness, and anxiety. Children in these settings can and often do become scapegoats, either as objects to be convinced and won over to the parent's side or as objects on which the parent projects and releases fears and dissatisfaction. Children who are constantly exposed to such strife are robbed of a sense of security and stability.[35]

Parents who are disproportionately affectionate with their children can create hostility and jealousy among siblings. Rivalry can result. Children who have to struggle for their needed affection may reach adulthood with a distrust of affection and with a view that all others are competitors.[10,16,34]

Inconsistent rewards. Parental methods of reinforcement can be irregular and contradictory. Some degree of inconsistency is of course inevitable. However, some parents display extreme inconsistency in their expectations and extreme unpredictability in their rewards and punishments. Children exposed to this cannot learn consistent ways of dealing with the environment. Often these children become immobile or noncommittal to avoid the suspense and anxiety of not knowing what the environment will produce next. Other children, adopting parental actions, display ambivalence and vacillation in feelings and actions.[6,15,35,36]

A slightly different twist to this inconsistency occurs when parents do not punish actions but expect performance before encouragement or rewards are given. The child is rewarded for exhibiting the behavior the parents like, but the child does not receive previous teaching from the parent regarding the action desired. Children reared under this type of parenting tend to be socially pleasant. By imitation of parental actions, they receive rewards from others. However, often they develop an insatiable and indiscriminate need for approval. Such contingent rewards appear to develop an excessive need for approval, making the child dependent on feedback from the environment.[17,35]

Biochemical factors

Bizarre behavior can also be the result of a change in the body's chemistry. Research has shown that the presence of some chemicals in the bloodstream, even in small amounts, can produce mental and behavioral changes. For example, LSD (lysergic acid diethylamide) and mescaline can lead to a temporary disorganization of thought processes. The effect of these two drugs, in producing a variety of psychotic-like behaviors, is so predictable that the behavior changes have been referred to as model psychoses.[11]

Neurotransmitters are the focus of much of the recent research dealing with bizarre behavior. They play an important role in the broad spectrum of physiological and behavioral activities. There is evidence that changes in these substances and alterations in the balance among them result in neurological dysfunction, which can lead to psychiatric disorders.[7]

The theories presented in recent literature center on (1) a change in neurotransmitter chemicals, (2) a change in amount and interaction of neurotransmitters, and (3) a disturbance in neuronal metabolism.

Change in neurotransmitters. In 1972 an enzyme was found in the human brain that can change transmitter chemicals, mainly serotonin, into hallucinogenic-like compounds.[24,33] Other scientists have hypothesized that the body manufactures an antibody, taraxein, that works against the neurotransmitters, interfering with the passage of information from cell to cell.[25,26]

Change in amount and interaction of neurotransmitters. In most areas of the brain, dopamine, one of the two main catecholamines in the brain, is the precursor of norepinephrine. It is transformed to norepinephrine by the enzyme dopamine β-hydroxylase, but in parts of the brain that lack dopamine β-hydroxylase, dopamine is presumed to be the neurotransmitter.[12,20,41]

One study reports that when synthesis of norepinephrine is decreased by the inhibition of dopamine β-hydroxylase, there is a shift in the catecholamine metabolism toward dopamine, which exacerbates bizarre behavior. Auditory hallucinations, delusional thinking, autism, depersonalization, confusion, forgetfulness, and impaired ability to calculate may occur. Physical changes such as hypertension, weakness, pallor, tightness in legs, chest pains, and shortness of breath also result.[38]

Another report gives evidence that when the excitatory effects of norepinephrine are blocked in the brain stem neurons, bizarre behavior decreases. This leads to the conclusion that when there is an overabundance of norepinephrine, there is an increased excitatory response in the neuron, which causes instability in neuron functioning. This can be seen in schizophrenia.[39]

Research findings also suggest that schizophrenics may suffer from irregularities in the functioning of the autonomic nervous system, which subject the individual to excessive or deficient arousal in response to stress. It has been found that in situations that cause only mild stress for normal subjects, arousal for schizophrenics is abnormally high. In response to situations that severely stress normal subjects, the schizophrenics' reactivity is often lower than the normal.[8,22]

In 1970 Fenz and Velner,[18] after reviewing the literature and conducting their own study, concluded that a common and basic deficit in all schizophrenics is the inability to modulate the level of autonomic response to variations in stimulation. When a healthy person is subjected to a constant level of intense stimulation of the nervous system, the protective process of inhibition occurs. This protective process reduces the person's general level of response. However, if intense stimulation continues, a change in the protective inhibition process occurs, and the relationship between strength of stimulation and response is reversed. Strong stimulation results in inhibition of the impulses in the nervous system, and weak stimuli elicit the response level of strong stimuli. This can cause the individual to have difficulty in separating relevant from irrelevant stimuli.[11]

There is also evidence that an imbalance of dopamine and acetylcholine in the basal ganglia of the brain can be related to bizarre behavior. This is supported by the finding that the administration of L-dopa, the precursor of dopamine, to a patient experiencing bizarre behavior aggravates the psychopathological symptoms already present.[3,4,41]

Norepinephrine is thought to inhibit dopamine production; the enzyme dopamine β-hydroxylase changes dopamine into norepinephrine. If the effectiveness of dopamine β-hydroxylase were decreased, less norepinephrine would be available to inhibit dopamine. As a result of this increase, the dopamine receptors would be flooded with dopamine, causing increased inhibition of those neurons inhibited by dopamine. There is further evidence that dopamine depletion can be compensated for by simultaneous norepinephrine depletion.[1,14,29]

On the basis of a pharmacological model in which bizarre behavior was induced by an amphetamine, it is proposed that the disturbance between transmitters consists of excess functional dopamine or related amines, excess serotonin or related amines, and excess acetylcholine. It appears that bizarre behavior may involve disturbances in a number of neurotransmitters and the effect each has on the others.[4,38]

Disturbance in neuronal metabolism. The nervous system requires high amounts of energy and a rapid turnover to maintain stable transmitter synthesis, release, and uptake.[20] Glucose and oxygen are the brain's primary sources of metabolic energy. The glucose and oxygen must pass from the blood to the brain via a blood-brain barrier. This membrane and others in the brain are made of lipids. Interference with the biosynthesis of the various lipids in the membranes can lead to alteration in neuronal sensitivity.[12,20]

Protein and amino acids in the brain function as enzymes, hormones, structural elements, and, probably, transport systems. Epinephrine, norepinephrine, dopamine, and serotonin are amino acid derivatives. Disorders of protein and amino acid metabolism may cause neurological dysfunction that can result in behavior problems and changes.[12,20] Such disorders can occur in anorexia nervosa; starvation; toxemia from mercury, lead, or other industrial toxins; and organic brain syndrome.

Vitamins and their derivatives function as cofactors for enzymes and enzyme metabolism. A vitamin deficiency, particularly of the B group, may interfere with neuronal functions and cause behavior changes.[20]

It is not yet clear whether biochemical factors are primary causes, secondary effects, or interactive factors. Neither is it clear how environment, stress, and development patterns relate to these biochemical factors. However, they all seem to participate in the production of bizarre behavior.

BEHAVIORAL DEFINITION

Bizarre behaviors emanate from alterations in the individual's perceptions, thought processes, and emotional expression.

Objective data

Altered perceptions. Any abrupt changes in the patient's behavior unexplained by environmental stimuli can indicate that either an illusion or a hallucination is being experienced. Nodding of the head, tilting it to one side, and talking to someone or something not present; being startled without apparent precipitation; and intent brushing of clothes and skin in quick, almost desperate, movements are all examples of objective behaviors that may indicate altered perception.

Hallucinations are sensory perceptions for which there are no external stimuli. An illusion is a misinterpreted sensory perception. Everyone at one time or another experiences illusion. For example, a woman walking down a dark street at night may think that the bush on the corner looks like a mugger, but as she gets closer, it is seen as a bush.

Illusions can be confronted in reality. For example, a patient may state that his father's picture is on the wall in a dimly lit room. However, on turning up the lights, the shadow, or "picture," disappears. Usually, reality can be manipulated to eliminate or cast doubt on illusions.

Hallucinations generate from an internal stimulus; they do not have any basis in reality. If the patient just described was experiencing a hallucination, the "picture" would have remained on the wall no matter how the environment was changed.

Although hallucinations and illusions can involve any of the senses, they are most often experienced in the visual and auditory modes. Hallucinations may be experienced in one or more modes. Illusions are most often experienced in only one mode.

Changes in posture, gait, or dress may indicate that perceptions of the self or body image have been altered. Body image is one's concept of the shape, size, mass, function, structure, and significance of the body and its parts. This image is the internalized picture of a person's physical appearance, movement, and space. It involves not only the physical, living body, but also inanimate objects such as eyeglasses, purse, cane, clothes, makeup, jewelry and other things that daily come into intimate contact with the person.

Behaviors indicative of possible body image alterations include appearing in public with no clothes or wearing two or three outfits at the same time. Other indications might be the change of not wearing any makeup by the woman who always does or the mask appearance of too much makeup. In addition to overuse or misplaced use of makeup, the person may wear an excessive amount of jewelry such as 25 bracelets, 10 necklaces, many pins, and 6 pairs of eyeglasses.

Altered thought processes. Changes in concentration, attention span, memory, judgment, speed of thinking, and content of thought may occur during bizzarre behavior. Disturbances in concentration will be exhibited by the patient becoming easily frustrated or bored with tasks that are in fact suitable to the patient's level of ability. Problems with concentration and attention span are to be expected when a task is beyond a patient's ability. Disturbances in attention span involve movement from one task to another in a flighty fashion but without the emotional overtones of frustration and boredom. Frustration is the feeling experienced when a person's expectations are not met. Increased uneasiness may turn into irritability or blossom into anger.[16] Boredom is the loss of interest in or the tiring of a task and is often accompanied by a desire to be elsewhere.

Disturbances in memory involve the inability to remember adequately what happened during any moment in the patient's past. The patient may not recognize a friend or family member. The patient may ask what the nurse's name is or who the patient's mother is. The patient may not know what day it is or what town the hospital is in.

Disturbances in judgment are demonstrated by indecision or by illogical problem solving. An example is the following decision regarding the purchase of a new car: "I owned a blue car that ran well. I like blue cars. There is a blue car for sale. I will buy that car."

Disturbances in speed of thinking are observable when the patient's speed of talking increases or decreases from the normal rate.

Disturbances in content of thought are indicated by the patient's use of circumstantiality, concrete thinking, flight of ideas, tangential thinking, word salads, ideas of reference, delusions, leveling of ideas, clang association, and thought blocking.

Circumstantiality occurs when the person is not able to separate the components of a situation but discusses all the things involved in detail. An example is seen in the following letter written by a patient: "Dear ____________, I am writing you a letter on a white paper with a yellow #2 pencil. The pencil has an eraser on the other end from the lead point. It is red. This pencil was made in the U.S.A. The paper is about 8 × 10 inches and sits on a brown desk top." The person exhibiting circumstantiality has difficulty separating the important content from the mundane.

Concrete thinking involves the inability to think abstractly. An example is found in the following conversation:

Nurse: Where did you come from?
Patient: My mother's womb.
Nurse: What brought you here?
Patient: A taxi.

This patient's thinking revolves around only the concrete, tangible facts of a situation.

Flight of ideas, tangential thinking, and word salads exemplify different degrees of disordered thought. In flight of ideas thoughts seem to take flight as the person jumps from one thought to the next with some connection in the sequence of the thoughts. The person may exhibit a continuous flow of speech that is not disjointed, for example, "My brother bought me a car. He likes to drive. Cars are very expensive." Tangential thinking is sometimes called looseness of association. The thoughts are loosely connected and difficult to understand, for example, "They came back. Tennessee comes first. X, Y, Z. God's wife will get you." Beyond this point the person may begin making up new words, called neologisms, in an attempt to communicate. An example of word salad is "Today is a good beeshevar in the bevoie with smigium."

Ideas of reference involve the patient thinking that all things have personal reference. Ideas of reference differ from delusions of reference. A delusion is a fixed false belief. The delusion may start as an idea, but it is ingrained in the individual's belief system. The difference is mainly one of degree. Ideas of reference are just that, ideas, whereas delusions involve beliefs. A person may notice that a woman is smiling and infer "She is laughing at me." The person experiencing this as an idea of reference could be helped with reality orientation or reality testing. The person experiencing the delusion believes it as a fact and cannot be dissuaded from this belief.

Leveling of ideas involves loss of the priority and value of things. The patient might speak about the speck of dust on the floor with the same emphasis and concern as he talks about his wife and children. The differences in meaning are lost.

Clang association involves the stimulation of a new trend of thought by external sound. It can involve a nonverbal or verbal reaction. For example, in a nonverbal response to a "bang" in the hall, a patient who had been talking about a dog may pretend to shoot a gun. A verbal clang response usually involves rhyming. After the "bang" the patient may start a "bang, clang, tang, glang, rang, bang, sang, gang" series until distracted by another sound. Sometimes in conversation the patient may take the last word of a sentence and create a stream of rhyme with it.

Thought blocking is evidenced by the patient stopping in the middle of a sentence and then not being able to finish the sentence even if reminded of what was being said.

Altered emotional expression. The person may exhibit a flat or inappropriate affect during a bizarre behavior episode. The person may not exhibit any emotional response, or, when affect is present, it may be inappropriate to the situation (e.g., laughing during a funeral).

Subjective data

Altered perceptions. Subjective behaviors that demonstrate altered perceptions in bizarre behavior include descriptions of the patient's perceptions. The following are some examples

Visual hallucination: "I am seeing God."
Auditory hallucination: "I heard a cannon go off!"
Tactile hallucination: "Get these snakes off me! They are crawling all over me!"
Illusion: After hearing a plane fly over the building, the patient said, "That was my mother yelling at me."

Disturbances in body image may be expressed as feelings about one's body. Depersonalization is the feeling of a loss of the boundaries between self and the environment. The patient may verbalize a sense of being outside of the self and watching events. Another expression of depersonalization is "I don't want to kill you. I think you are part of me." Other subjective behaviors that delineate altered perceptions of self are expressed as feelings of weightlessness or heavy body parts and a disturbed sense of time. The patient may relate feelings of being lost in time.

Altered thought processes. Subjective behaviors exhibiting altered thought processes include statements of feeling or awareness of what is happening. The following are examples:

Altered concentration: "I can't keep my mind on anything anymore."
Altered memory: "I can't remember things like I used to."
Decreased judgment: "I can't seem to make up my mind about anything."
Altered speed of thinking: "My thoughts are going so fast I can't keep up with them."
Flight of ideas: "My thoughts don't stand still, and I forget what I'm thinking."
Thought blocking: "Sometimes I have spells; my thoughts seem to disappear or be taken away."

Altered emotional expression. In many instances the person exhibiting bizarre behavior is unable to identify the emotions being experienced. The person may indicate that emotions are not experienced: "I don't feel anything." The person may also identify that the emotions expressed are opposite to those felt: "When I laugh, I want to cry, and when I cry, I want to laugh."

INTERVENING VARIABLES

The intervening variables that increase or decrease the person's ability to deal with reality are different for each individual, just as the antecedent conditions are different for each individual.

Present developmental stage

The present developmental level of the individual influences the expression of bizarre behavior. The young adult or adolescent will not have as many set patterns of behavior as an older adult; yet the adult may have a longer history of successful problem solving and functional living to draw on than the adolescent. Each developmental level provides both potential strengths and potential liabilities that may affect the bizarre behavior episode. Pains and inadequacies experienced during previous developmental stages may emerge, increasing the individual's anxiety about the present and possibly causing regression to an earlier, more secure developmental state. Persons who never learned to trust others, who are dominated by feelings of shame or doubt, are limited in the ability to deal with reality.

Stimuli

Although the person exhibiting bizarre behavior is very sensitive to both external and internal stimuli, the individual is usually not able to integrate these perceptions in meaningful or useful patterns. If external stimlui are so excessive that they become overwhelming, they often further confuse the patient and exaggerate the bizarre behavior. When there is not enough stimulation from external sources, the person may become overly attentive to internal stimuli. A seclusion room with nothing in it and no human contact for long periods can be as overwhelming as a noisy, crowded, television room. One patient's description of how this heightened sensitivity made him feel was "I'm too alert. Colors are brighter, noises louder, nothing ever stops. Everything is pouring in at once."

Motivation

The individual's personal level of motivation may influence the degree and length of bizarre behavior. For example, a woman who was admitted to the hospital with extreme bizarre behavior after her mother's death returned to reality in a short time because she said, "I have to go home and take care of my baby." Her motivation to get well was extremely high. Even when she seemed beyond the staff's reach, she would respond to her daughter's voice on the telephone. Another women admitted during the same week with a similar degree of bizarre behavior remained in her alternate reality for almost 2 months, and she needed to remain under hospital care in a long-term facility for 2 years. Her behavior was precipitated by a divorce. She had no one waiting for her at home.

Family myths and beliefs may also influence bizarre behavior. Some families (and cultures) believe that it is a "sin" to be "crazy" or that one who has been admitted to a hospital is "lost." These beliefs could affect not only when the person would seek help, but also how responsive the individual could be to treatment.

There are also more subtle myths. For example, when four brothers reached the age of 24, they were hospitalized for extreme depression and bizarre behavior. Each brother experienced the same type of behavior and was admitted to the hospital during the month after the twenty-fourth birthday. Their father, grandfather, great-grandfather, uncles, and great-uncles all had similar experiences. Not all had hospital admission records, but all had depression at age 24. After much discussion with the family, it was found that this family believed that one did not become a man unless one had experienced depression and that a boy was a boy until age 25. The behavior was precipitated by family expectations.

Family support

The family can help or hinder the individual's experience with bizarre behavior. If the family rejects the troubled individual outright, the patient's feeling of abandonment will be increased. If the family can accept the pain of the loved one and not look for blame, their visits, cards, and support can become positive reinforcement for getting well.

One man who had been hospitalized with bizarre behavior had finally progressed far enough to go home on his first weekend pass. During the weekend he learned that his wife had been unfaithful while he was in the hospital and that she did not want a "half-crazy man." He returned to the hospital exhibiting more bizarre behavior than he had on admission.

NURSING INTERVENTIONS—GOALS AND EVALUATION CRITERIA

The goal of nursing intervention for the person exhibiting bizarre behavior is to help the patient develop socially acceptable methods of coping with life's stress.

The following subgoals can assist in the achievement of this overall goal: (1) maintenance of physical safety, (2) development of trust, (3) increase of meaning of reality, (4) increase of recognition and verbalization of feelings, (5) increase of reality testing or validation. The methods used to achieve these subgoals often overlap. For example, interventions that help maintain the patient's physical safety may also form a basis for trust development. As trust evolves, the meaning of reality may increase. The intervention process is fluid, with these goals blending and building on each other.

Maintenance of physical safety

The degree of safety intervention required is dictated by the degree of aggression and projection of feelings. A person who is actively hallucinating needs constant supervision. There is no way of monitoring a patient's alternate reality except by observation. "Voices" and "visions" have commanded people to set fire to buildings and to harm themselves and others. Continued observation and the removal of potentially harmful objects are essential. Potentially harmful objects include sharp objects, matches, belts, breakable containers, bottles, freestanding lamps, and some types of furniture. Even the individual's clothing can be a potential source of harm. One individual who experienced bizarre behavior as a result of injection of phencyclidine (PCP) blinded himself with his own hands. Observation and alertness to abrupt changes in behavior are critical for safety maintenance with this type of patient. The patient may be safest without clothes in a seclusion room that has no furniture and is constantly monitored. A hallucination that creates fear without aggression may only require that the patient lie in bed in a quiet room with a nurse sitting within arm's reach or holding the patient's hand.

Safety for the patient experiencing bizarre behavior also involves control over stimuli in the environment. Radios, televisions, conversations, intercoms, bells, hall traffic, call lights and other common stimuli in the acute care setting could bombard the patient, thus making reality more confusing. The nurse should validate how much external stimulation is comfortable for the patient. This can be done nonverbally by observing the patient's agitation in response to different levels and types of noises.

When the patient does not need close supervision, frequent, intermittent monitoring can be used to maintain the patient's safety. When entering and leaving the patient's room, the nurse should speak directly to the patient, using eye contact or touch to emphasize the message of who the nurse is and what is going to happen.

Often the person experiencing an alternative reality loses the ability to meet the needs of bodily functions. The person is totally dependent regarding cleanliness and nourishment. The patient's fluid and nutrient intake must be monitored to assure adequate levels of ingestion. The use of finger foods may facilitate nutrient intake. This food form is easily eaten and does not necessitate the use of potentially dangerous plates or eating utensils.

The behavior indicative that this safety goal has been achieved is the absence of injury in the patient and others.

Development of trust

For trust to evolve beyond the "safety" stage the nurse must make contact with the patient in the individual's reality. This can happen if the nurse repeatedly tries to communicate with the patient and to understand the patient's attempts at communication. The nurse should talk to the patient at each encounter. Responses and questions should be direct, simply stated, and concrete. The patient experiencing bizarre behavior will have a decreased ability or inability to use abstract thought. The nurse should explore what the behavior means to the patient and clarify the meaning of the patient's statements. This should be attempted even if the patient does not seem to be in contact with the nurse. One should never doubt the patient's ability to communicate. If words are not effective, colors, pictures, music, or poetry can be used. Misinterpretation of patients' verbal and nonverbal messages by people not experiencing bizarre behavior is common. The risk is even greater when one person is responding to a reality that has no meaning to the other. The nurse should attempt to identify themes in the patient's behavior. Since the bizarre behavior may appear random, consistent recording, or documenting, of the behavior and the sequence of events involved may assist in the identification of themes in behavior patterns.

The following is an example of a nurse who succeeded in making contact with a patient who was lost in an alternate reality. A patient had been dangerously agitated on an evening shift and had to be held down on the bed for the nurse to inject a sedative. In the process of this struggle the patient's face was in his pillow for a short time. After this episode he frequently ranted about being smothered and that he was going to smother all of "them." In a team conference someone suggested that perhaps his preoccupation with smothering was related to his face being in the pillow during the injection 2 days earlier. When the nurse asked him, "Could it be that you felt smothered the other night when we had to give you that injection to calm you down and your face was covered by the pillow?" He stopped his bizarre ranting, calmly said yes, and then continued ranting. Then the nurse asked the patient whether he was mad at the staff for allowing that to happen. Again he stopped, calmly said yes, and then continued ranting. When asked whether the staff was the "them" that he wanted to smother in return, the patient again ceased his bizarre behavior long enough to firmly say yes, only to return to the previous behavior, but the smothering theme was eliminated.

Making such contact always involves some risk. The risk could be that of being wrong or that of lengthening the time that the patient spends in the other reality. However, somewhere the two realities must touch in order for the patient to return. The nurse can help bring this about.

Contact can be assisted by nonverbal behavior. This happened with a young woman who had been spending her days sitting Indian fashion on the floor of her room, rocking back and forth, and singing things that did not make sense. The nurse, who had been trying to make contact with this patient by spending time with her and talking to her, finally got down onto the floor. She sat directly across from the patient, also in Indian fashion, and began to sing questions and conversation to the patient. At first the patient only stopped singing. As the nurse continued to sit there, the patient stopped rocking. Over a period of days with the nurse repeating this approach the patient began to converse with the nurse in song while sitting on the floor. At first the patient spoke about herself only in the third person and only for short periods before she would begin to gibber. Gradually, further contact was made, and their relationship expanded.

Contact is the meeting of the patient's alternate reality and the reality of the nurse. Something is communicated and understood by both nurse and patient. Contact should recur and increase in frequency during the trusting phase. The nurse needs to be available and consistent for the patient to increase the frequency of contact. As contact occurs, communication will increase and trust will evolve.

During this time the nurse should approach the patient using everyday, present-oriented, nonthreatening topics. A time and place should be identified for consistent, predictable meetings between the nurse and patient. The nurse should remain with the patient during the time allocated for their meeting, even if the patient is silent during this time. The patient should understand that there is no obligation to talk during the meeting. Although the patient may not be capable of making decisions during this time, plans that include the patient should be discussed even if the individual does not respond to the communication.

As feelings of trust develop, the patient will increasingly share what is being experienced. This may occur via direct verbalization by questions about what should be happening or by attempts to include the nurse in the alternate reality.

Other behaviors evidencing growing trust are increased periods of contact, increased attention span during these contacts, and initiation of conversation by the patient. Increased responsiveness to questions; orientation to time, place, and person; and attempts to make wants known are further evidence of trust development.

Increase of meaning of reality

As the patient experiences increased trust in the nurse, the patient will increasingly accept the nurse's explanation of reality. However, before the patient will accept reality, the alternate reality and its meaning must be dealt with.

The verbal and nonverbal social interactions of the patient should be observed. These observations should be shared with the patient in a nonjudgmental way, for example, "This is what I noticed, and I was wondering if this is what you are feeling right now," and "You don't look upset, but if that happened to me, I'd be upset." The modeling of acceptable emotions and responses with and in front of the patient in daily activities provides suggestions regarding how to deal with reality.

If the patient is having dissociated thoughts, the nurse should talk about concrete realities of the present. The patient should be helped to focus on the immediate environment. No status or recognition is given to hallucinations. The nurse accepts that the patient is hearing voices but does not recognize that the voices are real, for example, "I do not hear any voices, but I believe you when you tell me that you do."

If the patient experiences hallucinations, delusions, illusions, or ideas of reference, the nurse should interpret reality and describe the behavior being exhibited. The focus should not be the altered perceptions because this may cause the patient to become more out of control as attention is directed to the bizarre behavior. Limits and controls such as a quiet room, walking with the patient, talking about the present, and focusing on concrete aspects of reality should be provided. Medication can be used to reduce anxiety if other measures do not bring relief. However, medication is for the patient's anxiety, not the staff's.

When the patient experiences ideas of reference, the basis for the feelings should be explored. Then the reality of the situation should be explained with clear, concrete statements. The nurse should look for stimuli that may be causing increased stress and explore these possibilities with the patient. When reality is too threatening, fantasy can provide a comfortable retreat. The patient's need for the fantasy may be accepted without supporting the context of it. For example, the statement, "Do you feel like you want to escape this situation?" focuses on the basis for the feelings, not the context of the fantasy.

Since fear can be experienced during episodes of altered perception, calm, simple, verbal reassurance is often needed. Touch should be used only if the patient is able to accept it.

Behaviors that evidence that reality is beginning to have increased meaning for the patient are the initiation of questions about how the nurse sees a situation, sharing feelings about the present reality, and accepting others' definitions of what present reality is. As the reality orientation progresses, the person learns how to dismiss hallucinations or decrease the use of fantasy when coping with stress.

Increase of recognition and verbalization of feelings

Recognition is cognitive awareness of a feeling, and verbalization is the identification of the feeling. A patient will experience increased recognition of feelings by watching the nurse model appropriate emotions and hearing the nurse identify and describe them. Verbalization takes place when the patient says, "I am angry," or "I feel sad." Often patients learn these skills individually. Recognition of feelings can be increased through consistent feedback.

The way that the patient's behavior affects others and is responded to by others should be discussed. The manner in which the patient's inappropriate behaviors alienate others should be identified in a nonthreatening way. Often friends and family members can be taught to give the patient feedback about their feelings regarding the patient and the patient's behavior.

The patient should be assisted in verbally identifying what is being experienced emotionally. The feelings should be discussed no matter how illogical they seem. Any expression of feelings, even negative feelings, should be given positive reinforcement. New ways to express feelings can be explored with the patient. For example, vigorous games such as handball or punching a bag could be used to express anger. Other alternatives include shouting in a seclusion room, singing, swearing, word confrontations, tearing up telephone books, and throwing sponges or bean bags. Exaggeration in such expressions can be expected as the individual practices these new behaviors.

The patient's behaviors should be described and discussed, and the feelings should be reflected, in a way that conveys understanding that such discussions are as difficult as developing new behavior patterns.

When the patient's statements contain irrational or nonsequential thoughts, the nurse should tell the patient which statements are confusing and seek clarification of their meaning.

Behavioral evidence of progress toward the achievement of recognition and verbalization of feelings includes the patient's ability to label feelings experienced. The individual will also begin to recognize and label feelings of others. Other behaviors indicative of progress include the use of nonverbal expressions that coincide with the verbalized feelings, identification of ambivalent feelings, and labeling of the ambivalent feelings.

Increase of reality testing or validation

Gradually the patient will spend more time in reality, eventually dismissing the alternate reality. This occurs as the person's ability to cope with the stress of everyday life improves. Decisions about the patient's welfare and activities that once had to be made by the nurse can now be made conjointly. The patient begins to use the nurse as a "ruler" to measure parts of reality.

It is a normal, everyday coping skill to test reality and validate what is perceived. Often a person who is going to lie in a hammock will test it first to see whether it is tightly hung. The individual sees the hammock hanging, yet tests that perception by feeling it and putting partial weight in it before climbing in. This is a simple example of reality testing. A young man who was just learning to test reality again after dismissing his alternate reality was pacing up and down the halls in a slow, pondering fashion. He stopped in front of a nurse and asked, "My pants are blue, my shirt is light blue, right?" She answered, "Yes." He then checked his perceptions of what had recently been happening to him.

The patient should be encouraged to share such thoughts and perceptions. The patient should also be encouraged to make more and more decisions. It is important at this point that whatever the consequences of an action are, the patient should have to deal with them. Gradually the patient should make more difficult or stressful decisions. An example was a young woman who had a tendency to change her mind a dozen times before doing anything. This was an indirect expression of her ambivalence, which repeatedly increased her anxiety when she had to make a decision. The anxiety then caused her to withdraw after reaching her decision. The nurse, wanting to help the patient express her ambivalence more openly, began discussing her decision-making patterns when there was no decision to be made. The nurse and patient set up a contract that the patient had one chance to make a choice and that she would have to stick by it. It was understood that if the patient did not believe she could make an immediate decision and stick to it, she would ask the nurse for some time within which to make it. At first, as a result of her anxiety from previous decisions, the patient would ask for 2 hours, which the nurse gave. Then the nurse began to shorten the time or to include a special bonus of some favorite reinforcement if the decision were made earlier than the time limit. This continued until the woman was asking for only 15 minutes in which to make the decision.

There were times when the patient would regress and change her mind. At this point the nurse would make her abide by her first decision, which at times was costly. One of her decisions involved whether to go to a picnic. The whole patient population was invited to a picnic, and this patient's first response was "I don't want to go." Later she changed her mind. However, the contract had been made to abide by her first decision, so the patient and the nurse were the only ones left behind when everyone else went to the picnic. The patient did get angry at the nurse but later agreed she was really angry with herself for her original decision.

Although this patient learned that one has alternatives, she also learned that one must deal with the consequences of a decision. After this incident she was able to reach decisions much more quickly with far less agonizing. The nurse helped the patient understand that reality has both limits and rewards. The patient found this out by testing reality.

As the patient is able to make more and more independent decisions, the nurse-patient relationship should gradually decrease in intensity. A summary of the progress of the nurse-patient relationship should assist in validating the reality of the relationship. Mutual feelings should be expressed to validate their existence and to demonstrate that this behavior is socially appropriate.

The individual should be encouraged to think about going home and to plan how to handle this change. The first change that must be faced is leaving the hospital. Often patients need the assistance of a transitional group or therapy forum during their move back into society. Examples of such assistance include a day hospital, family or marital therapy, recreation or work therapy, and vocational or rehabilitation counseling.

Behaviors that evidence the patient is validating reality include the ability to define reality in the present, cessation of bizarre behavior, increasingly seeking the company of others, and maintaining socially appropriate responses to the context of conversation.

CONCEPT OUTLINE

I. *Conceptual definition:* Bizarre behavior is a pattern of behavior that, although meaningful to the person exhibiting the behavior, does not have a recognizable meaning to persons observing it.

II. *Antecedent conditions*
   - A. Interpersonal factors
     1. Lack of learning opportunity
        - a. Parental rejection
        - b. Parental overprotection
        - c. Parental overindulgence
        - d. Absence of role models
     2. Inconsistent feedback
        - a. Conflicting communication
        - b. Inconsistent rewards
   - B. Biochemical factors
     1. Change in neurotransmitters
     2. Change in amount and interaction of neurotransmitters
     3. Disturbance in neuronal metabolism

III. *Behavioral definition*
   - A. Objective data
     1. Altered perceptions
        - a. Illusions
        - b. Hallucinations
        - c. Change in body image
     2. Altered thought processes
        - a. Concentration
        - b. Attention span
        - c. Memory
        - d. Judgment
        - e. Speed of thinking
        - f. Content of thought
     3. Altered emotional expression
        - a. Flat affect
        - b. Inappropriate affect
   - B. Subjective data
     1. Altered perceptions
     2. Altered thought processes
     3. Altered emotional expression

IV. *Intervening variables*
   - A. Present developmental stage
   - B. Stimúli
   - C. Motivation
   - D. Family support

V. *Nursing interventions—goals*
   - A. Maintenance of physical safety
     1. Removal of potentially harmful objects
     2. Control of amount of stimulation in environment
     3. Monitoring of patient and assistance with basic physical needs

B. Development of trust
   1. Exploration of meaning of patient's statements
      a. Speaking directly to patient
      b. Use of simple, concrete language
   2. Identification of themes in behavior
      a. Recording of sequence of events and patient's responses
   3. Establishment of predictable times to meet with patient
   4. Fulfillment of commitments
C. Increase of meaning of reality
   1. Sharing of observations regarding verbal and nonverbal interactions of patient
   2. Provision of nonjudgmental feedback
   3. Modeling of acceptable emotions and responses
   4. Conversation about concrete realities, no status given to hallucinations, and acceptance of patient in present state of experiencing hallucinations
   5. Interpretation of reality, no focus on altered perceptions, provision of limits, and use of medications if other measures do not reduce anxiety for patient experiencing delusions and illusions
   6. Exploration of basis for feelings, explanation of reality in clear, concete statements, identification of stress in the situation, and acceptance of patient's possible need for escape from reality for patient experiencing ideas of reference
   7. Provision of calm, simple verbal reassurance
   8. Use of touch when patient is able to accept it
D. Increase of recognition and verbalization of feelings
   1. Provision of consistent feedback
   2. Identification of how patient's behavior is affecting others
   3. Friends and family taught to give feedback
   4. Patient helped to identify feelings
   5. Positive reinforcement for expression of feelings
   6. Exploration of new ways to express feelings
   7. Clarification of confused statements sought
E. Increase of reality testing or validation
   1. Availability of "ruler" to help patient validate reality
   2. Patient encouraged to make decisions
   3. Patient exposed to consequences of decisions
   4. Validation of progress in patient-nurse relationship
   5. Patient helped to plan for return home
      a. Assistance in joining transitional groups

VI. *Evaluation criteria*
   A. Absence of injury
   B. Increased attention span
   C. Orientation to time, place, and person
   D. Increased responsiveness to questions
   E. Initiation of conversation by patient
   F. Patient's questions about reality
   G. Acceptance of others' definition of reality
   H. Decreased use of fantasy, illusions, and hallucinations
   I. Ability to label feelings
   J. Use of nonverbal expression that coincides with verbal communication
   K. Increased reality testing
   L. Use of appropriate responses in conversations
   M. Use of alternative methods of expression
   N. Increased socialization
   O. Cessation of bizarre behavior

REFERENCES

1. Antelman, S. M., and Caggiula, A. R.: Norepinephrine-dopamine interactions and behavior, Science **195**:646, 1977.
2. Baldessarini, R. J.: Biogenic amines and behavior, Annu. Rev. Med. **23**:343, 1972.
3. Ban, T. A.: Recent advances in the biology of schizophrenia, Springfield, Ill., 1973, Charles C Thomas, Publisher.
4. Bateson, G., Jackson, D. D., Haley, J., and Weakland, J.: Toward a theory of schizophrenia, Behav. Sci. **1**:251, 1956.
5. Bijou, S. W.: Reinforcement history and socialization. In Hoppe, R. A., Milton, G. A., and Simmel, E. C., editors: Early experiences and the processes of socialization, New York, 1970, Academic Press, Inc.
6. Biller, H. B.: Father absence and the personality development of the male child, Developmental Psychology **2**:181, 1970.
7. Brodsky, L.: A biochemical survey of schizo-

phrenia. Can. Psychiatr. Assoc. J. **15**:375, 1970.
8. Broen, W. E., Jr.: Schizophrenia: research and theory, New York, 1968, Academic Press, Inc.
9. Caplan, G.: Principles of preventative psychiatry, New York, 1964, Basic Books, Inc., Publishers.
10. Clausen, J. A.: Family structure, socialization, and personality. In Hoffman, L., and Hoffman, M., editors: Review of child development research, vol. 2, New York, 1966, Russel Sage Foundation.
11. Coleman, J. C.: Abnormal psychology and modern life, ed. 5, Glenview, Ill., 1976, Scott Foresman & Co.
12. Cooper, J. R., Bloom, F. E., and Roth, R. H.: The biochemical basis of neuropharmacology, ed. 3, New York, 1978, Oxford University Press, Inc.
13. Cortes, C. F., and Fleming, E. S.: The effect of father absence on the adjustment of culturally disadvantaged boys, J. Special Education **2**:413, 1968.
14. Crow, T. J., Johnstone, E. C., Deakin, J. F. W., and Longden, A.: Dopamine and schizophrenia, Lancet **2**:563, 1976.
15. Deur, J. L., and Parke, R. D.: Effects of inconsistent punishment on aggression in children, Developmental Psychology **2**:403, 1970.
16. Einstein, G., and Moss, M. S.: Some thoughts on sibling relationships, Social Casework **48**:549, 1967.
17. Feinsilver, D.: Communication in families of schizophrenic patients, Arch. Gen. Psychiatry **22**:143, 1970.
18. Fenz, W. D., and Velner, J.: Physiological concomitants of behavioral indexes in schizophrenia, J. Abnorm. Psychol. **76**:27, 1970.
19. Ferguson, L. R.: Dependency motivation in socialization. In Hoppe, R. A., Milton, G. A., and Simmel, E. C., editors: Early experiences and the processes of socialization, New York, 1970, Academic Press, Inc.
20. Gardner, E. D.: Fundamentals of neurology: a psychophysiological approach, ed. 6, Philadelphia, 1975, W. B. Saunders Co.
21. Grace, H. K., Layton, J., and Camilleri, D.: Mental health nursing: a socio-psychological approach, Dubuque, Iowa, 1977, Wm. C. Brown Co.
22. Gruzelier, J. H., Lykken, D. T., and Venables, P. H.: Schizophrenia and arousal revisited, Arch. Gen. Psychiatry **26**:427, 1972.
23. Haber, J., Leach, A., Schudy, S., and Sideleau, B.: Comprehensive psychiatric nursing, New York, 1978, McGraw-Hill Book Co.
24. Heath, R. G., Gruschwan, A. F., and Coffey, J. W.: Relation of taraxein to schizophrenia, Dis. Nerv. Syst. **31**:391, 1970.
25. Heath, R. G., Krupp, I. M., Byers, L. M., and Liljekvist, J. I.: Schizophrenia as an immunological disorder, Arch. Gen. Psychiatry **6**:1, 1967.
26. Himwich, H. E.: Study backs biochemical etiology in schizophrenia, Psychiatric News **5**:5, 1970.
27. Hoppe, R. A., Milton, G. A., and Simmel, E. C., editors: Early experiences and processes of socialization, New York, 1970, Academic Press, Inc.
28. Kantor, R. E., and Herron, W. G.: Reactive and process schizophrenia, Palo Alto, Calif., 1966, Science & Behavior Books, Inc.
29. Kety, S. S.: Current biochemical approaches to schizophrenia, N. Engl. J. Med. **276**:325, 1967.
30. Kneisl, C., and Ames, S. A.: Mental health concepts in medical surgical nursing: a workbook, ed. 2, St. Louis, 1979, The C. V. Mosby Co.
31. Lidz, T., Cornelison, A., Terry, D., and Fleck, S.: Intrafamilial environment of the schizophrenic patient. VI. The transmission of irrationality, Arch. Neur. Psychiatr. **79**:305, 1958.
32. Lu, Y. C.: Contradictory parental expectations in schizophrenia, Psychiatry **19**:231, 1956.
33. Mandell, A. J., Segal, D. S., Kuczenski, R. T., and Knapp, S.: The search for the schizococcus, Psychol. Today **6**:68, 1972.
34. Meissner, W. W.: Sibling relations in the schizophrenic family, Family Process **9**:1, 1970.
35. Millon, T., and Millon, R.: Abnormal behavior and personality, Philadelphia, 1974, W. B. Saunders Co.
36. Parke, R. D.: The role of punishment in the socialization process. In Hoppe, R. A., Milton, G. A., and Simmel, E. C., editors: Early experiences and the processes of socialization, New York, 1970, Academic Press, Inc.
37. Peterson, D. R., Becker, W. L., Hellmer, L. A., Shoemaker, D. J., and Quay, H. C.: Parental attitudes and child adjustment, Child Dev. **30**:119, 1959.

38. Sankar, D. V., editor: Schizophrenia: current concepts and research, Hicksville, N. Y., 1969, PJD Publications Ltd.
39. Simon, A., Herbert, C. C., and Straus, R., editors: The physiology of emotions, report, Springfield, Ill., 1961, Charles C Thomas, Publisher.
40. Singer, M. T., and Wynne, L. C.: Thought disorder and family relations of schizophrenics, Arch. Gen. Psychiatry **12**:187, 1965.
41. Snyder, S. H.: The dopamine hypothesis of schizophrenia: focus on dopamine receptor, Am. J. Psychiatry **133**:197, 1976.
42. Swensen, C. H., Jr.: Introduction to interpersonal relations, Glenview, Ill., 1973, Scott Foresman & Co.

CAROL A. WATSON

NANCY N. WYATT

Chapter 8

ALTERED LEVELS OF AWARENESS

I've entered
a world
with nothing to keep,
I'm
lost in wakefulness
robbed of sleep.

Time
a phantom
I never see,
Darkness
a fear
that wrestles me.

Trapped—
I run
with nowhere to go,
Events—
tugboats
with my feelings in tow.

My body
betrays me
My thoughts
fly away—
"Oh, please,
nurse . . . stay."

I'm in a place
where even you seem unreal
and things that aren't me
are all I can feel.

PAULETTE R. Di ANGI

CONCEPTUAL DEFINITION

Consciousness, broadly defined, is the awareness of oneself and one's environment. This involves the availability of stimuli, both interoceptive and exteroceptive; the reception of those stimuli; and the perception of their meaning and significance. Interference with any aspect of this process results in an altered level of awareness.[15,16]

An optimal range of internal and external stimulation is necessary for the maintenance of normal levels of awareness. If stimuli fall below the optimal level, an individual will seek alternative stimuli in an attempt to restore equilibrium. Sensory stimuli greater than levels normally tolerated precipitate attempts by the individual to decrease the amount of input by physically and/or psychologically retreating from the situation.[16]

Literally thousands of bits and pieces of information from sensory end organs are transmitted continually by the peripheral and autonomic nervous systems through the spinal cord to the higher brain centers. The spinal cord not only segregates incoming sensory information into tracks that go to the appropriate sites in the brain, but also regulates and maintains reflex activity.

The next level of integration occurs in the brain stem. It regulates many of the body's vital functions and contains the reticular formation, a diffuse network of neurons extending throughout its boundaries. The reticular formation activates, prepares, and alerts the rest of the brain for the reception of incoming sensory information.

The highest level of control occurs in the cerebral cortex, which processes incoming sensory information in such a way that appropriate responses occur. More than 99% of all sensory information received is discarded by the brain as unimportant and therefore requiring no action. For this reason one is able to wear clothing, for example, and not be continually distracted by its friction against the body.[6]

For an individual to maintain awareness, sensory stimuli must be available within a certain range of intensity. In addition, the individual must be able to receive, sort, integrate, and interpret this information. If alterations occur anywhere along this chain from available sensory material to the cerebral cortex, the individual's level of awareness will be altered.

ANTECEDENT CONDITIONS

Alterations in the sensory-perceptual environment, body chemistry, and neurophysiological processes are the three major causes, or antecedents, of altered levels of awareness.

Altered sensory-perceptual environment

The sensory-perceptual environment may be altered by restriction or overload. Sensory stimuli received through exteroceptive olfactory, auditory, gustatory, tactile, and visual channels must be maintained within an optimal range and be varied and meaningful in order for a normal state of awareness to be maintained. Sensory-perceptual restriction results from a diminished amount, variety or pattern of sensory input.[5,16,21] Restrictions can be induced in clinical situations when patients are placed in isolation, traction, or full body casts or when burn patients are encased in heavy dressings.[3,7,8,17] In addition, sensory overload can so markedly increase the amount or intensity of input that normal discrimination is lost. This often occurs in intensive care units, where lights are on for 24 hours a day, complex monitoring equipment is attached to the patient, and sleep patterns are disrupted.[9,14,22] However, the optimal range of sensory input appears to be different for each individual; what may appear to be a normal sensory environment may actually be overloaded or restricted.[16,19]

Altered body chemistry

The second major antecedent is altered body chemistry. The body's chemistry must be maintained in a specific range for neurons to function normally. Acid-base imbalance, fluid or electrolyte imbalance, changes in availability of nutrients, and pharmacological agents all can alter the body's chemistry and affect neuronal activity.

A lowering of the body's pH decreases neuronal transmissions, whereas a rise in pH results in hyperexcitability. Although many electrolytes influence the activity of the neuron, the most important electrolytes are potassium, sodium, and calcium. Elevated levels of sodium and potassium result in increased excitability of the neuron, and decreased concentrations result in diminished excitability. Increased calcium levels result in decreased neuronal irritability, and lowered calcium levels lead to neuronal hyperexcitability.[20]

Neurons must also receive a constant, ready supply of oxygen, glucose, and thiamine to maintain normal function. Although the brain accounts for only 2% of body weight, it consumes 20% of the body's oxygen supply. The nervous system cannot store oxygen and therefore functions ineffectively in anaerobic metabolism. The brain's circulatory system contains only 7 cc of oxygen at any one time, which is adequate for only 10 seconds of functioning. If the blood supply is totally cut off for only 5 seconds, consciousness is lost; and after 3 to 4 minutes of oxygen deprivation irreversible neuronal cell death takes place. Adequate cerebral circulation requires that systolic blood pressure of at least 70 mm Hg be maintained.[6]

Since the neuron can use only glucose as a source of energy and is unable to store it, an adequate supply is mandatory for the maintenance of neuronal functioning. The brain uses approximately 400 calories/day. In addition, although insulin is not needed to transport glucose across the brain cell membrane, thiamine must be present for glucose to be used.[6]

The exact action of pharmaceutical agents such as central nervous system depressants and stimulants on the nervous system is still unknown. It is theorized that they act in one of three ways: (1) by affecting some step in the production or action of neurohumoral transmitters, (2) by interfering with neuronal metabolism, or (3) by altering the rate of ion pumping.[13]

Central nervous system drugs affect the nervous system either by general depression, selective depression, or general stimulation. In addition, the effect of depressants and stimulants is additive to the state of the individual. For example, a general depressant would exert greater depressant effects in an individual who is psychologically depressed than would be expected in a nondepressed individual.[13]

General depressants exert their action by depressing the functioning of all central nervous system neurons. This group of drugs includes general anesthetic agents (e.g., nitrous oxide, halothane, thiopental [Pentothal] sodium), alcohol, and sedative-hypnotic drugs. When general depressants are used over an extended period, inducing a chronic state of depression, the sudden withdrawal of the medication will precipitate a prolonged state of hyperexcitability. However, hyperexcitability usually does not occur if the drug has been used for only a short time.[13]

Drugs that selectively depress specific areas of the central nervous system include antipsychotics (e.g., chlorpromazine hydrochloride [Thorazine], trifluoperazine [Stelazine], thioridazine hydrochloride [Mellaril]), anticonvulsants (e.g., primidone [Mysoline], diphenylhydantoin [Dilantin]), anti-Parkinson's agents (e.g., trihexyphenidyl [Artane], benztropine mesylate [Cogentin]), and analgesics and analgesic-antipyretics (e.g., narcotics, aspirin, acetaminophen [Tylenol]). These drugs are selective in that they might decrease the response to painful stimuli or reduce the body's thermal response, for example, but would not alter other avenues of neural response such as wakefulness.[13]

General stimulants of the central nervous system act by nonselective stimulation of all excitable neural tissue. Central nervous system stimulants are classified as either antidepressants (e.g., imipramine hydrochloride [Tofranil], amitriptyline hydrochloride [Elavil]), analeptics (e.g., strychnine), or hallucinogens (e.g., LSD, peyote, marijuana, hashish). Acute, excessive stimulation by these drugs is always followed by neuronal depression when the drug is suddenly withdrawn. This is due to neuronal fatigue as a result of exhaustion of neuronal metabolites and neurotransmitters.[13]

Altered neurophysiological processes

The third antecedent of altered levels of awareness is changed neurophysiological processes. Such alterations occur as the result of a neuropathological condition that is either peripheral, in the spinal cord, or in the brain. Peripheral lesions interfere with the reception of sensory stimuli by causing nerves to become either more or less sensitive to stimuli. Peripheral lesions are caused by conditions such as polyneuritis, diabetic neuropathy, and neuralgia. Lesions in the spinal cord affect reflex activity as well as the transmission of stimuli to the brain. Neuropathological conditions of the spinal cord include tumors, trauma, and demyelinating diseases. Lesions in the brain interfere with the processing of incoming information and the interpretation of its meaning. If disruption occurs in the brain stem and involves the reticular formation, the individual will become less responsive as the reticular formation becomes more involved. Neuropathological conditions of the brain include tumors, cerebrovascular accidents, infections, trauma, and congenital disorders.[6]

BEHAVIORAL DEFINITION

Objective data

Behaviors that substantiate an alteration in an individual's level of awareness cannot be observed in isolation but need to be related to each other, to the sensory and social environment, and to past behavior patterns.

Six general categories of objective behavior indicate alterations in awareness. First are behaviors demonstrating alterations in thought processes. As the individual's ability to test reality decreases, signs of impaired memory and judgment or perceptual distortions such as hallucinations, delusions, and illusions may be exhibited.[23] Associative looseness may also be exhibited, with varying loss of orientation to time, place, and person. Usually, alteration in awareness of time and sequencing of events is demonstrated initially, with subsequent disorientation to place and person as the individual's level of awareness decreases.[4,11] As the person's control and ability to test reality diminish, the individual may also become hypersuggestible, very willing to comply with the suggestions of others. This may become so extreme that side comments are interpreted as directives. For example, a comment from one staff member to another to "go jump out a window" might be perceived as a directive, and the patient may try to do just that—jump out a window.

The second behavior category involves changes in the individual's attention span, usually manifested as increased distractibility, inability to concentrate, or inability to follow the flow and meaning of a conversation.[4,11]

Lability in emotional expression comprises the third category. The individual may display extremes in feelings, ranging from euphoria to rage to fear. Rapid mood changes may occur. The patient may express ambivalent feelings as conflicting and vacillating emotions make it difficult to communicate feelings and make decisions. Conversely, emotional detachment and uninvolvement with associated flattened affect may be exhibited.

Behaviors primarily associated with depressed or confused states of consciousness, precipitated by disturbances in neurophysiological processes or body chemistry, often are accompanied by changes in vital signs. The disturbances usually indicate increased intracranial pressure or brain stem involvement. Increased intracranial pressure is characterized by a decrease in both pulse and respiratory rates and by a widening pulse pressure as the systolic pressure increases and the diastolic pressure remains unchanged or drops. Complaints of headache and nausea with episodes of projectile vomiting may accompany these pressure changes. Alterations in the brain stem may be manifested by hyperthermia or hypothermia.[6]

Changes in neuromuscular or neurosensory functioning may precipitate asymmetrical, uncoordinated, restless, or involuntary musculoskeletal activity. Involuntary movements may range from mild tremors to generalized seizures. Changes in body tone such as paralysis, muscular weakness, flaccidity, rigidity, or spasticity may be exhibited in all muscles or only in specific muscle groups. Loss of smooth muscle sphincter control may be manifested as fecal or urinary incontinence or both. The particular changes in body movement patterns and tone provide clues regarding the type and location of the antecedent condition.[6] Alteration in third cranial nerve functioning may be reflected by enlargement of pupillary size and decreased reactivity. An early indication of brain stem involvement is enlargement of one pupil and sluggish reaction of that pupil to light. As brain stem alterations increase, both pupils become fixed and dilated.[6]

The sixth category useful in the validation of changing states of consciousness involves changes in the individual's reaction to incoming stimuli. Persons may respond to stimuli in a nonpurposeful manner as the neuropathological condition advances. For example, painful stimuli may elicit no response or an exaggerated response. Deep tendon reflexes may become hyperreflexic or hyporeflexic. Speech disorders such as dysphasia and aphasia may also accompany these changes.[6]

Subjective data

In addition to these objective manifestations, a number of subjective findings may be present. Feelings of loss of control may be communicated by the individual experiencing altered levels of awareness. This behavior may originate in the individual's perceptual distortions, loss of orientation, and difficulty in distinguishing the real from the unreal.[16] Understandably, loss of control precipitates expressions of fear and helplessness.

The individual may also report changes in the meaning and significance of what is being observed and experienced. Commonly this involves an increased sense of personal significance with concurrent feelings of profound personal insight and truth. The person may express a sense of rejuvenation. New feelings of hope and rebirth or hyperacuteness may be related by the individual. These magnified perceptions can result in such disturbances as hallucinations, illusions, and delusions.[16,23]

Ineffability may also occur as the individual finds it difficult to describe the nature and essence of what is being experienced. The patient may express frustration regarding unsuccessful attempts to explain perceptions and experiences.

Expressions of altered body image are usually associated with depersonalization and the dissolution of boundaries. Body parts may feel weightless, disconnected, or unusually heavy. Neuropathological conditions with problems of blurred vision and musculoskeletal dysfunction may compound this type of body image distortion. Changes in perception of tactile stimuli may range from hyperesthesia to anesthesia.

INTERVENING VARIABLES

Extraneous conditions in any situation and individual characteristics influence the susceptibility of an individual to an altered level of awareness. These factors modify the effect of the antecedents, so all individuals do not react the same way to an antecedent's impingement.

An individual is better able to adapt to or cope with any impingement if other aspects of function are not also being stressed. Therefore the person who is physically and mentally healthy, well rested, and well nourished can withstand changes in stimulation levels much better than someone who is physically or mentally ill, fatigued, or malnourished.[19,21]

Anxiety level has a direct effect on awareness level. Elevated anxiety narrows one's focus, diminishing the amount and variety of stimuli to which the individual can respond. This can protect a person from sensory overload, or it can so restrict perception that reality orientation is decreased.

The developmental level of the individual affects how well alterations in sensory input are handled. The younger the individual, the more dependent on others for stimuli and the more reliant on external stimulation. Young children also have shorter attention spans and lose interest more rapidly than adults. On the other end of the age scale, the older individual's ability to respond to change or to adapt to or interpret environmental impingements such as temperature, noise, and activity level diminishes. This increases the potential of sensory restriction or overload.[9,19]

The environment to which one is accustomed has significant influence on the amount and variety of stimuli an individual can handle. Individuals used to a quiet environment may not be able to withstand increased amounts or changes in patterns of stimuli such as those encountered in a hospital setting. Conversely, individuals accustomed to an environment with high levels of stimuli or varied stimuli patterns have a greater risk of experiencing perceptual restrictions in a quiet, less varied environment such as that often found with isolation procedures used to control infections.[5,17]

Another major intervening variable that affects level of awareness is motivation. The demand characteristics of a situation affect how one is able to tolerate extremes of sensory input. Demand characteristics are the individual's expectations of the purpose or requirements of a situation. For example, an individual who is studying for a final examination the next day will be able to maintain long periods of intense concentration better than someone who is told to study the reasons for the Civil War for 5 hours just because that would be useful information. One's mental set in given situations can also influence reaction to a possible altered level of awareness. For example, an unwilling individual cannot be hypnotized.[16]

Another intervening variable is cultural expectations and beliefs. These play a major role in behavior because individuals tend to act in accordance with the expectations of their cultural group. Some cultures encourage strong, stoic behavior no matter what the situation, whereas other cultures allow and expect demonstrative behavior. These cultural factors determine to a great extent the behavior exhibited by an individual who is subjected to changes in sensory input or other antecedents of altered levels of awareness.

The rate of physiological change experienced also affects the awareness level. For example, a quick rise in intracranial pressure, which allows little time for adaptation, will produce rapid and possibly dramatic behavior changes. However, a gradual increase in pressure such as that brought about by some slowly growing tumors allows for adaptation to that pressure. In these instances changes in behavior or loss of function may occur so gradually that they go unnoticed.

An eighth intervening variable that must be used to assess the degree of alteration in the level of awareness is the individual's usual past pattern of behavior. Past personality, cognitive ability, and level of awareness must be used as a base line in the assessment of the degree of alteration.

NURSING INTERVENTIONS—GOALS AND EVALUATION CRITERIA

The general goal of nursing intervention is to support or increase the individual's level of awareness. This broad goal can be attained through the achievement of the following five specific goals: (1) fulfillment of basic needs, (2) maintenance of safety, (3) maintenance or restoration of sensory-perceptual functioning, (4) maintenance or restoration of identity control, and (5) maintenance or restoration of neurophysiological functioning.

Fulfillment of basic needs

A priority nursing care goal in dealing with altered levels of awareness is fulfillment of the individual's basic needs. Maintenance of a patent airway is of primary concern for a person with an altered state of consciousness. Individuals with severe neurophysiological disturbance caused by brain stem damage may require facilitation of respiration via a tracheostomy tube, administration of oxygen, mechanical ventilation, or suctioning. In situations of loss of consciousness the individual's head should be positioned so that secretions will not be aspirated and the tongue will not fall back and occlude the airway.[4]

Nutritional, fluid, and electrolyte status may necessitate parenteral fluid administration or nasogastric gavage. If intracranial pressure is increasing, fluid intake may need to be restricted.[4]

The nurse may need to restructure the environment or reduce environmental stimuli to help the individual rest adequately. This is particularly critical because fatigue contributes to increased disturbances in awareness.

As the patient's level of awareness decreases, the nurse will need to implement measures to maintain the individual's personal hygiene. Frequent eye, mouth, and skin care should be initiated. In addition, the secondary problems of immobilization (hypoxia, renal calculi, skin ischemia, pulmonary congestion, venous stasis, and contractures) must be prevented. (See Chapter 5.) Turning, deep breathing, and exercise regimens must be established. If the person is nonresponsive, these activities should be passively performed at least every 2 hours.[1,4]

The criteria used to evaluate intervention effectiveness relate specifically to the basic need being addressed. Effectiveness is usually indicated by balanced ingestion and excretion, decreased restlessness, and decreased levels of inflammation, edema, ischemia, and hypoxia.

Maintenance of safety

In addition to the safety aspects involved in meeting basic needs such as adequate oxygenation, other areas of safety must be monitored. Sharp objects, objects with temperature extremes, and objects that could be tripped on or stumbled over should be removed from the environment of persons with impaired judgment, muscle weakness, or decreased coordination. Safety maintenance may also include the use of side rails on beds or the application of restraints.[12] However, restraints should be used judiciously because they may add to the individual's confusion. Seizure precautions may be required for a person who has central nervous system pathology. Such precautions include elevated, padded side rails on the bed, nearby suction equipment, and an available airway. If side rails are used, the person's safety can be maintained without physical restraint in the event of a seizure. This is particularly important because the muscle movements during a seizure can be so strenuous that restraint of the movement could cause bone fractures.[4]

The evaluative criteria of effective intervention in this area relate to the absence of injury.

Maintenance or restoration of sensory-perceptual functioning

When attempting to restore or maintain sensory-perceptual functioning, the nurse can play a major role in increasing the meaning of environmental stimuli. An individual experiencing changes in level of consciousness requires structure in the environment. Structure can be provided by simple and concrete directions and explanations. The nurse can provide this type of clarification by interpreting such stimuli as sights, sounds, and smells in the patient's hospital surroundings. In addition, hospital routines, policies, and procedures should be explained. In some circumstances structuring requires limitation of the amount and type of sensory input the patient receives. All communication must be presented in such a manner that the person can comprehend and respond.

Reality orientation by frequent reorientation to person, place and time may also be necessary for the individual who experiences perceptual distortions. The nurse should take every opportunity to explain to the patient what is being done and why it is being done.[12,18]

When providing sensory input, the nurse should encourage the use of all the individual's senses. If the person has limited or absent function of one or more senses, the nurse can facilitate use of intact sensory mechanisms. Judicious use of television, radio, calendars, telephone, mobiles, wall decorations, newspapers, magazines, and books can provide meaningful sensory input. Verbal interactions as well as use of touch and eye contact are additional ways of providing meaningful auditory, tactile, and visual stimuli.[19]

Care must be taken to maintain meaning for the various stimulus patterns employed. This entails clarification of misperceived objects and events. The nurse can avoid entering the patient's perceptual distortions by helping the person to focus on concrete realities in the immediate environment. The nurse should explore with the person environmental factors that may be contributing to impaired perception. When reality becomes threatening for the individual, fantasy may provide a comfortable retreat that alleviates heightened anxiety. Although the patient's need for fantasy is accepted, its substance should not be reinforced.[10,17]

In dealing with perceptual distortions and associative looseness, the nurse needs to encourage description of both perceptions and related feelings by the patient. This intervention can include reflection of the person's feelings and the sharing of observations pertaining to the patient's behavior in a nonthreatening, nonjudgmental manner. The nurse must communicate understanding of the individual's difficulty in coping and encourage the patient to develop acceptable, alternative means of expression.[2] Family members often need help in learning how to respond to unusual behavior. The nurse's interaction with the patient can provide a role model for the family. A meaningful social contact with family members can facilitate the patient's taking an active role in interacting with significant others.

Behaviors that can be used to evaluate achievement of this goal of maintenance or restoration of sensory-perceptual functioning include the person's increased ability to test reality, with associated absence of such perceptual distortions as hallucinations and delusions; initial orientation to person, with subsequent orientation to place and time; demonstration of an intact and realistic body image; stabilization of emotional expression; increased attention span; active involvement of sensory mechanisms; and realistic perceptions of sensory input.

Maintenance or restoration of identity control

Maintenance or restoration of identity control comprises the fourth goal. All the previously mentioned nursing interventions can be instrumental in achieving this goal. Perhaps most important are the activities intended to enhance the individual's sensory-perceptual functioning. The patient with changes in awareness needs meaningful patterning of sensory stimuli. In this realm, social contact with significant others may be crucial. The nurse can play an instrumental role in facilitating the individual's use of sensory mechanisms by providing meaningful tactile, auditory, and visual stimuli.

The nurse can assist the individual who is threatened with loss of identity control by structuring and clarifying the environment. Provision of established routines and orientation to time, place, person, objectives, and events assist the individuals in maintaining an understanding of who and where they are. When exploring an individual's feelings, the nurse must convey acceptance of those feelings, regardless of how illogical they may appear. However, acceptance of feelings does not include their reinforcement. Anticipation of needs, with their subsequent fulfillment, will also communicate the nurse's acceptance of the patient as a person.

Behaviors used as criteria of this goal's achievement are (1) reorientation to time, place, person, objects, and events in the environment, (2) increased ability to use sensory systems, (3) increased ability to respond appropriately to the environment, (4) lowered anxiety levels, (5) expression of feelings related to changes in awareness state, and (6) increased decision-making capabilities.

Maintenance or restoration of neurophysiological functioning

Another area of nursing concern is the maintenance and restoration of the person's neurophysiological function. Most of the interventions in this classification are dependent insofar as they evolve from a medical therapeutic regimen. These nursing activities relate to correction or neutralization of the person's underlying neuropathological disorder. Hence the specific nature of the intervention depends on the type and extent of central nervous system pathology.

Correct administration of central nervous system medications falls in this category of nursing activities. In addition to knowledge related to the action and the therapeutic and side effects of these medications, the nurse needs to be aware of the specific influence the drugs have on awareness. It is also important to know which drug interactions, created by the combination of medications the patient receives, will affect the central nervous system.

Specific behavioral criteria of the effectiveness of this intervention are (1) restored optic nerve function as evidenced by a brisk and equal constriction of pupils in response to light, (2) return of the gag reflex, (3) restoration of symmetrical, coordinated, and purposeful body movements, (4) alleviation of headache, nausea, and vomiting, (5) absence of such body tone dysfunctions as muscular weakness, flaccidity, paralysis, and muscular rigidity, (6) return of past personality patterns.

CONCEPT OUTLINE

I. *Conceptual definition:* An altered level of awareness is a physical state in which mental functioning is impaired and normal responses to stimuli are decreased, increased, or absent.

II. *Antecedent conditions*
   A. Altered sensory-perceptual environment
      1. Sensory-perceptual restriction
      2. Sensory-perceptual overload
   B. Altered body chemistry
      1. Acid-base imbalance
      2. Fluid or electrolyte imbalance
      3. Hypoxia
      4. Glucose inadequacy
      5. Thiamine deficiency
      6. Use of drugs (depressants and stimulants)
   C. Altered neurophysiological processes
      1. Peripheral neuropathological condition
      2. Spinal cord pathological condition
      3. Cerebral and brain stem pathological condition

III. *Behavioral definition*
   A. Objective data
      1. Altered thought processes
      2. Decreased attention span
      3. Emotional lability
      4. Changes in vital signs
      5. Changes in neuromuscular or neurosensory functioning
      6. Changes in reactions to incoming stimuli
   B. Subjective data
      1. Feelings of loss of control
      2. Perceptual disturbances
      3. Increased sense of personal significance or insight
      4. Ineffability
      5. Altered body image

IV. *Intervening variables*
   A. Physical and mental health
   B. Anxiety
   C. Developmental level
   D. Environment
   E. Personal motivation
   F. Cultural expectations
   G. Rate of physiological change
   H. Past patterns of behavior

V. *Nursing interventions—goals*
   A. Fulfillment of basic needs
      1. Ensurance of patent airway
      2. Maintenance of nutritional balance
      3. Support of sleep patterns
      4. Provision of personal hygiene
      5. Maintenance of mobility
   B. Maintenance of safety
      1. Provision of safe environment
      2. Use of protective restraints
      3. Use of seizure precautions
   C. Maintenance or restoration of sensory-perceptual functioning
      1. Increase of meaningful stimuli
      2. Clarification of environment
      3. Facilitation of use of all sensory mechanisms
      4. Patient encouraged to verbalize perceptions and feelings
      5. Facilitation of active involvement
   D. Maintenance or restoration of identity control
      1. Enhancement of sensory-perceptual functioning
      2. Provision of environmental structure and clarity
      3. Patient encouraged to verbalize feelings
      4. Communication of acceptance of person
   E. Maintenance or restoration of neurophysiological functioning
      1. Support of medical regimen

VI. *Evaluation criteria*
   A. Balanced ingestion and excretion
   B. Decreased restlessness
   C. Decreased inflammation, edema, ischemia, and hypoxia
   D. Absence of injury
   E. Orientation to person, place, and time
   F. Increased testing of reality
   G. Decreased perceptual distortion
   H. Realistic body image
   I. Increased ability to use sensory systems
   J. Appropriate responses to environment
   K. Lowered anxiety
   L. Increased verbalization of feelings
   M. Increased decision-making ability
   N. Pupils equal and reactive to light
   O. Return of gag reflex
   P. Symmetrical, coordinated, and purposeful body movements
   Q. Alleviation of headache, nausea, and vomiting
   R. Absence of body tone dysfunction
   S. Return of past personality patterns

REFERENCES

1. Adams, N.: Prolonged coma: your care makes all the difference, Nurs. '77 **7**:20, 1977.
2. Burgess, A. C., and Lazare, A.: Psychiatric nursing in the hospital and the community, Englewood Cliffs, N.J., 1973, Prentice-Hall, Inc.
3. Campbell, E.: Nursing problems associated with prolonged recovery following trauma, Nurs. Clin. North Am. **5**:551, 1970.
4. Carini, E., and Owens, G.: Neurological and neuro-surgical nursing, ed. 6, St. Louis, 1974, The C. V. Mosby Co.
5. Chodil, J., and Williams, B.: The concept of sensory deprivation, Nurs. Clin. North Am. **5**:453, 1970.
6. Chusid, J. G.: Correlative neuroanatomy and functional neurology, ed. 16, Los Altos, Calif., 1976, Lange Medical Publications.
7. Downs, F.: Bedrest and sensory disturbances, Am. J. Nurs. **74**:434, 1974.
8. Eaton, P., and Heller, F.: Therapeutic care of orthopedic patients, Nurs. Clin. North Am. **2**:429, 1967.
9. Falk. S. A., and Woods, N. F.: Hospital noise: levels and potential health hazards, N. Engl. J. Med. **289**:774, 1973.
10. Gaarder, K., and Chase, C.: Control of states of consciousness. I. Attainment through control of psychophysiological variables, Arch. Gen. Psychiatry **25**:429, 1971.
11. Gardner, M. A. M.: Responsiveness as a measure of consciousness, Am. J. Nurs. **68**:1034, 1968.
12. Gerdes, L.: The confused or delerious patient, Am. J. Nurs. **68**:1228, 1968.
13. Goodman, L. S., and Gilman, A., editors: The pharmacological basis of therapeutics, ed. 5, New York, 1975, Macmillan Publishing Co., Inc.
14. Lipowski, Z. J.: Sensory and informational inputs overload: behavioral effects, Compr. Psychiatry **16**:199, 1975.
15. Ludwig, A. M.: Altered states of consciousness, Arch. Gen. Psychiatry **15**:225, 1966.
16. Ludwig, A. M.: Altered states of consciousness. In Tart, C. T., editor: Altered states of consciousness, New York, 1972, Doubleday & Co.
17. Meinhart, N., and Aspinall, M. J.: Nursing interventions in hypovigilance, Am. J. Nurs. **69**:994, 1969.
18. Morris, M., and Rhodes, M.: Guidelines for the care of confused patients, Am. J. Nurs. **72**:1630, 1972.
19. Myers, T.: Tolerance for sensory and perceptual deprivation. In Zubek, J., editor: Sensory deprivation: 15 years of research, New York, 1969, Appleton-Century-Crofts.
20. Rose, B. D.: Clinical physiology of acid-base and electrolyte disorders, New York, 1977, McGraw-Hill Book Co.
21. Solomon, P., and Rossi, A. M.: Sensory deprivation. In Howells, J. G., editor: Modern perspectives in world psychiatry, New York, 1971, Bruner Mazel Publishers.
22. Taylor, D. E. M.: Problems of patients in an intensive care unit: the aetiology and prevention of the intensive care syndrome, Int. J. Nurs. Stud. **8**:47, 1971.
23. Zuckerman, M.: Hallucinations, reported sensations and images. In Zubek, J., editor: Sensory deprivation: 15 years of research, New York, 1969, Appleton-Century-Crofts.

JOANN M. ELAND

Chapter 9

PAIN

a knot
which
has no
strings
with
which
to untie
it.

PAULETTE R. Di ANGI

CONCEPTUAL DEFINITION

Pain is a personal, private sensation of hurt that protects the body by signaling the presence of current or impending tissue damage.[59] It is individually experienced and often difficult to describe.

In 1965 Melzack and Wall[49] proposed what is now the most commonly accepted theory of the pain mechanism, the gate control theory. The model of this theory is exhibited in Fig. 3. According to this theory the body's interpretation of and response to painful stimuli are influenced by many neurological processes. A number of sites receive neurological messages about pain sensations. One is the substantia gelatinosa, which is located in the dorsal horn of the spinal cord. Two others, the cerebrum and thalamus, are part of what Melzack and Wall refer to as the central control processes.

Neuronal fibers have been classified into three groups, A, B, and C, according to size, action potential, and conduction rate. However, only A and C fibers transmit pain impulses. Class A fibers are large, myelinated, fast-conducting fibers with four subclasses: alpha, beta, gamma, and delta. The pain transmission of only alpha and delta fibers has been identified. The class A alpha fibers are cutaneous afferent

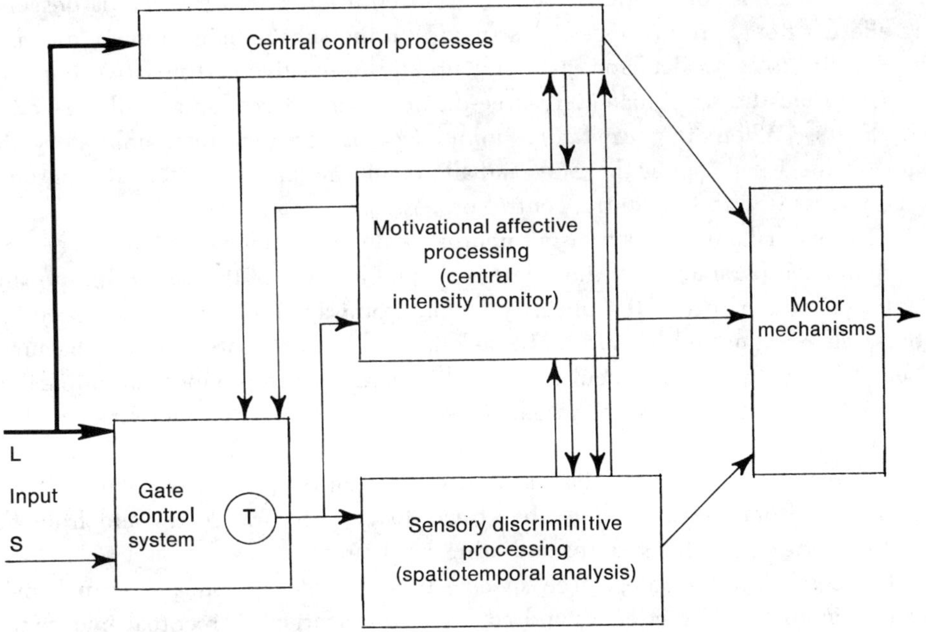

FIG. 3. Conceptual model of the sensory, motivational, and central control determinants of pain. (From Melzack, R., and Casey, K. L.: Sensory motivational and central control determinants of pain: a new conceptual mode. In Kenshalo, D., editor: The skin senses, Springfield, Ill., 1968, Charles C Thomas, Publisher.)

fibers. According to the gate theory these large-diameter inhibitory fibers modify and inhibit pain transmission in the substantia gelatinosa.[16]

Excitatory neurological messages of injury are carried to the substantia gelatinosa by A delta and C fibers. C fibers are small, nonmyelinated, slow-conducting fibers. Melzack and Wall[49] refer to them as small-diameter excitatory fibers. Class A delta fibers are usually associated with the first pain sensation at the site of an injury, whereas class C fibers usually convey dull, generalized sensations of pain.*

A specialized system of large-diameter A alpha fibers directly alerts central control processes to injury before information is processed in the substantia gelatinosa. Melzack and Wall[49] suggest that the medial lemniscus of the dorsal column and dorsal lateral systems are probably the specific large-diameter fiber tracts that trigger the early involvement of these central control processes. The special set of large fibers carries information about the nature and location of the stimuli and activates selective portions of central control, including memory of past experiences and response strategies.[46]

All other large and small A and C fibers terminate in the substantia gelatinosa. The substantia gelatinosa consists of seven layers, or laminae, in which pain impulses from small-diameter excitatory fibers (+) and large-diameter inhibitory fibers (−) and any inhibitory impulses (−) transmitted from central control via descending efferent fibers are processed. A structure in the substantia gelatinosa known as the T cell acts as a calculator that sums up all the positive and negative impulses received from the small-diameter, large-diameter, and descending inhibitory efferent fibers. When the excitatory input (+) is greater than inhibitory input (−), the T cell "opens the gate" and allows information about the pain sensation to be transmitted to the central control processes.

Neospinothalamic fibers transmit neurological information regarding the sensory discrimination parameters of time, intensity, and location of the pain from the substantia gelatinosa to the thalamus. A second pathway, the paramedial ascending fibers, also begins in the substantia gelatinosa and terminates in the thalamus. These fibers activate the reticular and limbic structures to produce the unpleasant affective quality of pain. This system is often referred to as the motivational-affective system.

The thalamus is a major relay station of the central nervous system. It relays information from the ascending fiber tracts to the cerebral cortex and from the cerebral cortex to motor systems and other brain areas.

The cerebrum evaluates three specific types of information: perceptual information, motivational tendency, and cognitive information. Perceptual information includes the sensory areas of location, magnitude, time, and place, whereas motivational tendency may be described as the tendency to escape or attack. Cognitive

---

*See references 7, 16, 21, 49, and 72.

information includes past experiences and various response alternatives. These three types of information interact and influence motor mechanisms, initiating the complex patterns of overt behavioral responses characteristic of pain.[46]

In summary, central control powerfully influences the mechanism of pain at three specific levels: (1) selective inhibition in the substantia gelatinosa before information is processed by the T cell, (2) selective inhibition in the substantia gelatinosa after the "gate" has been opened, and (3) influence of motor mechanisms or other brain areas to alter or stop pain.

The following two examples illustrate the operation of the gate control system. If an individual accidently closes a drawer on a finger, sustaining minor injury, the small-diameter excitatory fibers send a perceptual message of neurological damage to the T cell in the substantia gelatinosa. Common behavioral reactions to such injury include shaking the hand or grabbing the finger. These activities stimulate the large-diameter inhibitory fibers that terminate in the substantia gelatinosa. Simultaneously the special set of rapidly conducting large fibers transmits the information of injury to central control. Central control directs the eyes to look at the finger and recalls previous painful episodes. If little tissue damage is seen, central control mediates the neurological input of the small fibers by sending inhibitory messages to the T cell via descending fiber tracts. The T cell sums up the input from both the excitatory and inhibitory fibers, including central control's inhibitory fiber input. In this instance the gate, which is operated by the T cell, would most probably remain closed, and the pain would subside with no further behavioral response.

If, however, a nail was torn off and a deep laceration was sustained when the finger was slammed in the drawer, the individual's reaction would be different. The small-diameter fibers would conduct many excitatory messages at a rapid rate to the T cell. Initially, the person might grab the finger or shake it, stimulating the large-diameter fibers. When the individual looked at the finger and saw the blood and the hanging fingernail, central control would probably not send inhibitory messages to the T cell. In this instance the excitatory input would outweigh inhibitory input when summed by the T cell, and the gate would open, transmitting information about the time, intensity, and location of the pain to central control via the neospinothalamic tracts. Messages that would activate the unpleasant affective aspect of pain would be sent by the paramedial ascending fiber tracts.

Central control would collect and evaluate the data about the pain it received from the special large fibers, the sensory discriminatory messages brought by the neospinothalamic tracts, the unpleasant affective quality of pain that originated when reticular and limbic structures received impulses via the paramedial ascending fibers, and information stored in the memory about past experiences and response alternatives. After evaluating all the data, central control would activate motor mechanisms to decrease or eliminate pain. In this particular instance the motor mechanisms might include bandaging the wound, visiting a physician for suturing, taking analgesics, and elevating the hand.

A more detailed discussion of the physiological and psychological mechanisms involved in the gate control can be found in Melzack's book, *The Puzzle of Pain*.[46]

It is thought that with chronic pain the input from the large-diameter fibers to the substantia gelatinosa is minimized or even eliminated, leaving the gate permanently "open." Any time the chronic pain stimulus occurs, the pain messages transmitted to the gate are referred to the central control processes because there are no inhibitory messages to prevent the gate from opening. In addition, the central control processes of the person with chronic pain provide painful memories of the suffering and relief failures experienced over an extended period. The dormancy of the large fibers plus the central control's painful memories will maximize the pain's intensity.[46] Unfortunately, persons suffering chronic pain do not become accustomed to the sensation of pain. Indeed, they may suffer more with the passing of time as physiological and mental depletions occur.[5]

Pain threshold and tolerance

Two of the most frequently misused and misunderstood words that refer to pain are threshold and tolerance. Pain threshold refers to the intensity of a noxious stimulus that is necessary for a person to perceive pain.[56] More simply stated, the pain threshold is the point at which warmth begins to burn or touch begins to hurt. Research[8,22-25,61] has found that most people's pain thresholds are similar. Tolerance refers to the duration or the intensity of a stimulus above the pain threshold that a person can experience before making verbal or other overt responses to the pain.[59]

One device used to measure pain threshold and tolerance looks like a pair of pliers with a manometer attached. The "pliers" are applied to the fingernail of a research subject, and the subject is asked to tell the investigator (1) when the pinching begins to hurt (threshold) and (2) when the pain can no longer be endured (tolerance). The point at which subjects indicate the sensation is beginning to hurt (threshold) is similar, but the point at which each individual subject requests the investigator to stop (tolerance) varies.

In experimental laboratories it has not been overly difficult to measure pain tolerance and threshold.* Some researchers have also attempted to produce laboratory experiences similar to clinical pain.[58,60] However, many problems are encountered when attempts are made to measure threshold or tolerance in a clinical setting. The reason for this difficulty is that central control receives and processes three types of information about pain from three sources:

1. *Perceptual information:* brought by neospinothalamic tracts.

---

*See references 45, 51, 53, 61, and 67.

2. *Motivational tendency:* brought about by the paramedial ascending fiber tracts activating reticular and limbic structures to produce unpleasantness.
3. *Cognitive information:* stored in central control.

Since all three areas contribute to the experience of pain, the physiological parameters of threshold and tolerance have limited clinical predictive value unless motivational tendency and cognitive information are also measured. A person's tolerance to pain is altered by changes in motivational tendencies as well as by changes in cognitive information about the pain experience.

Since pain is such a individualistic and subjective experience, there are two possible explanations for behavior indicating a person is experiencing a degree of pain greater than usual for a given situation. Pain is a protective signaling mechanism. An inordinate amount of pain may be an indication of the presence of an unidentified pathological condition such as masked infection, hemorrhage, or embolus. The second explanation relates to the protective function of pain tolerance. Since the pain response is influenced by the person's perceptions of the meaning of the pain, exaggerated behavior may indicate that the pain experience is very stressful to the individual.

ANTECEDENT CONDITIONS

One of the questions about pain that remains unanswered is how a specific stimulus causes the sensation of pain. There is general agreement that chemical irritation of small fibers will result in pain. However, there is no agreement about why pressure, electrical insult, and thermal changes cause pain. One hypothesis is that these stimuli injure cells, thereby releasing irritating chemicals such as histamine, prostaglandins, and bradykinin.

Wall[65] has divided antecedent conditions that cause pain by the release or production of irritating chemicals into three categories: (1) pain of the initial injury, (2) pain of delayed onset, and (3) pain as a result of secondary effects of tissue damage.

Pain of initial injury

Pain associated with initial injury is triggered by such stimuli as pressure, temperature, electrical current, and partial nerve transection, which initate the firing of A delta fibers.

When stimuli such as electrical current, thermal change, and pressure are gradually increased, the neurological response sequence of the small and large fibers appears to be similar. Initially, the large fibers are stimulated, but as the intensity of the stimuli increases, the small fibers begin to fire. When the intensity of the small fiber firing is greater than that of the large fibers, pain is experienced. For example, most people agree that massage and vibration are pleasant sensations, but when such pressure sensations increase in intensity, they become painful. Although thermal stimuli over a wide range are perceived to be uncomfortable, most persons agree that temperatures greater than 45° C and less than 0° C are pain producing. The specific manner by which these stimuli precipitate cell injury is explained in the discussion of inflammation (Chapter 10).

Pain of delayed onset

Pain of delayed onset can be affected by the processes of sensitization, inflammation, and complete transection and partial destruction of nerves.

Sensitization is a process that alters the pain threshold of the tissue. The specific physiological changes that occur in this phenomenon have not been identified. Sensitization frequently occurs after tissue denudation of injury that exposes nerve endings. After sensitization a small, innocuous stimulus that would usually not produce pain does produce pain. For example, pouring warm water over the knee usually does not cause pain; yet, if the knee has been scraped, this stimulus is painful.

When inflammation occurs, cells are injured, and this process is accompanied by vasodilation, swelling, and pain. The mechanism that generates pain in an inflamed area is thought to be a combination of sensitization, pressure, temperature changes, and chemical release from the cells. The direct pressure on the irritated nerve endings may further irritate the fiber, and this pressure also increases the release of chemicals from the injured cells. Vasodilation and the resultant elevated temperature increases the rate of the chemical changes.

When nerves are completely severed, as in the case of amputation, the frequent result is a delayed development of severe pain. This pain is commonly referred to as phantom pain. The patient has a sensation of severe pain, which seems to arise from and be located in the amputated part. It is thought that this painful condition is due to severed large fibers, neuroma formation on small fibers, abnormal sympathetic activity, and, to some extent, emotional responses.

Partial destruction of a nerve, as in diabetic neuropathy, alcoholic neuropathy, or herpes zoster, can also affect delayed pain. Again the exact mechanism is unknown, but in all three diseases there is thought to be a selective destruction of large fibers. In the case of diabetic neuropathy the large fiber destruction appears to be followed by small fiber destruction.

Pain as result of secondary effects of tissue damage

Pain of either peripheral or visceral origin can cause muscle spasms. For example, when a bone is fractured, muscle contractures and spasms are an immediate response of the surrounding muscle. When a kidney stone becomes lodged in a ureter, the surrounding viscera contracts around the stone. Although the mechanisms that precipitate these reflex muscle contractures have not been identified, it does appear that the stimulus of pain precipitates the contractions. Also, the more intense the pain, the more severe the contractions. When the muscles' metabolic demands exceed the vascular supply, anaerobic metabolism occurs. The resultant buildup of lactic acid in the tissue causes further pain. Such secondary effects of initial tissue damage cause further irritation to the small-diameter fibers.

Autonomic reflexes can also precipitate pain sensations as secondary effects of tissue damage. An example of such a reflex is the condition of causalgia. Causalgia is a severe burning pain, characteristically associated with bullet injuries that have quickly and violently partially severed nerves. The affected part usually appears cold and discolored and often drips with sweat. Temperature changes, light pressure, and vibrations from loud noises can produce severe pain in the affected part. Although the specific cause of the pain is unknown, relief is frequently afforded by surgical interruption of the sympathetic innervation to the painful part.

Referred pain is a third type of pain experienced as a result of secondary effects of tissue damage. Referred pain is pain in a body part that has not sustained tissue damage. An example is the arm and shoulder pain experienced during a myocardial infarct. The tissue damage occurs in the heart, but the crushing chest pain radiates over the shoulder and down the arm.

It is thought that referred pain occurs because small fibers from several body areas converge on a single cell in the spinal cord. When severe pain impulses are transmitted to that cell, the result is the experience of pain in all the areas from which fibers converge on that single cell. In the case of cardiac pain the small fibers from the heart wall enter the spinal cord at the same location, cervical vertebra 6, as the small fibers from the arm.

Relationship of location of source to pain experience

The location, or site, at which the pain stimulus contacts the body affects the character of the pain experience. Pain experiences are influenced by the type and number of nerve tracts that innervate different tissues. The broad categories of tissue types include cutaneous, or superficial, tissue; deep somatic tissue; and deep visceral tissue.

Cutaneous pain. Cutaneous, or superficial, pain can have two distinct qualities that reflect the A delta and C fiber involvement. The A delta fibers, associated with the first pain sensation, elicit sharp, tingling, or stinging sensations. The C fibers are activated after the A delta firing and convey feelings of dull, generalized pain.

Deep somatic pain. Deep somatic pain is aching, boring, and dull and often is not as localized as cutaneous pain. The vagueness of the pain response and the patient's inability to identify the specific site of the pain reflect the fact that fewer small fibers innervate deep structures and that C fibers predominate in these tissues. Generally, the deeper the affected tissue, the more widespread and diffuse the pain sensation.

Deep visceral pain. Pain of visceral origin is poorly localized at onset. However, when it is present for a long period, it can become localized. Viscera, like deep somatic structures, are sparsely innervated. This accounts for the initial localizing difficulty. Nerve fibers that innervate viscera run parallel to the sympathetic nerves, which provides a partial explanation of the autonomic symptoms that often accompany visceral pain. Visceral pain has been characterized as vague, dull, aching, or burning, but can become sharp when visceral lumens are obstructed. When obstruction occurs, as with a renal stone in a ureter, pain is characterized as gripping, cramping, or twisting. Pain associated with obstruction is cyclical, and the patients' behavior will correlate with the changing sensations. When the pain is dull and aching, the patient is often quiet or curled up in a knee to chest position. When the pain becomes gripping or cramping, the patient becomes restless and frequently uses a rocking motion.

BEHAVIORAL DEFINITION

Objective data

Physiological responses. The initial physiological response to the experience of acute pain is activation of the body's fight or flight stress response. The blood shifts from visceral and superficial vessels to organs essential for flight (the skeletal muscles, heart, lungs, and central nervous system). Levels of circulating blood glucose and epinephrine increase, sustaining sympathetic activity.

When the pain is intense but of short duration, a brief parasympathetic response may occur as a compensatory reflex. When the pain persists, the body begins to adapt and decrease its sympathetic response. Although parasympathetic symptoms usually appear only during chronic pain or after brief episodes of intense pain, it is not unusual for such parasympathetic activity as nausea and vomiting to occur dur-

TABLE 1. Physiological parameters affected by pain*

Response	Sympathetic stimulation	Parasympathetic stimulation
Pupil size	Dilated	Constricted
Perspiration	Increased	No effect
Rate and force of heart rate	Increased	Decreased
Blood pressure	Increased	Decreased
Depth and rate of respiration	Increased	No effect
Urinary output	Decreased	No effect
Peristalsis of gastrointestinal tract	Decreased	Increased
Basal metabolic rate	Increased	No effect

*From Johnson, M.: Assessment of clinical pain. In Jacox, A., editor: Pain: a sourcebook for nurses and other health professionals, Boston, 1977, Little, Brown & Co.

ing episodes of acute pain. Table 1 identifies the physiological parameters that are most commonly affected during experiences of acute pain.[24]

Body posture and movement. Four major types of body posturing or movement accompany experiences of acute pain: protective movements, rhythmic or rubbing movements, immobilization, and restless or purposeless movements.

Pain is a protective mechanism, a signal of pending or present damage. When superficial pain occurs, the body's reflexive reaction is to move away from the pain stimuli. The hand quickly withdraws from the hot stove; the foot jumps off the tack. It takes a great conscious effort to inhibit the involuntary removal of the body from a stimulus producing pricking, burning, or extreme pressure sensations. A child may aggressively strike out, hitting or biting those perceived to be inflicting pain. Even adults may push people away, refusing help as they attempt to flee from the pain.

A person in pain may also use rhythmic movements, holding, rubbing, or massaging a part to decrease pain sensations. Such activities often stimulate large-diameter fibers, inhibiting pain. A man who hammers his thumb almost reflexively shakes his hand to lessen the pain. When the pain is very intense, the person may hold the injured part or an adjunct part very tightly until the external pressure sensation overrides the pain sensation. When deep pain is experienced, the person may rub or massage the part. The first sign that a young child has an acute ear infection is often the child's continual pulling or rubbing of the ear. Such movements provide cues to the location of the stimulus. Often children in pain, and even many adults, find the touch of another comforting. They may cling to another's body, tightly grip hands, or have the other person rub or stroke the pained part.

Body posturing and immobilization of the injured part are also used to reduce pain sensations. Such positioning often reduces the tissue movement around the painful area and decreases tension on the painful site. Examples of such posturing are the drawing of knees to the chest when experiencing abdominal cramping, bending forward when ambulating after abdominal surgery, limping on a sprained ankle, or reduced chest expansion with respirations following thoracic surgery. Splinting activity may involve the whole body. The body may be held rigid with the hands tightly clenched. The muscles of the jaw may be tightened, the eyes either widely open or tightly closed. The teeth may be tightly closed or biting on the lower lip, and a variety of facial contortions may occur.

The fourth type of movement is associated with episodes of very intense severe pain such as colic that has generated excessive energy. The movement may include frequent changes of position. These position changes are often so abrupt that the body appears as if it is being tossed from spot to spot. Trembling and rocking motions may occur, and purposeful actions may become inaccurate. Furniture may be bumped, and objects dropped or knocked over.

Vocalization. It is not uncommon for pain to elicit crying, sobbing, gasping, or screaming. Sounds such as crying may be the child's only way of communicating that pain is being experienced. Such sounds may be almost involuntary when the pain is unexpected and severe.

Subjective data

Pain is a subjective response to a noxious stimulus. Since the objective data present during pain experiences are often typical of other stress experiences or of bizarre behavior, their clinical usefulness is limited to signaling the possible existence of pain. The only way to determine the quality, intensity, extension (location), and duration of pain is through the person's description of the experience. The majority of adults are able to describe these four dimensions of pain when they are requested to and assisted in doing so. Children, however, because of their cognitive development, may find this very difficult. The lack of vocabulary to describe pain or discomfort as well as fear of health professionals and of the injections that follow complaints contribute to this difficulty. The painful experience children most commonly associate with physicians and nurses is that associated with injections. When 186 hospitalized children between the ages of 4 and 10 were asked "Of all the things that have ever hurt you, what hurt you the worst?" 49% replied an injection or needle. It is particularly interesting that in the group who answered injection or needle there were six children who each had undergone 25 or more surgical procedures.[15]

In a study conducted by Jacox and Stewart[32] adult patients were asked whether they liked discussing their pain with others. Some patients described how helpful it was to discuss their pain, but many preferred not to discuss it or gave ambivilant replies. The most frequently given reasons for not discussing pain included the belief that people were generally not interested in hearing about another's pain and the belief that complaining about pain had a negative social value.

Quality and duration of pain. The sensations of pricking and burning are characteristic of cutaneous, superficial pain, whereas a duller, aching pain is more characteristic of the pain that does not arise from surface structures.[19,41,68] Terms used to describe the quality of pain often infer a time dimension. The adjectives sticking, flashing, shooting, and stabbing describe momentary pricking sensations of varying severity. Adjectives implying longer duration are burning, aching, throbbing, boring, pressing, and crushing. However, the terms "soreness" and "tenderness" relate to pain that is accentuated by pressure or motion. Melzack and Torgerson[48] have identified a series of words that are used in describing the sensory, affective, and evaluative qualities of pain (Table 2).

These words reflect the three categories of data processed by central control: perceptual (sensory), motivational (affective), and cognitive (evaluative). The words have been ranked in subgroups according to intensity. For example, with temporal

TABLE 2. Classes and subclasses of pain descriptors as rated by patients*

Class	Descriptors
Sensory	
Temporal	Flickering
	Quivering
	Pulsing
	Thumping
	Throbbing
	Beating
	Pounding
Spatial	Jumping
	Flashing
	Spreading
	Radiating
	Shooting
Punctate pressure	Pricking
	Boring
	Drilling
	Stabbing
	Lancinating
	Penetrating
	Piercing
Incisive pressure	Sharp
	Cutting
	Lacerating
Constrictive pressure	Pinching
	Nipping
	Tight
	Squeezing
	Pressing
	Binding
	Gnawing
	Biting
	Cramping
	Gripping
	Crushing
Traction pressure	Tugging
	Pulling
	Wrenching
Thermal	Hot
	Burning
	Scalding
	Searing
Brightness	Tickling
	Tingling
	Itchy
	Smarting
	Stinging
Dullness	Dull
	Sore
	Numbing
	Hurting
Dullness	Aching
	Drawing
	Blurred
	Steady
	Heavy
Sensory miscellaneous	Tender
	Taut
	Rasping
	Splitting
	Tearing
Affective	
Tension	Nagging
	Fatiguing
	Tiring
	Exhausting
	Dragging
Autonomic	Nauseating
	Sickening
	Suffocating
	Choking
Fear	Fearful
	Frightful
	Terrifying
	Dreadful
Punishment	Racking
	Punishing
	Gruelling
	Cruel
	Vicious
	Killing
	Torturing
Affective-evaluative-sensory: miscellaneous	Grinding
	Wretched
	Awful
	Blinding
	Wicked
Evaluative	Annoying
	Bearable
	Troublesome
	Miserable
	Distracting
	Agonizing
	Ugly
	Intense
	Intolerable
	Unbearable
	Savage
	Violent

*Modified from Melzack, R., and Torgerson, W. W.: Anesthesiology 34:54-55, 1971.

pain, flickering represents the least amount of pain, and pounding represents the most intense pain.

These lists can be useful in helping patients describe their pain. The number of words chosen from an overall category can provide insight into the nature of the patient's pain as well as the intensity of that specific component.

Extension or location of pain. Body outline drawings may be useful for adult patients who have difficulty telling a nurse where their pain is located. It may be easier for patients to locate the pain on drawings because a sophisticated vocabulary is not required. In addition, patients experiencing pain in private areas such as the breast, rectum, or genitalia may find communication via body outline drawings more acceptable than verbalization. The size of the painful area and whether and where it radiates are two subdimensions of the location of pain.[37]

A series of recent studies with children has found that children are also able to identify the location of their pain using body outlines.* When children under 7 years of age are questioned about their pain, the most frequent response is silence. It is far beyond a young child's cognitive abilities to verbally relate sensory, affective, and evaluative feelings. However, when questions about the location of pain are asked in a way the child can understand, a child can locate and describe pain intensity.

Children given body outlines and crayons are able to color where they hurt on the drawings. After coloring the hurt, the child can be asked about the coloring, for example, whether a specific area hurts now or hurt earlier in the day or why the child hurts. Research has found that children can show where they hurt, identify areas of current hurts, and frequently give explanation as to why they hurt.[13,15,42,57]

A 4-year-old boy who had undergone a nephrectomy colored his incision, several venipuncture sites, his intravenous site, and a skin breakdown on his heel. When questioned about the coloring, he said that the venipucture sites hurt only when "the lab stuck you, unless they left a bump [hematoma]," that the intravenous site hurt when the needle was "put in" but after that "if you held real still it didn't hurt," that his heel hurt a little, but that his worst hurt was "where I had my surgery." The child could tell when something hurt, exactly where it hurt, and which pain was the worst.

A 4-year-old boy with an immune deficiency had been hospitalized for 2 months for treatment of an infection of the left leg extending from ankle to groin. His condition became stable, and he was allowed to go home. After 2 weeks at home he was readmitted for what was thought to be either a deep vein thrombus of the left leg or another leg infection. When he was first asked to put Xs on a body outline to show where he hurt, he placed a deep red X over the abdomen, but would not explain why. The physicians stated there were no clinical signs or symptoms to explain the child's coloring. The child was taken to the operating room 15 hours later with a small bowel obstruction. When the child was interviewed a second time, 24 hours after surgery, he colored the antecubital fossa, which was bruised from venipuncture. He also drew a line across both legs just above the knees and colored both legs below the line. He said that his arms hurt because of needles and that his left leg hurt because of the plaster splint he was required to wear at night to prevent contractures. He refused to say why he colored the right leg. Interestingly, he did not color the two intravenous sites, the incision location, which began at his sternum and ended at the symphysis pubis, or the surgical drain locations. During the third interview he colored one small area in the right groin but refused to talk about it. His right leg developed a cellulitis and began draining yellow-brown exudate 3 days after the second interview. This 4-year-old child on two separate occasions identified hurts before he had any other signs or symptoms of pathology. However, he also verbally denied pain because, no matter how intense his pain, he did not want an injection.

Intensity of pain. The neospinothalamic fibers transmit information pertaining to the time, intensity, and location of pain, and the paramedial ascending fibers transmit information regarding the unpleasantness of the sensation. There are therefore two dimensions of intensity. One dimension relates to the degree of the sensation, and the other to the distress produced by the sensation. Johnson[34,35] has developed two scales that measure the amount of sensation as well as the amount of distress, and in addition indicate how these feelings have changed with time.

Stewart[63] developed another method to assist patients in describing the intensity of pain. Five hundred adults experiencing short-term surgery, long-term pain, and pain of malignant origin were given a chromatic array of yellow-orange-red-black and asked to indicate the color that best represented their pain. The short-term surgical group consisted of patients who had undergone appendectomy, hernia repair, or cholecystectomy. Patients in this group frequently selected yellow or orange to represent their pain. People suffering from rheumatoid arthritis frequently chose red or red-violet as being representative of their long-term pain. Pain of malignant origin was represented by red, violet, or black. Unlike other measurement tools, which measure only one aspect of the pain experience, Stewart found that color includes both pain intensity and the affective component.

In 1975 I adapted Stewart's color scale for use with children. Five studies using this scale have found that children between the ages of 4 and 10 can also use color to describe pain.* The children in these studies represented a wide range of socioeconomic status; a wide variation in diagnosis, including burns, bone marrow aspiration, and a wide range of medical and surgical problems; both inpatients and outpatients; and five different geographical locations (Missouri, Washington, Ohio, Kansas, and Iowa).

In the early studies using color, children were presented with eight crayons

---

*See references 13, 15, 29, 42, and 57.

(black, brown, purple, blue, red, green, yellow, and orange) and asked to choose a color that was "like hurting." Red, black, and purple were frequently chosen by the 342 children to represent their pain.[13,15,29]

I interviewed hospitalized children between the ages of 4 and 10 on three successive days. The children's color choices changed from day to day, as did the way in which they colored the body outline. On certain days a red crayon might be chosen, with the child coloring very dark over the area of hurt. The following day the child might choose a yellow crayon and barely press the crayon to the paper. It was concluded that these changes represented both changing intensity and affective changes.[13,15]

In an attempt to learn whether day-to-day color changes reflected alterations in the nature of pain, Loebach[42] and Schroeder[57] had their subjects construct their own color scales. Each child identified which color represented the most hurt, second worst hurt, and so forth. Again, red and black were most frequently identified as representing the most hurt. Loebach[42] found that immediately after a bone marrow aspiration children would frequently choose the color they had identified as representing the most hurt. With the passage of time, the child's color choices indicated lessening amounts of hurt.

Schroeder[57] interviewed burned children on three specific occasions: (1) after a dressing change, (2) after a venipuncture, and (3) at a time not associated with procedures or stressful events such as a parent going home for the day. Colors chosen by the children changed with the situation. Dressing changes were identified by all children as representing the most pain. Second most painful was the venipuncture. During the interview that took place at a time perceived as minimally stressful, color choices varied. Some children chose the colors that represented little or no pain, whereas others still chose colors associated with pain.

Hester[28] developed a poker chip tool to help children describe pain intensity. The child uses one to four poker chips to quantitatively represent pieces of hurt.

Recently, picture projection techniques have also been used to help children express the degree of pain being experienced. Eland,[11,12] Ward,[66] and Hester[28] used line drawings of a cartoon animal in four painful situations, whereas Alyea[1] used four line drawings of a face. Children between the ages of 4 and 10 were asked to rank the pictures in order of pain. After the ranking was completed, the children were asked to identify the picture that was most similar to the way they felt. Although ordering of pictures in the various studies varied, the children were capable of ranking the pictures and identifying which one was most like their current pain.

These recently developed and tested assessment tools have considerably expanded the health professional's ability to communicate with children about pain. However, it must be stressed that repeated success of such assessment tools requires that the subsequent intervention be acceptable to the child. Injections or suppositories are frequently not acceptable interventions to children less than 7 years of age. If unacceptable interventions follow the reporting of pain via these assessment tools, it can be expected that the child will soon not cooperate with the repeated use of these tools.

Chronic pain. Verbal reports of acute pain usually correspond with the present pathological condition as well as with overt bodily responses and physiological changes. Such responses may or may not be present during chronic pain. It is possible for an individual in chronic pain to describe calmly the agonizing pain being experienced, without exhibiting the usual behaviors or physiological signs associated with pain. The verbalization and the absence of observable pain behaviors may seem contradictory. It is unlikely that an individual in chronic pain would have the characteristic rapid pulse, elevated blood pressure, rapid respiration rate, or perspiration associated with acute pain. The body simply cannot maintain the stress response over long periods.[37] In addition, overt pain behaviors over prolonged periods are not seen as appropriate. Many people with chronic pain exert considerable effort to eliminate overt pain responses to become more socially acceptable. The patient's definition of the pain experience is particularly crucial in the assessment of chronic pain because overt behavioral responses and physiological responses to pain have often been eliminated.[14]

INTERVENING VARIABLES

All the intervening variables that will be discussed have the potential of altering a person's tolerance to pain. Central control evaluates perceptual, motivational, and cognitive information and directs pain responses on the basis of that evaluative process. The meaning of pain, past experiences, future expectations, physiological alterations of pain threshold, and communication patterns can all influence the evaluation of pain and, in turn, influence pain responses.

Meaning of pain

The meaning that pain has for the individual flows from cultural, religious and social expectations, past experiences, and future expectations.

Cultural, religious, and social expectations. Culture and ethnic origin are two variables that influence pain behavior. Pregnant women in some African cultures work in the fields until it is time to give birth. With the onset of labor the husband goes to bed and may remain there for 3 or 4 days, behaving as though he were experiencing severe pain. After delivery the woman bundles the child and retuns to work. Zborowski[70,71] pioneered the systematic study of the pain responses of ethnic groups. He found that wide variations in overt pain behaviors evolve from ethnic expectations and hold consistent to second- and even third-generation immigrant groups. Zborowski[71] extensively outlined the sociocultural attributes characteristic of the following four major cultural groups: Old American, Jewish, Irish, and Italian. This work provides a general idea of how the four groups of people usually respond to pain. Any patient from a specific cultural group could, of course, have all, part, or none of the behaviors usual to the group. However, the behavior typical of the groups provides an indication of the meaning of pain in the different cultures.

A member of the Old American group is typically white, protestant, born in the United States, and with no ties to a foreign group. The Old American will attempt to give an efficient description of pain but otherwise will remain nonexpressive. Behaviors such as crying, moaning, or groaning are avoided because they will do no good. Also, the Old Americans will deny the existence of pain so that they may stay productive. To them being ill means being unable to fulfill their expected social role. When these persons are in severe pain, they usually choose to be alone.

Jewish people have been described as having a low tolerance for pain and a tendency to use dramatic adjectives such as intolerable and excruciating in describing their pain. Jewish patients are also concerned with the significance of the current pain on their future. Verbalization such as crying and moaning is acceptable part of the pain experience and is needed to alert others to assist the patient. When in severe pain, the Jewish person does not want to be alone. Families are expected to become very involved in the illness and to care for the one who is suffering.

The Italian also believes that it is natural to express pain, even if it involves crying, moaning, or complaining. Members of this group want people around during the pain episode. They use the presence of friends or involvement in work to divert the mind from the pain. However, pain is viewed in terms of the significance of the current sensation and not future implications. Therefore these patients seek immediate pain relief even if it is only temporary.

Irish and Old American patients are similar in their calm and unemotional responses to pain. Irish patients will not complain about severe pain. They will be reluctant to discuss it and may even withdraw from significant others. They do not mind admitting the suffering, but they want to suffer alone. In contrast, the Old American does not admit to suffering because this implies helplessness. Irish patients view pain in terms of future expectations and are proud of their ability to fight and endure pain. For this reason they are slow to seek medical attention.

A patient's religious beliefs also have the potential to influence the meaning of pain. Illness may be viewed as a punishment for sins or misdeeds.[69] An example is the 55-year-old woman who came to a neurosurgery clinic with complaints of tic douloureaux, a neuralgia of the second and third branches of the trigeminal nerve. She believed that God had given her the neuralgia as punishment for eating and talking too much. Initial attempts to help this woman accept treatment failed. It became apparent that the health team was going to have to work within this belief system in order to assist her in accepting the surgical intervention that would relieve her pain.

Children also view pain as punishment. This is particularly true of children in the "magic thinking" years of 4 to 7. This view can be reinforced by some parent behaviors during illness experiences. An example is the mother who threatens the child by saying, "If you don't behave, I'll have the nurse give you a shot."

In Western culture the accepted sex role behavior requires men to be stoic, brave, and silent when experiencing pain.[46] An example of a response to this expectation is a 6-year-old boy who received a skull fracture, fractured femur, multiple lacerations and contusions when struck by a car. The child was interviewed in the hospital 5 days after his injury, when his father was present. At that time the boy denied having experienced any pain since admission to the hospital. The child was again interviewed the following day, when his aunt and grandmother were in the room. When asked about pain, he broke into tears. In front of his aunt and grandmother he was able to say that he was currently experiencing pain and had been in pain on many occasions since the time of the accident.[12]

This particular child's behavior is consistent with his age group's desire to please. He attempted to emulate behaviors he thought were acceptable to his father. In his father's absence he was able to express his pain and distress in the presence of an aunt and grandmother who were accepting and sympathetic.

Past experiences. Because of central control's ability to store and recall information about prior painful experience, an individual's past experience influences current responses to pain.[47] It is possible, for instance, for a person who has had numerous hospitalizations to have established effective methods of coping with pain. In contrast, another individual who has had frequent hospitalizations may wonder how much more pain can possibly be endured. On a previous admission the pain may have been so intense and the interventions so unsuccessful that the person psychologically lost control. Anticipated pain can become an overwhelming threat to this individual.

Children in the process of developing a cognitive background on which to base interpretations of experiences do not have, as most adults have had, friends who have described pain experiences. The child who comes to an emergency room after sustaining a small laceration illustrates the difference in responses based on past interpretations. It is not at all uncommon for a physician to be able to suture a laceration with minimal complaints from a child. After quietly undergoing suturing, the child may become extremely distressed, cry, and kick when the nurse appears with an injection of tetanus toxoid. The child had not had prior experiences with suturing and did not expect that it should hurt. However, there was no doubt about injections. They had been experienced, and they hurt.

The child has limited ability to communicate pain because of developing cognitive processes and a limited vocabulary. When the stimulus is a needle, the child's perception of it is similar to the adult's, and, initially, the motivational tendencies may be similar; but the similarity between the responses of adults and children stops here. The child's central control usually has a limited amount of information from past experiences except in the area of injections. A child's past experience tells him "injections hurt," and central control's message to motor mechanisms is "escape." The body's normal response to a prickling or pressure sensation is to withdraw or pull away. When central control processes this limited amount of information, the response to injection if predictable. Children less than 6 often view an injection as punishment for misbehaving. For these children two events are related if they occur in close time proximity. If a child's action just before the injection was eating a banana, it is predictable that eating bananas will cease. The success of injection of an analgesic is further negated by the time of the onset of the medication's effect. For the child with no time concept, the alleviation of pain seems to be unrelated to the injection. An explanation to a young child at the time of injection about the necessity of an analgesic is not processed by central control with future expectations. The nurse explaining the analgesic's effects to a child may confront at least four problems: (1) the child's past experience says shots are awful, (2) injections are frequently perceived as hostile acts by the nurse, (3) the child cannot be expected to compare the pain of a surgical incision with that of an injection, and (4) the child's time concept prevents connection of the two events. Children quickly learn not to complain of pain because complaints of pain are followed by injections. The two are related because of time proximity—if you complain of pain, you get an injection; therefore do not complain, and, if necessary, deny all pain.

Difficulties in communication. Difficulties in communication can occur at any age, but they consistently occur with children. Children are developing their cognitive information base and accordingly are in the process of learning words to express the way they are feeling. Early in this process a child may complain of a headache in the knee or stomach.

Nausea, like pain, is a subjective response to a stimulus, but unlike pain, it frequently has an objective consequence—vomiting. Parents insist that even young children understand the concept of "tummyache" that leads to vomiting so that the event will take place at the appropriate location. The child, attempting to please the parents, usually learns at an early age what a "tummyache" is and responds appropriately. The child processing the events is essentially saying, "Oh, I just threw up; the way I felt just before throwing up must be a 'tummyache' (because Mom said so)." Repeated episodes of nausea and vomiting reinforce the child's learning of the sensations associated with nausea. Unfortunately, no such mechanism helps the child understand the concept of hurting.

A second difficulty encountered in learning correct labels is the character of sensations that accompany pain: sensory, affective, and, to a lesser extent in children, evaluative. Melzack and Torgerson[48] have identified 144 words that are used to describe pain of varying intensity. How difficult it must be for young children to attribute the throbbing and pounding sensations of headache and the sharp, smarting pain of a skinned knee to the same word label!

In the past it has been easier for nurses to deny the possibility of the existence of pain and to attribute pain behavior in children to emotions such as fear, anxiety, separation, high temperature, sadness, or anger. In a study of 25 children between the ages of 5 and 8 who had undergone surgery it was found that these children collectively received a total of 13 doses of nonnarcotics and 11 doses of narcotics for pain relief during their entire hospital stay.[11] These children, all hospitalized at a tertiary care center, had undergone surgical procedures such as spinal fusion, nephrectomy, traumatic amputation, atrial septal defect repair, and palatoplasty. No medication for pain relief was received by 13 of the children. There were p.r.n. orders for the administration of analgesics for 21 of the 25 children. However, the nursing staff had not identified a need for these analgesics.

A follow-up study matching adults with similar diagnoses to 18 of the above children revealed differences in analgesic use.[15] The 18 adults collectively received 372 doses of narcotic analgesics and 299 doses of nonnarcotics, making the total number of doses 671! It appeared that pain was a consideration in the care of these adult surgical patients because analgesics were administered freely. However, when the same surgical procedures were performed on children, the situation was drastically different. The pain-producing stimulus was identical for each subject pair. However, the child had limited ability to verbally communicate about and interpret pain. In addition, the child may have feared the injection that follows pain complaints.

It has been shown by 13 separate research studies in five different geographical locations that an average of 62% of over 600 hospitalized children between the ages of 4 and 10 never received any analgesics. All these children underwent procedures that are perceived to be painful for adults. In one sample of 22 burned children at a regional burn center only 2 children (9%) received analgesics during their hospital stay.[57]

The older adult, unlike the developing child, has had the cognitive ability to communicate and process painful stimuli, but because of developmental decline may no longer be capable of doing so. A 70-year-old woman with a fractured hip illustrated some of these communication difficulties. During an evening shift report Miss K. was identified as a 70-year-old woman with a fractured hip who was confused and disoriented. All four of her extremities had been restrained to prevent her from getting out of bed. When the night nurse entered her room, the patient demanded that the restraints be removed. All but the one on the arm with the intravenous administration site were removed. It was explained that the restraint would help the patient remember to keep the arm still. On examining the patient's thigh, the nurse noted frequent muscle spasms. When the patient was asked if she hurt or was having pain, she replied no to both questions. Such an inconsistent response to severe muscle spasms prompted the nurse to ask the patient how her leg felt. She replied, "Oh, it's very sore." When asked if she would like to have the soreness go away, the woman responded, "Can you do that?" The patient had received no analgesics since her injury. Intramuscular analgesics were administered at 3-hour intervals throughout the 11-to-7 shift. By morning the woman who had been identified by the evening nursing staff as being confused and incoherent and requiring restraints knew where she was, that she had fallen and broken her hip, that she was going to have surgery, and that the night nurse had "gotten rid of the soreness." Throughout her hospitalization "soreness" was the only word that she ever used to describe her pain.

Future expectations. The future meaning of pain can also alter a person's pain threshold. During the Second World War an anesthesiologist named Beecher[2] observed that only one in three severely wounded soldiers complained of enough pain to require morphine. Most of the soldiers either denied the existence of pain or had so little pain that they did not want morphine. These soldiers were not in a state of shock. For these severely wounded men the wounds that physically removed them from a life-threatening situation meant that they would not be returning to the front lines, and usually meant that they would be sent home. Beecher's explanation was validated after the war when he examined the responses to pain of a group of civilian men hospitalized with surgical wounds similar to those of the men wounded in battle. These civilians regarded major surgery as a depressing, calamitous event. In contrast to the wounded soldiers, four out of five civilian men complained of severe pain and pleaded for morphine.[2,3]

The pain associated with childbirth is usually viewed as transient, with the result well worth the effort. In contrast, pain indicative of carcinoma has a very different significance. This is particularly true in Western society, in which the word "cancer" is considered synonymous with pain and death. The meaning of pain for an individual who has a long-standing carcinoma is undoubtedly different than that for a person whose cancer has been recently diagnosed. Patients may view their pain as an inability to fill social commitments such as attending a son's wedding, or as an inability to fulfill the social role of being able to work and lead a "productive life."[10]

The loss of identity control affects an individual's response to pain. People who are hospitalized may believe that they have no control over things that are happening to them, and hospital routines and procedures may support this perspective. The fear and anxiety that accompany the feelings of loss of control over one's destiny can increase the distress associated with a pain experience.

Physiological alterations of pain threshold and tolerance

Changes in a person's concentration or attention focus may unpredictably alter an individual's pain threshold. The threshold can be lowered by traumatic denudation or injury of tissues that exposes nerve endings. Ordinarily nonnoxious stimuli may become very painful. An example is the change in the skin's response to touch after sunburn. Anesthesia, analgesia, or sedation, in contrast, can raise the threshold and tolerance by altering a person's affective response to a painful stimulus.

Alterations in level of awareness, caused by such a wide variety of physiological changes as cerebral trauma, electrolyte or fluid imbalance, hypoxia, or sleep, will also change the person's response to pain. The greater the alteration, the less capable is the individual to respond to stimuli.

When a person is fatigued, there is less energy available for coping strategies. Fatigue also decreases a person's mental ability; mental processes decelerate, and the person has difficulty focusing attention. In such instances fatigue may alter the pain threshold through misperception or misinterpretation of stimuli. However, usually fatigue has a greater impact on pain tolerance than on pain threshold.

NURSING INTERVENTIONS—GOALS AND EVALUATION CRITERIA

Nursing interventions directed at the relief of pain have two primary goals. The first goal is to alter central control's perception of the meaning of the pain. The second goal is to alter the sensory messages transmitted to the T cell. The specific subgoals that contribute to the achievement of these two goals include (1) increase of cognitive control, (2) decrease of motivational-affective distress, (3) reduction of small-diameter fiber irritation, and (4) increase of large-diameter fiber transmission.

Alteration of central control's perception of meaning of pain

Increase of cognitive control. Information is particularly important to patients who are strangers to the hospital environment and its procedures. Patients need to know what is going to happen to them, what the activities will involve, what will be expected of them, and what the nurse will be able to do to help them during difficult or painful times.

One important reason for obtaining information by the nursing history about past experiences is to provide a base line for comparison of present pain experiences. When a nurse discusses past pain experiences with a patient, the similarities or differences of the present situation can be identified. The patient can also identify which interventions have alleviated pain in the past and which have not worked. This information can be used to plan interventions for the current situation.

The following example illustrates the strength of the influence of cognitive understanding on the response to pain. During a 3-week hospitalization an 8-year-old boy experienced a wide variety of uncomfortable procedures in preparation for surgery. These experiences included venipunctures, intravenous therapy, enemas, x-ray examinations, and the insertion of a nasogastric tube, a subclavian catheter, and a sigmoidoscope. Prior to each of these experiences the nurses had explained to the child what was going to happen and how he would feel. He was cooperative with the staff during every procedure. The night before surgery he was to receive an antibiotic intravenously and an intramuscular injection, and an intravenous catheter was to be inserted. When the physician began these activities before explaining what was to be done, the child became frightened, protested, and then physically fought the physician.

Many research studies have investigated a phenomenon called the placebo effect. In one such study by Beecher,[3] 35% of the subjects reported pain relief from placebos. Placebos are inactive substances that resemble medications. The effect of placebos illustrates two dimensions of cognitive control. The first dimension relates to the influence of positive suggestions (e.g., "This pill will take away your pain") on central control processes. The second dimension of this effect relates to the power of central control over the person's evaluation of the pain being experienced.[2-4,38,55]

When a medication administration is accompanied by information to the patient regarding the action and timing of the drug and a positive suggestion that the medication will work, two dimensions of cognitive control are made available to augment the pharmaceutical action of the drug. An example of such positive information giving is the nurse who enters the patient's room with an analgesic and says, "The medication I'm going to give you is a strong analgesic called morphine. You can expect to receive some benefit in 15 to 20 minutes, and you will feel much better in 45 minutes. I will be back so the two of us can evaluate how well the medication worked." This nurse also conveyed an additional message in this communication, that the nurse cared about the patient's pain and that together they would evaluate the medication's effectiveness.

On some occasions the administration of a placebo is ordered. It may be a glucose tablet or an injection of sterile water or saline. Often such substances will effectively relieve pain when they are administered with a convincing explanation that includes (1) this new medication, which has worked very well in the past, has been ordered by the physician, (2) this medication is stronger than the previously used analgesics, (3) the medication will start working quickly, and (4) the nurse is convinced it will work for the patient.

The patient benefits from a placebo because of the positive suggestion. The patient usually wants to believe that this medication will work. The pain that has been experienced is frightening and real, and the patient will do almost anything to get rid of it. When the nurse appears with a new medication after the others have not worked and says everything the patient wants to hear, the person wants to believe it. The problem with placebos is that they have no physiological effect on pain. Only the suggestion affects the pain. If the patient finds out that a placebo is being used, the trust in the nurse-patient relationship is undermined. It is unlikely that the patient will trust the staff in the future, and the patient may become skeptical of all future treatment modalities.

When patients gain cognitive control regarding expected pain experiences and intervention modes, fear of the unknown decreases and central processes become susceptible to suggestion. The patient becomes more willing to participate in and be cooperative with needed activities that are uncomfortable. The sensations experienced may still be uncomfortable or painful, but feelings are described in sensory terms rather than affective terror terms.

When central control is able to use suggestion, the change in pain behavior occurs quickly. The relief should coincide with the suggested timetable. A reduced need for vigilance will be evidenced by the patient's reduced comments of worry and increased ability to relax, rest, and sleep.

Decrease of motivational-affective distress. Johnson[34,35] and Johnson and Rice[36] have found that persons who have received information about the type of sensation that will be experienced during a specific procedure have lower fear, anxiety, and distress levels during the procedure. Pain stimuli remain constant, but central control has altered the patient's response to pain.

Another intervention that alters both motivational and cognitive influences on central control is relaxation. Emotions such as anxiety, fear, and fatigue contribute to muscle fatigue and tension. When a patient with tissue injury such as a surgical incision experiences these feelings, a pain cycle is initiated. The incisional pain increases anxiety and fear. These emotions tense muscles, which put stress on the incision, resulting in more pain, which increases anxiety, and so forth. Several basic comfort measures promote relaxation and can help break such a cycle of pain. The nurse can suggest that the patient pretend to be a container full of water with a leak, and that slowly every drop of water is dripping out. The patient can then substitute tension for the water and let the tension run out. Other techniques include selective tightening and relaxing of specific muscle groups.[31]

Relaxation of muscles can also be facilitated by a back rub, a warm bath, clean, smooth bed sheets, and comfortable room temperature. In addition to the relaxing effects of these comfort measures, the patient receives the message that the nurse is interested and concerned.[26] This perception often decreases a patient's need for vigilance.

Patients need adequate sleep and rest to help withstand the stress of pain. In addition, the body's energy needs to be conserved for repair processes. When a patient is experiencing fatigue, any task becomes more difficult; and when energy is mobilized and focused in the motivational-affective and cognitive domain in response to pain, energy available for repair processes is reduced.[14] Night sleep is often facilitated by duplicating the patient's usual nighttime routine whether it involves brushing teeth, going to the bathroom, having a cup of coffee, or taking a warm bath. Straightening sheets, scheduling procedures during waking hours, repositioning the patient, back rubs, analgesics, hypnotics, and sedatives can be critical in ensuring a good night's rest.

Although it is not often used in acute pain situations, progressive relaxation can help individuals cope with pain. Patients who use biofeedback, yoga, or transcendental meditation in their daily life frequently find these techniques an effective means of coping with pain.*

Two important things that can be done for patients in pain are to listen to them and to stay with them. Pain is not as terrifying and all-encompassing when another person is present. The value of touch in pain relief cannot be underestimated.[26] The nurse who holds a patient's hand during a procedure that is particularly difficult or painful, who places a hand on the patient's arm during the sharing of a frightening experience, or who gives the patient a back rub to facilitate relaxation is nonverbally saying, "I care about you. The way you feel is important to me."

Analgesics, including codeine, meperidine, and morphine, affect central control's perception of pain. Patients receiving these analgesics report that pain is still present but that they are no longer bothered by it. The most probable explanation for this selective inhibition or motivational affective alteration is the opoid action in the limbic system.[20] Unfortunately, children do not find injections acceptable, regardless of their benefit. Codeine is the only analgesic that is close to being equally efficacious in oral and intramuscular form.[20]

Both nurses and patients need to understand that if pain reaches a high intensity level before the medication is administered, a therapeutic dose of a potent narcotic may not effectively relieve it.[44] A second dose of the same narcotic 3 to 4 hours later or a smaller amount administered in a shorter time may be necessary before the distress is reduced. When an initial dose is not effective, the patient should be told why the first dose did not relieve the pain before the person's central control processes become convinced that the medication is not powerful enough. When a patient waits until pain is very intense before requesting an analgesic, the very mechanics of locating the narcotic keys, drawing up the medication, and signing it out, as well as interruptions by other personnel, may delay the administration enough that the pain becomes so severe that one dose of the analgesic will not alleviate it. Patients should be told to request analgesics before the pain becomes severe.

Nurses should take the initiative to assess pain status and not just wait for patients to complain of pain. The patient's pain complaint is frequently transmitted to the nurse by a nursing assistant or an intercom message to the nursing station. The nurse should personally assess the patient's status before initiating specific interventions. Such assessments are crucial to pain management and particularly important at times such as just before meal breaks or at change of shift when less people are in the clinical area.

Nurses should also anticipate painful episodes and intervene before their onset. An example is the patient who experiences abdominal surgery. It is inevitable that

*See references 6, 17, 39, 52, and 62.

pain will occur with getting out of bed or with coughing. Before such activities, the nurse should check when the last analgesic was given. An analgesic should be received at least 45 minutes before activity initiation to allow ample time for onset of action. The nurse who does not anticipate and intervene in such situations can expect less than adequate coughing or ambulation by the patient. A child in pain can be expected to be completely uncooperative in such treatment endeavors.

The patient with an acute onset of back pain who is scheduled to go to the x-ray department for a myelogram is another example of needed anticipatory intervention. It should be anticipated that 45 to 60 minutes of lying on a hard, cold x-ray table for someone with back pain, even without the discomfort associated with a myelogram, will severely aggravate existing pain. If a preprocedure medication has not been ordered, the most potent analgesic that has been ordered for the patient should be administered at least 45 minutes before the procedure is started.

During the night patients often awaken with pain and request an analgesic. After the few minutes required to bring the analgesic to the bedside, the nurse may find the patient dozing again. It is frequently assumed that the patient was really not experiencing severe pain or the patient would not have fallen asleep. The patient, however, has likely just dozed off into a light sleep and will soon be awakened again by the pain. The nurse in this situation should awaken the patient, validate that pain is being experienced, and administer the analgesic. In addition, the patient may need a sedative or hypnotic as well as other comfort measures to increase the possibility of returning to a deep sleep. When the nurse does not administer the analgesic, such patients often reawaken in a short time with pain so intense that one dose of the analgesic may not effectively relieve it.

Nurses are often hesitant about administering narcotics to patients because of fears about addiction and drug tolerance. In acute pain experiences such as those associated with surgery the most severe pain occurs in the first 3 postoperative days. When pain has been controlled from onset, the patient's need for medication will decrease within the first 3 days and the number of pain complaints initiated by the patient will also decrease. In addition, when a patient's pain is controlled, the patient is less likely to develop complications associated with immobility.

After the third postoperative day the patient should not require narcotics for pain control on a regular basis. However, analgesics will still be required to control the pain associated with such physical exertion as ambulation, respiratory therapy, and physical therapy. Drug addiction or tolerance during such episodes of acute pain is unlikely.

Patients can also be helped to cope with both acute and chronic pain by changing the focus of central control from pain to another stimulus. The needed intensity of the competing stimulus varies with pain intensity and the patient's ability to concentrate. Marathon runners use this technique by focusing on their goal or the runner ahead of them instead of focusing on fatigue, sore muscles, and various aches and pains experienced during the race.

Patients can be helped to cope with pain by using the same technique.[54] Television programs, radios, and hospital visitors can keep central control preoccupied during what otherwise would be painful periods. Distraction can also be an effective intervention while the patient is waiting for an analgesic to take effect or during a painful procedure. A method that can be used at such times is to ask the patient to relate in as much detail as possible a pleasant day from the past. The memory of a special day and good times can help the person escape the reality of the present situation. Scrapbooks and photograph albums may help people with failing memories recall their pleasant days.

When the motivational distress of a pain episode is decreased, the patient's anxiety symptoms should reduce. Skeletal muscles should become more relaxed, attention span should increase, and diversion of the mind to topics other than the pain should be possible. Pain references in conversations should be reduced or absent. Although the pain sensation may still be present, it is described in sensory terms rather than affective terror terms.

Alteration of sensory messages transmitted to T cell gate

Reduction of small-diameter fiber irritation. Although analgesics alter central control's perception of pain, some analgesics such as aspirin and codeine and some anti-inflammatory agents such as phenylbutazone (Butazolidin) and corticosteroids also work at the level of the cell to decrease chemical irritation to the small-diameter fibers.*

Aspirin remains one the the best anti-inflammatory and analgesic agents available. Aspirin works at the level of the cell to decrease chemical irritation by reduction of tissue pressure and by suppression of the production of prostaglandins.[65] However, for effective pain management the blood level of aspirin must be maintained. This requires ingestion at regularly scheduled intervals even after the pain sensation has diminished.[20] The use of aspirin for pain management does have two disadvantages related to the influence of central control: aspirin is relatively inexpensive, and it is a readily available substance. This medication's side effects and risk level are so low that it does not require a prescription. Central control often believes that if a drug is cheap and does not require special handling, then it must not be very strong. If it is not strong, it will not work. Unfortunately, aspirin will probably not relieve the pain of a person who believes that.

Barbiturates have a recognized role in providing sleep and rest; they also have specific action sites that make them particularly useful for patients in pain. There is some evidence that barbiturates physiologically alter the transmission of input

*From Tourville, J.: Personal communication, 1977.

from the peripheral fibers to T cells.[18,30,50] Barbiturates also diminish the electrical activity in the midbrain reticular areas, which in turn alter the pain-transmitting abilities of the substantia gelatinosa. Inhibitory messages are sent from the midbrain reticular areas to the substantia gelatinosa by descending fibers from the brain.[33]

With knowledge of specific action sites of pharmacological agents that have been ordered prn, a nurse who desires to relieve severe pain and provide sleep could administer a combination of medications such as the following: (1) aspirin to decrease small-diameter fiber irritation,[65] (2) morphine to alter pain perception and to stimulate large fibers,[27] and (3) a barbiturate to interrupt transmission from peripheral fibers to the T cell and directly alter the gating mechanism itself.[18] Administration of pharmacological agents with different action sites, when combined with other nursing measures such as a back rub, maximizes the potential for pain relief. The risk of administering a narcotic, a barbiturate, and a nonnarcotic analgesic depends on each of the drugs' action sites.

Applications of heat and cold to an injury site can also assist in decreasing small-diameter fiber irritation. In an acute injury such as an ankle sprain the initial pain caused by the twisting and tearing of tissue is increased by the tissue swelling. The pressure of the edema in the injured area may cause the damaged cells to release more chemical irritants such as bradykinin. The edema also places direct pressure on the small fibers. Application of ice to the area precipitates vasoconstriction, reducing edema and thereby reducing pressure on the small fibers. In addition, cold decreases the speed at which impulses are transmitted to the spinal cord.

Heat applications precipitate vasodilation. When heat is applied approximately 72 hours after the initial injury, vasodilation facilitates removal of debris and fluid, thereby reducing pressure in the tissue.[40] Vasodilation precipitated by heat can also relieve the pain of muscle spasm or muscle tension by facilitating aerobic metabolism.

Muscle tension and external body pressure can also be relieved by repositioning of body parts to reduce tissue pressure and tissue tension areas. Topical applications such as powder or cornstarch can effectively lessen mechanical friction to the body's surface.[40]

When these nursing interventions successfully neutralize or reduce the chemical irritation of small-diameter fibers, the sensation of pain will be reduced or removed. The timing of such relief, however, is related to the time of the onset and/or peak of the chemical neutralization. A delay in onset is expected. The patient should report a reduction or absence of the sensation. Soreness and tenderness should be reduced or absent. Activity levels should increase, and mobility become more fluid. Pain posturing should be eliminated.

Increase of large-diameter fiber transmission. One of the newest unexplored areas of nursing intervention for pain relief takes the form of stimulating large fibers to increase their input to the substantia gelatinosa to override small fiber input.

Pain relief associated with massage of painful body parts or back rubs is thought to be explained by altered sensory component of pain via stimulation of large fibers in addition to altered cognitive information. Probably the best example of large fiber stimulation is when an individual strikes an elbow on an immovable hard object, hitting what is commonly referred to as the "crazy bone." The pain is sharp and frequently radiates down the forearm because of the A delta innervation of the periosteum. Some pains feel better when rubbed, and this is clearly one of those examples. The immediate action after striking the elbow is to grab it and rub the area. Rubbing or vibrating increases the action of large-diameter fibers, but the problem of such intervention is in finding large fibers and vibrating only the large fibers. The large fibers running parallel to lumbar nerves are buried beneath fat and muscle, but fibers on the elbow, wrist, and knee are superficial and are fairly easily stimulated.

It is thought that acupuncture assists in relieving pain because the needles (1) cause a change in central control's focus, (2) stimulate large fibers, and/or (3) stimulate the sympathetic nerves that supply the painful area.

Vibrating pillows and hand vibrators can effectively relieve some acute pain, but difficulty arises in locating the inhibitory fibers. When pain becomes chronic, it is thought that large fibers become inactivated by an unknown mechanism. The result is that no competing stimuli enter the substantia gelatinosa, so the gate is always open. Central control's cognitive and motivational interpretation only makes the situation worse. The use of transcutaneous nerve stimulators and implantable nerve stimulators represents a refinement in inhibitory fiber stimulation. The electrical impulses from these devices cause the inhibitory fibers to fire, in many cases with enough activity to close the gate.[64] However, because of cognitive and motivational influence on central control, these devices may not be successful. The patient's past experience with the unpleasant affective state of pain may override these inhibitory messages. Unfortunately, the study of large fiber stimulation is too new to prescribe interventions other than to suggest massage and vibration. It is not currently known with which disease entities, surgical conditions, or locations this is most effective.

When the stimulation of large fibers reaches an intensity that overrides small fiber input, the patient's activity level usually increases. Posturing becomes more relaxed. Attention is focused on other interests and activities. It even becomes possible for the patient to fall asleep. The patient often denies that the pain has been relieved. The sensation of pain is still there, and the patient may indicate that the intervention does not appear to be working. If the intervention is stopped and the pain stimulus is still present, the patient will often state that the pain is still there but subdued or covered up. When the intervention is initiated, changes in behavior should occur fairly soon. However, the patient may not be aware of changes in pain behavior until they are identified by another person.

CONCEPT OUTLINE

I. *Conceptual definition:* Pain is a personal, private sensation of hurt that protects the body by signaling the presence of current or impending tissue damage.

II. *Antecedent conditions*
- A. Release or production of irritating chemicals
  1. Pain of initial injury
     a. Pressure
     b. Temperature
     c. Electrical current
     d. Partial nerve transection
  2. Pain of delayed onset
     a. Sensitization
     b. Inflammation
     c. Complete nerve transection
     d. Partial nerve destruction
  3. Pain as result of secondary effects of tissue damage
     a. Muscle contracture or spasm
     b. Autonomic reflexes
     c. Referred pain
- B. Relationship of location of pain source to pain experience
  1. Cutaneous pain
  2. Deep somatic pain
  3. Deep visceral pain

III. *Behavioral definition*
- A. Objective data
  1. Physiological responses to acute pain
     a. Increased heart rate, respirations, and blood pressure
     b. Perspiration
     c. Increased metabolic rate
     d. Dilated pupils
     e. Increased urinary output
     f. Decreased peristalsis
  2. Body posture and movement
     a. Protective movements
     b. Rhythmic or rubbing movements
     c. Immobilization
     d. Restless or purposeless movements
  3. Vocalization
     a. Crying
     b. Sobbing
     c. Gasping
- B. Subjective data
  1. Quality and duration of pain
     a. Perceptual terms
     b. Motivational terms
     c. Evaluative terms
  2. Extension, or location, of pain
  3. Intensity of pain
     a. Degree of sensation
     b. Degree of distress
  4. Chronic pain
     a. Contradictory verbalization and objective behaviors

IV. *Intervening variables*
- A. Meaning of pain
  1. Cultural, religious, and social expectations
  2. Past experiences
  3. Difficulties in communication
  4. Future expectations
- B. Physiological alterations of pain threshold and tolerance
  1. Sensitization
  2. Altered levels of awareness
     a. Anesthesia, analgesia, and sedation
     b. Cerebral trauma
     c. Electrolyte or fluid imbalance
     d. Hypoxia
     e. Sleep
     f. Fatigue

V. *Nursing interventions—goals*
- A. Alteration of central control's perception of meaning of pain
  1. Increase of cognitive control
     a. Information distribution
     b. Placebo effect
  2. Decrease of motivational-affective distress
     a. Information distribution
     b. Relaxation
     c. Comfort measures
     d. Duplication of nighttime routines
     e. Progressive relaxation, biofeedback, and meditation
     f. Touch
     g. Listening
     h. Analgesics
- B. Alteration of sensory messages transmitted to T cell gate
  1. Reduction of small-diameter fiber irritation
     a. Analgesics
     b. Anti-inflammatory agents
     c. Barbiturates
     d. Heat and cold
     e. Positioning of body
  2. Increase of large-diameter fiber transmission
     a. Massage
     b. Rubbing

c. Acupuncture
d. Vibrators
e. Nerve stimulators

VI. *Evaluation criteria*
A. Relaxation of skeletal muscles
B. Decreased use of affective descriptors
C. Increased activity level
D. Elimination of pain postures
E. Decreased complaints of pain
F. Increased attention span
G. Focus of attention on topics other than pain
H. Reduced complaints of soreness and tenderness
I. Increased ability to rest, relax, or sleep
J. Absence of pain sensations

REFERENCES

1. Alyea, B. C.: Child pain rating after injection preparation (thesis), University of Missouri at Columbia, 1978.
2. Beecher, H. K.: Pain in men wounded in battle, Ann. Surg. **123**:96, 1946.
3. Beecher, H. K.: Measurement of subjective responses: quantitative effects of drugs, New York, 1959, Oxford University Press.
4. Billars, K. S.: You have pain? I think this will help, Am. J. Nurs. **70**:2143, 1970.
5. Bonica, J. J.: Fundamental considerations of chronic pain therapy, Postgrad. Med. **53**:81, 1973.
6. Budzynski, T. H.: Biofeedback procedures in the clinic. In Jacox, A., editor: Pain: a sourcebook for nurses and other health professionals, Boston, 1977, Little, Brown & Co.
7. Burgess, P. R.: Patterns of discharge evoked in cutaneous nerves and their significance for sensation. In Bonica, J. J., editor: Advances in neurology, vol. 4, New York, 1974, Raven Press.
8. Clark, W. C., and Mehl, L.: Thermal pain: a sensory decision theory analysis of the effect of age and sex on d′, various response criteria, and 50% pain threshold, J. Abnorm. Psychol. **78**:202, 1971.
9. Collins, L. G., and Stone, L. A.: Pain sensitivity, age, and activity level in chronic schizophrenics and in normals, Br. J. Psychiatry **112**:33, 1966.
10. Copp, L. A.: The spectrum of suffering, Am. J. Nurs. **74**:491, 1974.
11. Eland, J. M.: Children's communication of pain (thesis), The University of Iowa, 1974.
12. Eland, J. M.: Children's experience of pain: a descriptive study, Unpublished data, 1976.
13. Eland, J. M.: The experience of pain in children, paper presented at the Mid-America Sigma Theta Tau Research Conference, Kansas City, MO., Aug. 1976.
14. Eland, J. M.: Living with pain, Nurs. Outlook **26**:432, 1978.
15. Eland, J. M., and Anderson, J. E.: The experience of pain in children. In Jacox, A., editor: Pain: a sourcebook for nurses and other health professionals, Boston, 1977, Little, Brown & Co.
16. Erlanger, J., and Gasser, H. S.: The action potential in fibers of slow conduction in spinal roots and somatic nerves, Am. J. Physiol. **92**:43, 1930.
17. Fordyce, W. E.: Behavioral methods for chronic pain and illness, St. Louis, 1976, The C. V. Mosby Co.
18. French, J. D., Verzeano, M., and Magoun, W. H.: A neural basis of the anesthetic state, Arch. Neurol. Psychiatry **69**:519, 1953.
19. Gasser, H.: Pain-producing impulses in peripheral nerves, Res. Publ. Assoc. Res. Nerv. Ment. Dis. **23**:44, 1943.
20. Gebhart, G. F.: Narcotic and non-narcotic analgesics for relief of pain. In Jacox, A., editor: Pain: a sourcebook for nurses and other health professionals, Boston, 1977, Little, Brown & Co.
21. Hallin, R. G., and Torsbjork, H. E.: Activity in unmyelinated nerve fibers in man. In Bonica, J. J., editor: Advances in neurology, vol. 4, New York, 1974, Raven Press.
22. Hardy, J. D., Wolff, H. G., and Goodell, H.: Pain threshold in man, Res. Publ. Assoc. Res. Nerv. Ment. Dis. **23**:1, 1943.
23. Hardy, J. D., Wolff, H. G., and Goodell, H.: Pain sensations and reactions, Baltimore, 1952, Williams & Wilkins Co.
24. Hardy, J. D., Wolff, H. G., and Goodell, H.: Pricking pain threshold in different body areas, Proc. Soc. Exp. Biol. Med. **80**:425, 1952.
25. Haslam, D. R.: Age and the perceptions of pain, Psychonomic Sci. **15**:86, 1969.
26. Hays, J. S., and Larson, K. H.: Interacting with patients, New York, 1963, Macmillan Publishing Co., Inc.
27. Herz, A., Albus, K., Metyz, J., Schubert, P., and Teschemacher, H.: On the central sites

for the anti-nociceptive action of morphine and fentanyl, Neuropharmacology **9**:539, 1970.

28. Hester, N. K.: The preoperational child's reaction to immunization, Nurs. Res. **28**:250, 1979.
29. Hester, N., Davis, R., Hanson, S. H., and Hassanein, R. S.: The hospitalized child's subjective rating of painful experiences (unpublished manuscript), University of Kansas, 1978.
30. Hillman, P., and Wall, P. D.: Inhibitory and excitatory factors influencing the receptive fields of lamina 5 spinal cord cells, Exp. Brain Res. **9**:284, 1969.
31. Jacox, A.: Pain alleviation through intervention, DHEW, PHS Grant Number NU. 00467-3, Washington D.C., 1976.
32. Jacox, A., and Stewart, M.: Psychosocial contingencies of the pain experience, Iowa City, 1973, The University of Iowa.
33. Jaffe, J. H., and Martin, W. R.: Narcotic analgesics and antagonists. In Goodman, L. S., and Gilman, A., editors: The pharmacological basis of therapeutics, ed. 6, New York, 1979, Macmillan Publishing Co., Inc.
34. Johnson, J. E.: Effects of structuring patient's expectations on their reactions to threatening events, Nurs. Res. **21**:499, 1972.
35. Johnson, J. E.: The effect of accurate expectations about sensations on the sensory and distress components of pain, J. Pers. Soc. Psychol. **27**:261, 1973.
36. Johnson, J. E., and Rice, V. H.: Sensory and distress components of pain, Nurs. Res. **23**:203, 1974.
37. Johnson, M.: Assessment of clinical pain. In Jacox, A., editor: Pain: a sourcebook for nurses and other health professionals, Boston, 1977, Little, Brown & Co.
38. Knowles, J. B., and Lucas, C. J.: Experimental studies of the placebo response, J. Ment. Sci. **106**:231, 1960.
39. Kroger, W. S., and Fezler, W. D.: Hypnosis and behavior modification: imagery conditioning, Philadelphia, 1976, J. B. Lippincott Co.
40. Lehmann, J. F., Warren, C. G., and Scham, S. M.: Therapeutic heat and cold, Clin. Orthop. **99**:207, 1974.
41. Lewis, T.: Pain, New York, 1942, Macmillan Publishing Co., Inc.
42. Loebach, S.: The use of color to facilitate communication of pain in children (thesis), University of Washington, 1979.
43. McCaffery, M.: Nursing management of the patient with pain, Philadelphia, 1972, J. B. Lippincott Co.
44. McCaffery, M., and Hart, L.: Undertreatment of acute pain with narcotics, Am. J. Nurs. **76**:1586, 1976.
45. McCarty, D. J., Gatter, R. A., and Phelps, P.: A dolorimeter for quantification of articular tenderness, Arthritis Rheum. **8**:551, 1965.
46. Melzack, R.: The puzzle of pain, New York, 1972, Basic Books, Inc., Publishers.
47. Melzack, R., and Scott, T. H.: The effects of early experience on the response to pain, J. Comp. Physiol. Psychol. **50**:155, 1957.
48. Melzack, R., and Torgerson, W. S.: On the language of pain, Anesthesiology **34**:50, 1971.
49. Melzack, R., and Wall, P. D.: Pain mechanisms: a new theory, Science **150**:971, 1965.
50. Mendell, L. M., and Wall, P. D.: Presynaptic hyperpolorization: a role for fine afferent fibers, J. Physiol. **172**:274, 1964.
51. Mills, R. J., and Rentiew, S.: Measurement of pain threshold by thermal contact, Lancet **1**:738, 1971.
52. Putt, A.: A biofeedback service by nurses, Am. J. Nurs. **79**:88, 1979.
53. Ryan, E. D., and Kovacic, C. R.: Pain tolerance and athletic participation, Percept. Mot. Skills **22**:383, 1966.
54. Sadler, T. G., Wiedland, B. A., Mefferd, R. B., Benton, R. G., and McDaniel, C. D.: Modification in autonomically mediated physiological responses to cold pressor by cognitive activity: an extension, Psychophysiology **4**:229, 1967.
55. Schapiro, A. K.: The placebo response. In Howell, J. G., editor: Modern perspectives in world psychiatry, New York, 1971, Brunner/Mazel, Inc.
56. Schludermann, E., and Zubek, J. P.: Effect of age on pain sensitivity, Percept. Mot. Skills **14**:295, 1962.
57. Schroeder, P.: Use of Eland's color method in pain assessment of burned children (unpublished research in progress at Shriner's Burn Hospital), Cincinnati, Ohio.
58. Smith, G. M., and Beecher, H. K.: Experimental production of pain in man: sensitivity of a new method to 600 mg. of aspirin, Clin. Pharmacol. Ther. **10**:213, 1969.
59. Sternbach, R. A.: Pain: a psychological analysis, New York, 1968, Academic Press, Inc.
60. Sternbach, R. A., Murphy, R. W., Timmer-

mans, G., Greenhoot, J. H., and Akeson, W. H.: Measuring the severity of clinical pain, Adv. Neurol. **4**:281, 1974.
61. Sternbach, R. A., and Tursky, B.: Ethnic differences among housewives in psychophysical and skin potential responses to electric shock, Psychophysiology **1**:241, 1965.
62. Stewart, E.: To lessen pain: relaxation and rhythmic breathing, Am. J. Nurs. **76**:958, 1976.
63. Stewart, M. L.: Measurement of clinical pain. In Jacox, A., editor: Pain: a sourcebook for nurses and other health professionals, Boston, 1977, Little, Brown & Co.
64. Sweeney, S., Johnson, M., and Eland, J. M.: Pain associated with neurological conditions. In Jacox, A., editor: Pain: a sourcebook for nurses and other health professionals, Boston, 1977, Little, Brown & Co.
65. Wall, P. D.: Physiological mechanisms involved in the production and relief of pain. In Bonica, J. J., Procacci, P., and Pagni, C. A., editors: Recent advances on pain, pathophysiology and clinical aspects, Springfield, Ill., 1974, Charles C Thomas, Publisher.
66. Ward, B.: Externally observed pain (thesis), University of Kansas, 1975.
67. Wolff, B. B., and Jarvik, M. E.: Factor analysis of human pain responses: pain endurance as a specific pain factor, J. Abnorm. Psychol. **78**:292, 1971.
68. Wolff, H. G.: Some observations on pain, Harvey Lect. **39**:39, 1943-1944.
69. Wu, R.: Behavior and illness, Englewood Cliffs, N.J., 1973, Prentice-Hall, Inc.
70. Zborowski, M.: Cultural components in response to pain, J. Social Issues **8**:16, 1952.
71. Zborowski, M.: People in pain, San Francisco, 1969, Jossey-Bass, Inc.
72. Zotterman, Y.: Touch, pain and tickling: an electrophysiological investigation on cutaneous nerves, J. Physiol. **95**:1, 1939.

PAULA CORNETT MOBILY

CARMELA ANN REHTZ

Chapter 10

INFLAMMATION

CONCEPTUAL DEFINITION

Inflammation is a defensive response against cellular injury wherein the body attempts to restrict the injurious agent, neutralize it, and repair damaged tissue. Cellular insult, or damage, can result from a variety of causes, but regardless of the causative agent, the essential dynamics of the inflammatory reaction remain constant.

Restriction of the injurious agent

The initial reaction to cellular injury is a microvascular response. After transient vasoconstriction, which may signify the body's earliest attempt to restrict the spread of cellular injury, the arterioles, venules, and capillaries dilate, rapidly increasing the blood flow to the injured part. Concomitant with the increased circulation, permeability increases in the vascular network and surrounding tissues, resulting in exudation of fluid and cells to the site of injury. Components of the fluid and cellular exudate serve to contain the inflammatory response via three basic mechanisms: formation of a fibrin barrier, migration of white blood cells to surround the agent, and restriction of vascular and lymphatic circulation. These dynamic reactions occur in the course of the inflammatory response regardless of the causative agent. They are of obvious value when cellular damage is secondary to the chemical insult of toxins released by invading microbes. However, this restriction is also valuable in situations lacking a microbial antecedent because it restricts the possible opportunistic entry of pathogens.

Fluid exudate. Fluid exudate is formed by the interaction of two factors. Increased blood flow to the site of injury increases the hydrostatic pressure in the vessels, forcing fluid from the vessels into the involved tissue space. Permeability of the vascular membrane is also increased. Normally the endothelial cells that line the vessels are contiguous with one another. During the inflammatory response these endothelial cells separate, allowing leakage of plasma proteins into the surrounding tissues. This is thought to occur in two phases, initially from the venules, and later, in a more prolonged phase, from the capillaries.[9,29] As the plasma proteins leak into the tissue, the osmotic pressure of the tissue increases, pulling fluid from the blood to form the fluid exudate.

The protein meshwork that supports the cells of the injured area fosters the formation of fluid exudate. As the meshwork becomes more fluid, tissue tension decreases. This change allows exudate to diffuse more readily into the injured area.[29] This fluid exudate is rich in a variety of substances important to the inflammatory response. The exudate contains antibacterial substances such as antibodies and may contain medication that is circulating in the plasma. Most medications readily diffuse into interstitial fluid except in the cerebral extracellular space and cerebrospinal fluid. Thus fluid exudate will transport antibiotics to inflammatory sites in most of the body. However, only lipid-soluble antibiotics cross the blood-brain barrier.[6]

The fluid exudate also contains fibrinogen, which, when converted to fibrin by tissue thromboplastins, leads to formation of a fibrin network.[2,14,29] This network serves to restrict the injurious agent by walling off the injured area.

Cellular exudate. The inflammatory response also causes vascular changes that promote restriction of the injurious agent. As the plasma constituents of the blood exude out of the vessels, the viscosity of the circulating blood in the vessels increases, causing decreased blood flow and eventual stasis. Concurrent with this, the white blood cells marginate to the endothelial lining of the surrounding vessels and begin to adhere to this lining in a process called pavementing. The exact mechanism that causes this adherence of white blood cells to the endothelial lining is as yet unknown.[26]

After pavementation occurs, the white blood cells penetrate the membrane of the vessels, move into the fluid exudate, and mass at the site of injury. This massing of cells is known as aggregation. The focus of the inflammatory response is surrounded by white blood cells as well as a fibrin barrier, which together serve as a restricting network.

Formation of a fibrin barrier and aggregation of white blood cells are the major forces for the restriction of the agent, but another mechanism may be involved. Clot formation in the minor vessels and clotting of the extracellular and lymphatic fluid proximal to the area of injury also serve to restrict the agent to the area of injury. As the white blood cells are marginating in the blood vessels, the red blood cells stream to the middle of the vessel, where they clump together. Platelets begin to adhere to these red blood cells and to cause clot formation in the minor vessels.[20,26] A similar process occurs in the lymphatic vessels and extracellular fluid. During formation of the fluid exudate, coagulation factors are released from the vascular system into the inflammatory site. Tissue injury causes release of tissue thromboplastin, which initiates the extrinsic clotting mechanism,[29] ultimately resulting in a fibrin clot in the extracellular fluid and local lymphatic circulation.[10]

Although the dynamics of the described changes are well documented, the exact mechanisms that mediate each of these processes have not been validated in vivo. Most investigators believe that these reactions are mediated by chemical agents released from damaged tissue. The primary mediators of the hemodynamic and permeability changes are believed to be histamine, kinins, prostaglandins, lysosomal enzymes, and components of the complement system.[27,29] Histamine, kinins, and prostaglandins are either released from the injured cells or produced by a process initiated by the cellular injury.[25,29] Lysosomal enzymes are released from neutrophils that have undergone lysis at the inflammatory site. The complement system consists of 11 sequentially interacting serum proteins[23] that are activated either by cell damage or by the formation of antigen-antibody complexes.[29] Because these chemical substances are either released or activated by cell damage, the degree of hemodynamic and permeability changes is proportional to the amount of tissue destruction or cellular damage elicited by the inflammatory antecedent.

The process of white blood cell aggregation at the inflammatory site is not completely understood. It is believed to occur in response to chemical mediators that are released at the site of injury. A number of substances have been identified as possible mediators. Neutrophils are attracted to certain complement components, products of collagen destruction, substances released from fibrinogen, components of the kinin system, and substances released from certain viruses and bacteria. Monocytes and macrophages are believed to be attracted by bacterial substances, certain complement components, and substances released from neutrophils and lymphocytes. Although these and a number of other substances are possible mediators, they have yet to be definitively validated.[26]

Neutralization of the injurious agent

Neutralization of the injurious agent is a vital component of the inflammatory response and must occur before tissue repair can progress. This neutralization is brought about by the activity of the fluid and cellular exudate just described. Whereas the fluid exudate dilutes any irritants or toxins, the components of the cellular exudate are the prime factors of the neutralization process. The key to neutralization is the phagocytic process of the white blood cells, which engulf and attempt to destroy the inflammatory antecedent. This destruction is believed to be caused by a number of factors, including an acidic pH, lysosomal activity, and production of hydrogen peroxide in the phagocyte.[26,27]

Phagocytosis is carried out by the leukocytic cells in the cellular exudate. Since neutrophils are smaller, more motile, and more prevalent in the bloodstream than other leukocytes, they are the first phagocytic cells to move into an injured area. The neutrophil is capable of phagocytosing 5 to 25 bacteria before dying.[10] These cells are followed by monocytes, which are referred to as macrophages once they migrate out of the involved venules and capillaries. After 2 to 3 days macrophages outnumber neutrophils at the site of injury. This is thought to occur because they have a longer life span and are able to survive in the more acidic pH that occurs in inflammatory tissues secondary to the accumulation of lactic acid.[26] Each macrophage is capable of engulfing as many as 100 bacteria prior to death.[10]

The leukocytes involved in the initial phase of the inflammatory reaction are recruited from those currently in the bloodstream. As the inflammatory response progresses and the circulating cells are depleted, the bone marrow is activated to produce and release more leukocytes. The stimulus for this response is thought to be a globulin substance, leukocytosis-promoting factor, that is liberated from the injured cells.[10] Others factors such as protein derivatives liberated from necrotic cells and bacteria may also stimulate the production of leukocytes.[26]

When the neutrophils and macrophages are not able to neutralize the antecedent through their phagocytic activity, lymphocytic cells help promote the phagocytic action. Lymphocytes play a vital role in the body's immune response, which works in concert with the nonspecific inflammatory response to neutralize the injurious agent. The immune system has two components: a humoral and a cell-mediated response.

In the humoral immune response, lymphocytes are transformed into cells known as B lymphocytes. Through a complex series of events these cells produce immunoglobulins, or antibodies. Antibody production is stimulated by the presence of foreign substances known as antigens. The antibodies produced are specific to the antigen encountered. These antibodies attach themselves to the antigens and inactivate them by agglutination, precipitation, neutralization, or lysis.[10]

The humoral immune system is capable of both a primary and secondary antibody response. The primary response occurs after an initial contact with an antigen, and the peak titer of circulating antibodies is not achieved for approximately 2 weeks.[25,29] However, in subsequent encounters with the same antigen, the secondary response will elicit a specific and more intense antibody production within 2 to 3 days of the encounter. Production will remain at the peak level for a period of weeks and then slowly decline.[25] This rapid, intense response is attributed to immunological memory, by which cells formed during the primary response "remember" the antigen and subsequently react more rapidly to produce the antibody.

In the cell-mediated response T lymphocytes are transformed from lymphocytic stem cells. These T lymphocytes are sensitized by contact with the specific antigens that can stimulate the cell-mediated response. On subsequent contact with the antigen these T lymphocytes eliminate the antigen either by direct attack or by release of factors that recruit additional macrophages to the area. In addition, the factors released by the sensitized T lymphocytes activate these macrophages, making them highly phagocytic and microbicidal.[21,24]

Another mechanism involved in neutralization of the injurious agent is activation of the complement system. This system is activated when antigens and antibodies combine.[10] The activated complement system will then form enzymes that will cause lysis, opsonization and phagocytosis, chemotaxis of additional neutrophils and macrophages, and agglutination and neutralization of viruses.[10]

Phagocytosis is enhanced by additional factors. The fibrin barrier of the inflammatory exudate traps the inflammatory agents, allowing the phagocytes to engulf them. Elevated body temperature and the local increase in heat at the inflammatory site caused by local hyperemia enhance phagocytosis.[26] This elevation in temperature causes an increase in metabolic processes, including those of the phagocytes.

Resolution and tissue repair

The third and final component of the inflammatory response is tissue repair. Although repair begins during the initial phase of the inflammatory response, it cannot be successfully completed until all debris left in the area from cellular injury and the previous phases of the inflammatory response are cleared. As in the neutralization process of the inflammatory response, phagocytosis is the primary method used to remove debris from the tissue. The lysosomal enzyme of the neutrophil can liquify many types of biological material. However, these small cells are incapable of digesting large particulate matter,[2] and their activity decreases as the tissue pH drops.[26] Because of these neutrophil limitations, the larger macrophage is the major cell involved in the digestion of degenerate fibrin, dead cells, necrotic tissue, and other cellular debris.[29]

If the debris is too large for the macrophages, large phagocytic cells known as foreign body giant cells may be formed. These cells are capable of digesting foreign bodies such as sutures, wood, glass, and steel. The exact origin of these cells is not certain, but it has been postulated that they are formed by fusion of macrophages.[25,29]

As with the inflammatory reaction, the sequence and results of the repair process depend on the location and extent of the cellular damage. When little or no destruction of underlying tissue occurs, the fluid exudate formed during the inflammatory response is reabsorbed via vascular and lymphatic circulation. The remaining cellular exudate and debris are phagocytosed by the macrophages, allowing the tissue to return to the functioning level it had prior to injury. This healing process is called resolution.

When a high concentration of neutrophils accumulates in tissues and the process of resolution cannot keep pace with exudate production, a process known as suppuration occurs. The suppurative exudate, or pus, that is formed contains viable and nonviable polymorphonuclear neutrophils, liquified digestion products of underlying tissue, the fluid exudate of the inflammatory process, and, usually, a bacterial invader.

When suppuration occurs in solid tissue, the exudate is collected in pocketlike areas called abscesses. Increase in the amount of exudate raises the pressure against the surrounding solid tissues. When an area of tissue with less resistance is found, the exudate will break through this tissue, forming sinus tracts. This allows the exudate to exit from the abscess to the skin surface or into a body cavity.

When tissue destruction occurs, the nature of the reparative process is dependent on the regenerative capacity of the cells adjacent to the damaged tissue. Epithelial, lymphoid, and hematopoietic cells have tremendous regenerative capacity. When destruction of these cells occurs, complete functional regeneration is possible. Other cells such as those found in the glands of the body can regenerate functional cells provided the basic framework, the supporting stroma, of that tissue is intact and some portion of the original parenchymal tissue remains. Other cells such as neurons have no regenerative capacity once their cell body is destroyed. Tissue that cannot regenerate is repaired by replacement with connective tissue, with subsequent scarring. In most instances a combination of regeneration and replacement by connective tissue occurs during the repair process. The manner in which this process proceeds relates to the extent of the wound and the possibility of reapproximating the wound edges. A clean surgical incision is an example of a wound that can heal by primary union, often also referred to as primary intention. Although the incision may be deep, little tissue is lost, and the separated edges of the wound can be brought together and the edges opposed. When greater tissue destruction occurs and the wound edges widely separate, creating a large tissue defect, healing must occur by secondary union, or secondary intention. Since the wound edges cannot be brought together, regeneration of parenchymal tissue or production of connective tissue is necessary to fill the tissue defect. The extent of healing needed is what differentiates these two types of wounds; the difference in their repair is essentially quantitative, whereas the dynamics and sequence of the process are the same.

Basically there are three phases of wound healing, or repair. The first phase, often termed the "lag," or "catabolic," phase, occurs concomitantly with the initial inflammatory response. This phase, usually lasting from a few hours to several days depending on the nature of the antecedent and the extent of tissue damage, is primarily concerned with the collection of cells and nutrients needed for repair. If epidermal damage has occurred, the wound will gap in the direction of muscle tension on the wound margins. Components of fluid and cellular exudate move into this tissue defect and combine to produce two structures that enhance the repair process. Superficially the red blood cells and plasma proteins dehydrate, forming a protective crust called a scab to seal the wound. Below this surface a fibrin meshwork develops to bridge the subepithelial wound space and serve as a structural scaffold for future connective-cell activity. Epithelialization, the migration of epithelial cells across the wound, can then begin.

Epithelialization can be initiated by and extend from only epithelial tissue. Usually epithelial cells are located at the edges of the wound; however, in the skin these cells are also present in epidermal appendages (i.e., hair follicles, pilosebaceous glands, and sweat glands). If part of these appendages remains in the wound, the migration of epithelial cells can also begin from these points.

Before epithelial margination can occur, the tissue to be covered must be free of debris and the formation of underlying granulation tissue must have begun. Granulation tissue is composed of capillary buds and fibroblasts, precursors of collagen synthesis.

Migration of epithelial cells has been observed as early as 12 hours after surgery, with a single layer of cells covering a primary union within 48 hours.[5,26] Once epithelial cells seal a wound, the loss of fluids and proteins and the entry of microbes are prevented.

The second phase of healing, often called the proliferation phase, begins approximately 5 days after injury and continues until the fourteenth or fifteenth day.[5,12] During this phase three important events occur: (1) there is a rapid proliferation of granulation tissue, (2) contraction pulls the edges of the wound toward each other, and (3) collagen is synthesized, increasing the wound strength.

Granulation tissue begins filling the subepithelial area, providing an underlying support structure for re-epithelialization. Since granulation tissue is impervious to bacterial invasion, it helps protect the wound until epithelialization is completed.[29] The degree of the proliferation of granulation tissue that occurs relates to the amount of tissue loss. Therefore the greater the deficit, the longer this process occurs.

Contraction of the wound is also important in the repair of large defects. Contraction is the force that pulls the edges of the wound together by inward migration of normal tissue, thereby decreasing the wound size. This phenomenon particularly facilitates the repair of surface wounds. Although the exact mechanism of this process is not clear, it is believed to be a function of the fibroblasts of the granulation tissue.[5]

Biosynthesis of collagen is the third important event of this phase. Collagen, the wound-healing factor that binds the tissues together, is synthesized from fibroblasts in a complex process that requires adequate amounts of vitamin C, protein, and other nutrients. As the collagen is formed, the tensile strength of the wound rapidly increases. (Tensile strength is defined as the force needed to cause separation of the wound.)

Although it is agreed that tensile strength increases rapidly during this phase, there has been no consensus on the exact amount of tensile strength recovered. Estimates range from 10% to 100%.[4] Most authors agree that tensile strength increases rapidly for approximately 60 to 100 days and then builds gradually for about 2 years, until it plateaus at approximately 70% to 90% of the tissue's original strength.[5,12]

Only a gradual increase in tensile strength occurs during the third and final stage of wound healing, which can be called the maturation, or remodeling, phase. This remodeling is characterized by reorientation of the collagen fibers and is thought to last approximately 2 years.[4,12] During this time collagen fibers realign themselves in the direction of greatest tension on the wound, increasing the wound's stability.[5]

Maladaptive effects of inflammation and wound healing

Although inflammation and wound healing are protective and adaptive responses, they can result in undesirable sequelae. Nonadaptive aspects of this process can be exemplified in simple form by a sprained ankle. The antecedent of the inflammatory response in this case is mechanical trauma to the cells of the ankle musculature and soft tissue. However, the ensuing inflammatory reaction soon becomes the primary antecedent of tissue damage. The fluid and cellular exudate produced result in edema, which in turn causes further cellular destruction, so the inflammatory process begins to cause more damage to the cells than the original trauma.

Other examples of this nonadaptive response are allergic and hypersensitive reactions, autoimmune disease, the irritation of a blood vessel that causes thrombus formation secondary to phlebitis, destructive changes in joints secondary to release of neutrophil lysosomal enzymes, and renal failure secondary to progressive glomerular fibrosis. In these instances a relatively harmless substance has been misinterpreted as a harmful invading antigen. Cellular damage occurs as a result of the inflammatory response or the phagocytosis of the body's own cells.

The dynamics of wound repair can also result in nonadaptive sequelae. When tissue damage occurs near a joint, the contraction phenomenon, while decreasing the size of the wound, can pull the tissue together in a manner that results in the loss of joint function. In addition, the collagen that binds the wound's edges together may also bind the healing tissues to adjacent tissues, decreasing motility. An example of this process is the postoperative binding of the gastrointestinal tract to the peritoneal cavity. Such binding, or adhesion formation, not only decreases motility, but can eventually obstruct the gastrointestinal tract by the retracting scar formation.

ANTECEDENT CONDITIONS

Inflammation occurs whenever an encounter between an agent and a cell results in cellular insult, or injury, or when the body interprets an encounter as having the potential to cause injury. Infectious agents are often thought of as the antecedent condition of inflammation. There are, however, many other causative agents. A common classification of origins of cellular damage includes mechanical, thermal, and chemical categories. These categories are not mutually exclusive. Frequently, in a given situation, there is an overlap of insult origin.

Mechanical injury

Mechanical agents cause cellular damage by direct and often forceful interruption of cellular continuity. Objects that lacerate, abrade, contuse, or incise will initiate cellular damage.[13] Whenever cell membranes are torn, cut, or scraped, the body's risk of invasion by infectious agents through these portals of entry is increased significantly. Injuries to the vascular and nervous systems have perhaps the greatest potential for systemic as well as local effects.[7]

Thermal injury

Excessive temperature, electrical stimuli, ultraviolet light, and ionizing radiation can cause thermal damage to cells. The application of excessive heat to a cell results in both protein denaturation and enzyme inactivation. Whether tissues coagulate, desiccate, or carbonize depends on the intensity and length of exposure. However, even short exposure to a moderately elevated temperature of 42.0° C (107.6° F) will disrupt cellular metabolism.[15]

The scope of cellular damage caused by cold parallels the effects of heat. Freezing of intra- and extracellular fluids and small vessel occlusion are the most probable mechanisms of cell injury produced by cold. Resulting ischemia and crystallization produce changes ranging from mild blistering to necrosis and gangrene.[3,17,26]

Electrical current will alter the polarity of membranes, cause marked shifts of ions intracellularly, and seriously impair the selective permeability of membranes. When electrical energy is converted to heat, thermal damage occurs.[13] It is important to note that the external, visible damage that results from electrical stimuli may be slight, masking possible severe and progressive internal, systemic tissue damage.[11] The extent and location of cellular damage induced by electricity depend on such factors as the type of current, the amperage and voltage, the pathways of the current, and the physiological integrity of the individual.[11]

Ultraviolet light in the form of direct, intense sunlight or reflected light can injure the epidermal prickle-cell layer. When overexposed, these cells liberate chemicals that diffuse and relax the walls of the blood vessels in the dermis, causing erythema. When severely injured, the prickle cells may die, whereupon white blood cells invade the area, serum accumulates, and blisters form.[18] The formation of blisters is succeeded by drying and scaling of outer layers of the epidermis, escape of imprisoned fluids, and regeneration of the epidermal cells.[7] When injury from overexposure to ultraviolet light is severe, toxic products are produced by the disintegration of proteins, with subsequent precipitation of systemic symptoms.

Ionizing radiation in natural or synthetic forms produces varying degrees of cellular injury. High radiation doses of 10,000 rad or more will destroy cells regardless of their stage in the mitotic cycle. Lower doses inhibit DNA synthesis and delay mitosis. After exposure, when DNA synthesis is resumed, mitosis may not occur, which results in giant nuclei formation. If mitosis does occur, various chromosomal aberrations become apparent. Breaks in chromosomes occur, with fragments reuniting in an abnormal way or joining other chromosomes. Sometimes these abnormalities are incompatible with life, and the cell dies.[29]

Cellular sensitivity to radiation relates to the stage of the mitotic cycle the cell is in when contacted by radiation. In most cell types maximum sensitivity occurs during mitosis. Tissues with a high mitotic rate are more sensitive than those in which mitosis rarely or never occurs. The severity of the body's reaction to ionizing radiation is dependent on the dose, the time between exposures, the number of exposures, the amount of tissue exposed, and the type of tissue exposed.[29]

Chemical injury

Most chemicals do not injure by hyperthermic activity; rather, they create tissue injury by protein coagulation or dissolution, precipitation of chemicals in the cell, severe cellular dehydration, or protoplasmic poisoning.[14] Typical responses of tissues affected by chemicals are (1) physical solution of the cell membrane, (2) dissolution of the lipids of the cell membrane, with accompanying changes in the surface tension of cells, (3) modification of osmotic pressure between the cell and its environment, (4) alteration of the electrical potential of the cells, (5) absorption of chemical substances by the colloids of the cells, and (6) alteration of the natural colloidal state of proteins of the cells by liquefaction or precipitation.[7]

An important consideration related to the outcome of contact with particular chemical agents is that some chemicals produce a local as well as a systemic effect. For example, the formic acid of a bee sting introduces a chemical inflammant of extrinsic origin. This agent has the potential of precipitating a systemic anaphylactic response as well as a local effect. Likewise, chemicals produced in the body by extrinsic infectious agents may produce systemic results.

Chemical inflammants can also be of intrinsic origin. These agents can be derived as a result of (1) misplaced or improperly activated enzymes, (2) toxins produced by necrotic and degenerating tissues, or (3) altered metabolism such as uric acid excesses associated with gout.[13]

Bacteria, viruses, and fungi are among the most common infectious agents capable of inducing cellular damage. The basic requirements for the occurrence of an infection is that the organism be able to adhere to, colonize, or invade the host and proliferate.[24] Since interstitial fluid is gellike, molecules can travel through it only by diffusion. It is almost impossible for agents such as bacteria to move through this fluid without first liquifying it by enzymatic action.[10] The specific manner in which these organisms cause cellular injury is not yet fully understood. However, it is known that some bacteria liberate exotoxins capable of causing injury at a distance from the site of the bacterial implantation. Other infectious agents may elaborate endotoxins that are released only on disintegration of the organism. In addition, cellular damage may occur through the elaboration of a variety of enzymes such as lecithinase, which is capable of destroying cell membranes, or the hemolysins produced by the beta hemolytic streptococci, which are capable of lysing red blood cells.[26]

Viruses are considered obligate intracellular parasites composed of genetic material that are capable of inserting themselves into host cells. These host cells are subsequently injured by the new genetic information being expressed in an altered state of cellular function. One expression of this new genetic content is the replication of additional infectious viruses, which may be accompanied by lysis of the host cell. However, the host cell could be altered without precipitation of its death. In fact, the cell may be stimulated to proliferate, as noted with virally induced tumors. Viruses may also injure host cells by evoking a variety of tissue-damaging immunological reactions.[24]

Fungi represent another type of infectious agent capable of producing cellular injury. Damage to cells results from allergic necrosis caused by sensitization to fungal proteins.[3]

Although the immune response is designed for protection of the individual, this same response may also initiate tissue damage. There are four commonly identified ways by which the immune response may be deleterious to the individual. First is the immediate hypersensitive homocytotropic reaction. This reaction is seen in anaphylaxis, in which antigen-antibody interactions involve the release of chemical mediator products from target cells to effect local and systemic allergic symptoms.

A second humoral immune response, known as a cytotoxic reaction, creates tissue damage by the action of the immunoglobulin G (IgG) antibody. Circulating IgG binds to cell surfaces in response to the presence of specific antigens. Coating of these target cells with antibody renders these cells more susceptible to lysis. An example of this complement-dependent, antigen-specific reaction is a blood transfusion reaction. Symptoms of this type of reaction vary, depending on the kind of cell bearing the antigen, the kind of antibody reacting with that antigen, and the interaction of complement components with the antigen-antibody complex.[16]

A third humoral immune reaction involves the immune complex mechanism. This mechanism for initiating tissue injury is typified by the Arthus reaction, in which several hours pass before symptoms fully develop. The reaction is mediated by IgG or IgM antibodies. These antibodies combine with antigens in tissue spaces, forming a complex. Complement then adheres to this complex and in turn attracts polymorphonuclear cells to invade the target tissue. Subsequently there is a release of toxic products into these tissues, initiating a severe inflammatory response.[16]

The fourth type of mechanism by which the immune system may produce cellular injury is demonstrated by delayed hypersensitivity reactions. These reactions involve a situation in which there is an increased reactivity to specific antigens not mediated by antibodies but by sensitized lymphocytes. When these sensitized small lymphocytes combine with antigen in the tissue, there is a release of lymphokines and local activation of macrophages, which leads to the characteristic symptoms of hypersensitivity.[8] Misdirected cellular or humoral immunity responses often result in significant and long-lasting tissue damage.

BEHAVIORAL DEFINITION

Objective data

The local signs of inflammation were recognized by Celsius and Galen nearly 2000 years ago. They include heat (calor), redness (rubor), edema (tumor), pain (dolor), and loss of function (functio laesa). These are often referred to as the cardinal signs of inflammation and are usually associated with acute inflammation or an active phase of chronic inflammation. The vasodilation and resultant hyperemia associated with the initial reactions to cellular injury produce heat and redness at the inflammatory site. Localized edema results from the formation of the fluid and cellular exudate secondary to the increase in capillary pressure and permeability. The localized pain is a subjective symptom. The possible causes of pain are considered in the discussion of subjective data. Loss of function may be caused by the tissue injury, or may be secondary to voluntary immobilization because of the pain or the edema. It may also occur because of enzymatic or metabolic activities that inhibit the tissue's function.

The systemic manifestations of inflammation may occur with either acute or chronic inflammatory reactions of local or systemic nature. The degree and occurrence of these signs depend on the extent and severity of injury rather than on its localization. Objective systemic manifestations of inflammation are elevated temperature, elevated white blood cell (WBC) count, and elevated erythrocyte sedimentation rate (ESR).

A temperature greater than 37° C (98.6° F) is a reliable index of a systemic inflammatory reaction. This elevation occurs secondary to release of pyrogens into the bloodstream; they trigger the thermoregulatory mechanisms of the hypothalamus. Although it has not been validated, it is thought that these pyrogens are released endogenously from neutrophils and monocytes and exogenously from bacterial invaders.

In most instances the elevated WBC count is caused by the increased production and liberation of neutrophils. The increase is often achieved by the release of more immature neutrophils from the bone marrow. However, in allergic inflammatory reactions and parasitic infections eosinophils and basophils may be the primary elevated components of the WBC count. In instances in which bacterial, viral, rickettsial, or protozoal invasion is overwhelming, it is possible that the WBC count will decrease (i.e., the white blood cells will be destroyed faster than the body can produce them). This condition is called leukopenia.

The ESR measures the speed of separation of cellular components from the plasma. The reason for a rise in the ESR during inflammation is not clearly understood, but it is believed to occur because the inflammatory response causes an increased concentration of fibrinogen in the blood. As fibrinogen coats the red blood cells, they clump together and settle out of the blood faster than normal.[22]

Because formation of exudate is an inherent component of the inflammatory reaction, the type of exudate produced provides a valuable indication of the extent of injury, permeability of capillaries, and progression of the body's defenses. There are essentially five types of exudate: serous, purulent, catarrhal, fibrinous, and hemorrhagic. Although these are the usual five classifications, a combination of these exudates may occur during an inflammatory reaction.

Serous exudate is a clear, watery, or pinkish-yellow substance formed when the fluid component of the inflammatory exudate is greater than the cellular component. It consists primarily of protein that has leaked from the blood vessels. This exudate occurs early in the course of the inflammatory response and is characteristic of situations in which only minor tissue damage has occurred (e.g., a blister).

Purulent exudate, often called pus, occurs when the inflammatory reaction involves organisms known as pyogens. These include staphylococci, *Escherichia coli*, *Klebsiella pneumoniae*, *Proteus* strains, *Pseudomonas aeruginosa*, meningococci, gonococci, and pneumococci. Purulent exudate is composed of leukocytes, inflammatory enzymes, bacteria, necrotic tissue, and other inflammatory debris. The specific color and odor of this type of exudate are reflections of the invading agent. A sweet white or yellow purulent exudate is characteristic of streptococcal or staphylococcal invasion. *Pseudomonas* characteristically produces a green purulent exudate, and *E. coli* has its own distinctive putrid odor.

Catarrhal exudate is produced by mucous membranes or mucus-secreting cells. This exudate is usually clear and is exemplified by the exudate associated with a cold and a "runny nose."

Fibrinous exudate occurs when the vascular permeability increases, allowing the larger particles of fibrinogen to escape. The precipitate in the injured area produces fibrin. This exudate has a sticky, gray, stringy appearance and is commonly seen with chronic inflammatory reactions involving serous membranes such as the pleura of the lungs, the peritoneum, or the pericardium.

Hemorrhagic exudate occurs secondary to severe vascular damage and bleeding. This type of exudate is common in some meningococcal and rickettsial infections, which cause necrosis of small blood vessels. This type of exudate is also common with tuberculosis and lung cancer.[29]

A biopsy of the inflamed tissues can provide additional indication of the phase of the inflammatory response as well as possible antecedents. For example, the predominant cells present during an acute response are neutrophils and macrophages. During chronic responses, or when viral or rickettsial antecedents are present, lymphocytes and plasma cells dominate. Also, if the inflammation has been precipitated by parasites or an allergic response, there should be an increased number of eosinophils in the tissue.

Subjective data

The origin of the subjective symptoms (anorexia, headache, joint ache, malaise, and fatigue) that accompany the inflammatory process is not clearly understood. Robbins and Angell[26] suggest that production of humoral substances during the febrile response may be one source. Another possible cause is the toxins released by some pathogens. A third possible cause is the great energy demands made on the body during the inflammatory process by phagocytosis, leukocytic production, collagen synthesis, and cellular proliferation.

The only local subjective symptom is pain at the site of insult. Although the mechanism of the stimulation of this pain has not been clearly delineated, the pressure of the edema is believed to be one cause. In addition, chemical mediators such as histamine and kinins released from the injured cells, and the increased acidity of the tissues as a result of the inflammatory process[24,26] are other possible pain stimuli.

INTERVENING VARIABLES

Characteristically the inflammatory response is swift, vigorous, and efficient as the body reacts to a traumatic cellular incident. The ability of the body to marshall and sustain an effective inflammatory response is determined by the interplay of many intrinsic and extrinsic factors active in each such situation. These intervening variables can be classified as agent- or host-related.

Agent-related variables

Agent-related variables characterize both the agent and the agent-cell encounter. These variables include the type; potency, or virulence; and amount of the agent. In addition, the duration of encounter with the host, extent of the cellular insult, and the site of the insult are also included in the group of variables.[1,19]

The relationship between the potency and amount of the injurious agent affects the degree of cellular insult. The correlation between these variables is not always directly proportional. For example, a large number of minimally potent organisms could exert a minimal impact on cell injury, or a small number of very potent organisms could cause a substantial injury. The virulence of the agent is the key variable influencing the extent of cellular injury.

The duration of exposure to an agent may influence the degree of cellular trauma, the body's ability to sustain a response to the insult, and the body's ability to respond to other cellular demands. The effect of the exposure time is related to the virulence of the agent as well as to the site of injury. For example, an electrical contact of brief exposure can be much more traumatizing to the cell than longer contact with a less intense agent such as the sun's rays.

In different tissue sites the degree of threat to the body may differ even more dramatically. For instance, there is much greater threat to the body from tissue damage in the myocardium than from tissue damage of the same size on the epidermis of the hand.

Host-related variables

Host-related variables define the individual's competence to respond to cellular insult. General health status is usually the first host-related intervening variable that is identified in a discussion of inflammation. This variable, however, is an ill-defined, weak index of individual competence. General health status represents a combination of all other host-related variables. The various components that contribute to health status define how this status intervenes in the inflammatory response. An optimum state of health is, of course, an advantage in coping with a traumatic event.

The variable of age influences other host-related variables such as immunocompetence and vascular integrity. The newborn has immature inflammatory capabilities. A mature immune system is not completely developed until the child is between the ages of 4 to 6. On the other end of the age continuum a progressive loss of immunological vigor occurs. Both the humoral and cell-mediated responses decline with advancing age. This decline is associated with increased incidence of cancer, susceptibility to microbial invasion, and frequency of autoimmune and allergic responses.[8]

Vascular competence is a variable that is linked to other host factors such as tissue type, nutritional balance, and age. Vascular competence incorporates structural adequacy and circulatory efficiency. Cellular and fluid access to and from the site of cellular insult is critical for the activities of the inflammatory process. The more vascular the tissue, the greater the access to the site of injury. In conjunction with this access advantage is the disadvantage of greater potential for the invading agent to be spread systemically through the circulation. For this reason tissue on the ends of the continuum of vascularity is at a disadvantage. The blood has excellent access to cellular and fluid compartments but almost no restrictive abilities. Therefore septicemia (bacteria or toxins in the blood) usually has a grave prognosis.

Tissue morphology, in conjunction with vascular competence, can either facilitate or inhibit inflammatory activities. When tissues are densely packed and vascular access is good, these activities are facilitated. A tissue with dense, compact cells inhibits the spread of infectious agents through the tissue by the resistance offered by the cells' close contact. In loose tissue such as that in the blood or the peritoneal cavity this cellular compactness is not present, and the ability of pathogens to spread freely through the area is evident.

Nutritional balance is another key intervening variable. Nutritional balance is a state in which the body has an adequate store and supply of vitamins and nutrients, fluids and electrolytes are balanced, and positive nitrogen balance exists.[18] During the inflammatory process the production of white blood cells requires the availability of protein and vitamin B. An adequate level of fluid is necessary to dilute toxins, and vitamin C and proteins are necessary for collagen formation and cell proliferation. In addition to these essential substances, the body also needs a caloric reserve or supply to support the high level of energy expenditures that occur during phagocytosis, leukocytic production, collagen formation, and cellular proliferation.

Metabolic balance also plays a pivotal role in sustaining inflammatory activities. Metabolic efficiency is in part affected by age, hormonal activity, and nutritional status. Metabolic rate, for example, can be reduced 20% to 30% in prolonged malnutrition.[10] Furthermore, faulty glucose metabolism can significantly limit the energy produced by cells. This can greatly reduce the high energy activities of phagocytosis. In addition, hyperglycemia will elevate the glucose level of the inflammatory exudate, making it an excellent medium for bacterial growth.

The momentum of the inflammatory response can be significantly altered when hormonal balance is disrupted. For example, pituitary and adrenal pathologies can critically modify adrenocortical influences on inflammation. The anti-inflammatory effects of cortisone could be greatly intensified by an adrenal dysfunction, or the metabolic rate could be markedly reduced by a pituitary or thyroid dysfunction.[10]

Hormonal balance acts as a physiological barometer of individual capabilities to meet the challenges of cellular insult. The compromised host, one who has been continually bombarded by stressors, is often in jeopardy. Selye[28] suggests that when the entire organism is experiencing stress, local effort is diminished.

NURSING INTERVENTIONS—GOALS AND EVALUATIVE CRITERIA

The goals of intervention regarding inflammation address the basic protective, adaptive, and restorative functions of this process. The four major goals of intervention are (1) elimination of the causative agent, (2) support of the inflammatory process, (3) facilitation of tissue repair, and (4) protection from further insult.

Elimination of causative agent

The initial goal in the management of cellular insult is elimination of the causative agent. This goal is attained by the following three types of activities: (1) identification of the injuring agent, (2) complete removal of the offending agent, and (3) effective control of local and systemic effects. Knowledge of the origin of the insult is essential to the provision of adequate and appropriate intervention.

Mechanical trauma. When cellular injury is of mechanical origin, it is vital that the agent and all agent fragments be extricated as soon as possible. This retrieval should be carried out gently through the entry tract. Minimal manipulation of affected and adjacent tissue will help prevent extension of the trauma and field of contamination. With direct removal of penetrating objects, bleeding may ensue from the entry tract. A free flow of blood may be beneficial in that it provides a means of flushing tissue remnants and foreign body contaminants from the injured site.

A thorough cleansing of the injured area and the surrounding tissue should by carried out to assist in the removal of wound contaminants and cellular debris. One of the least traumatizing approaches to loosening and removing products of cellular trauma is copious irrigation of the site with water or normal saline solution. Also, careful washing of the affected area with a mild soap can reduce the surface tension of the contaminants, thereby assisting in dilution and removal. Antiseptics should never be introduced into a wound because they have the ability to chemically injure tissue.

Thermal trauma. The elimination of thermal agents is aimed at neutralization, containment, and reversal of the thermal action. In situations involving heat exposure, action should be directed at arresting heat penetration. The most obvious way to accomplish this is removal of the heat source. For a superficial injury the immediate application of cold or ice inhibits progression of the injury to deeper tissue. Cold application also helps retard inflammatory edema formation and reduces sensations of pain. The parameter to use to determine the amount of time that cold should be applied is absence of pain and edema formation when the cold application is removed from the site.

The effects of cold exposure or tissue freezing can be reduced by immersion of affected parts in water of a temperature only slightly greater than that normal for the body (37.8° to 40.6° C [100° to 105° F]). This temperature decreases the degree to which the cells' homeostatic mechanisms are stressed. Of equal importance is the need to handle the injured tissues as gently as possible. This is essential because crystalized tissues are extremely fragile.

The key to the control of the effects of thermal agents such as ultraviolet light is early recognition of actual or potential damage. Whether the source is natural or reflected light, the evaluation of contact time, the appreciation of subtle, initial tissue changes, and the understanding of symptom lag time is important to the determination of when protection or removal from the light sources is needed. If exposure appears to have potential for damage, immersion in a cool bath (32.2° to 35.0° C [90° to 95° F]) may help reduce some of the thermal damage. This action is most effective before burn symptoms become evident.

Removal of the source of electrical trauma must be accomplished before touching the victim. If the electricity cannot be turned off, it is essential to use nonconductive materials such as wood to free the affected individual from the electrical source. The individual's cardiopulmonary functioning should be assessed immediately after removal of the electrical source.

As with electrical trauma, the removal of an individual from radiation sources should be carried out only after protection is ensured for the individual rendering care. Since the impact of radiation is dependent not only on dose but also on distance from the source and duration of exposure, these variables should be used to contain or reduce the effects of exposure. Persons working with radiation sources should continually monitor their cumulative exposure level.

Chemical trauma. Chemical agents have both immediate and long-term effects. Identification of the specific causative agent will facilitate the use of appropriate retardants. In all external contacts with chemicals immediate, copious lavage with water can dramatically reduce the chemical's effects. This washing action not only dilutes the noxious agent, but also removes it from the site. Internal or systemic effects must be controlled through the use of appropriate neutralizing or emetic agents.

Pharmaceutical agents such as antibiotics and sulfonamides are used to eliminate infectious agents. The maintenance of appropriate drug blood levels is particularly essential to the effectiveness of these pharmaceutical agents. Absorption requirements, excretion routes, interactive effects, and the timing of drug administration are variables that affect this maintenance. When infectious agents or their toxins are topical, lavage and tissue débridement can be used to remove the contamination mechanically.

Increasing fluid intake aids in diluting toxins by limiting the local and systemic effects of infectious agents. This measure is facilitated if fluid ingestion is greater than 2000 ml/day.

When tissue damage is precipitated by the body's immune response, the primary approach to removal of the causative agent is to neutralize or suppress the inflammatory response by means of anti-inflammatory and immunosuppressant pharmaceutical agents and/or the application of cold.

Evaluation criteria. That invisible agents or fragments of an agent have been eliminated must be inferred from local and systemic signs and symptoms. If the injury to the tissue has been limited, the pain, swelling, and redness at the site of injury will subside rather quickly after removal of the agent. When exudate continues to form and pain or loss of function accelerates, either the agent has not been completely removed or the cellular trauma has been extensive. The absence of growth of infectious agents in tissue or blood cultures is an indication of their elimination.

Support of the inflammatory process

The essential activities of the inflammatory process can be successfully mobilized and sustained when an individual's physiological and psychological supports are maximized.

Nutritional support. Nutritional stability contributes in several ways to the protective, adaptive, and restorative functions of the inflammatory process. Vitamin B, vitamin C, and proteins are essential to white blood cell production, collagen and fibrin formation, and cellular rebuilding, respectively. Nutritional deficiency can severely retard the body's ability to mount and sustain the inflammatory process. Early detection and correction of nutrient deficiencies are imperative to the support of this process. Use of vitamin supplements along with an enriched-protein and enriched-carbohydrate diet will aid in meeting the demands and replenishing depleted stores of these nutrients.

Fluid balance also is an integral part of nutritional stability. In the inflammatory process, fluid promotes the dilution and removal of systemic toxins. The elevation of body temperature also causes an increased demand for fluid to replace the increased insensible loss of fluid. Barring contraindications such as decreased renal function, cardiac overload, or cerebral edema, fluid ingestion should be increased above the normal 2000 ml/day intake requirement.

Meeting energy expenditures. Another variable closely linked to nutritional factors is the energy expended by the inflammatory process. Phagocytosis creates an intense and persistent need for energy. Moreover, elevation of body temperature increases the metabolic rate, which further elevates the body's energy needs. The degree to which an individual is able to adapt to specific energy requirements depends on the person's nutritional reserves and available energy sources.

Increased energy needs can be attended to in a variety of ways. Nutrient support in the form of increased intake of carbohydrates is one means of increasing energy production. However, while energy reserves are being rebuilt, other energy requirements should be kept to a minimum. Decreasing activities by means of bed rest or immobilization of the affected part reduces energy demands. A lowered activity level should be maintained past the time when inflammatory symptoms such as elevated temperature are diminished. Prolongation of resting can assist in preventing a relapse. The stringency of the rest regimen should parallel the degree of insult and the vigor of the inflammatory process.

General personal hygiene comfort measures can also help reduce the energy expended by an individual dealing with everyday stresses. The comfort and relaxation accomplished by such measures as bathing, oral hygiene, back rubs, or the straightening of linens should not be underestimated. Physiological comfort promotes relaxation and facilitates resting, thus reducing energy expenditures. In some situations it is also necessary to assess the patient's hormonal balance in conjunction with the energy demands of the inflammatory process. The appropriate level of hormonal replacement should be administered as needed.

Reduction of temperature elevation. Hypothermic agents such as aspirin, environmental temperature in the comfort range, and topical application of cold can help diminish the energy-depleting effects of an elevated temperature. Hypothermic agents must be continually evaluated in terms of overall effectiveness and long-range implications. For example, if hypothermic drugs are used too early in the inflammatory process, they may mask important diagnostic symptoms.

Evaluation criteria. Support of the inflammatory process is evidenced by a gradual reduction of the reaction's intensity. The elevated temperature, ESR, and WBC count begin moving back to their normal range. The person is able to rest comfortably and has the energy for things such as ingestion of adequate nutrients and performance of personal hygiene activities. As the energy demands of the inflammatory process decrease, the person can sustain a greater focus of attention and range of activities. Symptoms such as anorexia, fatigue, headache, and joint ache decrease. Measurement of fluid and dietary intake will provide an indication of their adequacy.

Facilitation of tissue repair

The goal of tissue repair facilitation can be accomplished by the following subobjectives: (1) assisting the body to clear the wound of debris and (2) assuring an adequate supply of the nutrients for tissue rebuilding.

Débridement. Cellular replacement cannot occur until the wound area is cleared of the products of cellular injury. This aspect of resolution can be facilitated by mechanically debriding the injured area. The most vigorous approach to wound débridement involves cutting away cellular debris and necrotic tissue. A gentler approach is the use of a mechanical washing action such as flushing the wound area or immersing the part in turbulent water such as a whirlpool.

Oxidizing agents such as hydrogen peroxide can also provide a gentle debriding action. However, care must be taken when using oxidizing agents because they can oxidize the protein of healthy tissues as well as that of debris. Wounds should always be flushed with a solution such as normal saline solution after oxidizing agents are used in débridement. Wet dressings and immersion soaking of an affected part assist in softening and/or liquifying the debris, which ultimately facilitates its removal. Exposure to such fluid environments must be limited, however, so that surrounding healthy tissue will not begin to macerate. Close observation of tissue status is critical.

Gentle débridement may be carried out by the use of dressings. The fibers of fine mesh gauze that has been smoothly laid over and gently pressed into the débridement area will adhere to the debris as the dressing and exudate dry. Removal of the fine mesh gauze will directly lift away the adhering debris. The drier the dressing when removed and the more fibers in contact with the tissue surface, the more vigorous the debriding action of the dressing.

Dressings that have a cotton or paper filler should never be placed in direct contact with the wound's tissue base because these fillers adhere to the tissues, adding to the debris of the wound. When these filler dressings are used to cover an open wound, fine mesh gauze should be placed between the wound and the dressing.

Nutritional support. Vitamin C and protein are essential to the formation of collagen and the repair of tissue defects. Dietary supplements of these substances may be needed to replenish the stores of these nutrients as they are depleted by the demands of tissue repair and replacement. Since vascular competence influences the transport of these nutrients to the repair site, measures to increase circulation should further assist the reparative process. Local circulation can be improved by the application of heat to the injured area, and the efficiency of systemic circulation can be improved by increased muscular activity such as ambulation.

Evaluation criteria. Facilitation of tissue repair is accomplished when the area of insult demonstrates recovery. Open wounds should evidence clean, viable tissues. The primary index of tissue rebuilding is the emergence of granulation tissue in the injured site with progressive epithelial margination. Sealing of an incision line is evidenced by the absence of tissue separation, purulent drainage, or odor. Pain at the site will be less intense and will gradually be replaced by a feeling of soreness. This soreness dissipates gradually, along with the local signs of heat, swelling, and redness. Greater freedom in movement of the affected part and advancing tolerance for activity are further evidence of tissue repair.

Protection from further insult

The momentum of cellular recovery advanced by the achievement of the previously discussed goals can be assisted by protecting the injured area from further insult. The success of this goal directly relates to the achievement of the following four subobjectives: (1) prevention of additional contamination, (2) prevention of dissemination of contaminants from the injury site, (3) reduction of mechanical trauma to injured tissue, and (4) maintenance of the integrity of the surrounding tissue.

Prevention of additional contamination. The additional stress caused by contamination of injured tissues by another infectious agent may decidedly reduce the recovery rate of this already compromised area. Consistent use of aseptic practices is the key to the achievement of this objective. The easiest, most basic, yet most often neglected aseptic practice is hand washing before and after caring for a patient's injured tissue areas. The use of aseptic technique can be facilitated by teaching the patient and family members how important this goal is and how aseptic practice can reduce further contamination of the patient's injured area.

One of the functions of a dressing is to keep the injured area clean by protecting it from airborne contamination. To maintain the effect of this protective function, the dressing must be dry because moisture assists bacterial entry through dressings via capillary action. This is one of the primary variables that should be used to determine how often a dressing should be changed. Protective dressings should be kept dry.

The patient should be isolated from all known sources of contamination such as another patient with a wound infection. There should be no direct or indirect contact between these patients or their environments.

Prevention of dissemination of contaminants from the injury site. Asepsis is also the key to accomplishing the objective of preventing dissemination of infectious agents from the area of injury. A containment cleansing routine for the infected patient and the environment should be organized so that the patient is not reinfected by contact with areas previously contaminated. The organization of such cleansing activities should include equipment items, clothing, dressings, linens, and bathing facilities.

In addition, minimizing the manipulation or massage of the infected area helps limit the spread of organisms to surrounding tissues. Active movement of the affected part should be avoided. The morphology of the tissues and the mobility of the affected part provide parameters regarding how immobilized the affected part should be. The looser the tissue and the greater the muscle activity necessary for the part's mobility, the more restrictive the immobilization should be.

Reduction of mechanical trauma. The injured site can be protected from mechanical trauma in a number of ways. Dressings not only protect the site from airborne contaminants, but also can absorb some of the force tissues receive when they come in contact with objects. A light dressing is adequate to keep the area clean. However, a bulky, cotton-filled dressing will provide a thick protective padding for a wound and absorb heavy production of exudate. The benefit of bulky dressings must be balanced with the risk of affording a warm, dark, moist area conducive to bacterial growth. Keeping the dressings dry reduces this risk.

The sutures used to close the surgical incision assist in keeping the wound edges approximated until an adequate amount of collagen is formed to provide the tensile strength for this task. The absorption rates of plain catgut, chromic catgut, and new chromic catgut are approximately 10, 21, and 90 to 180 days, respectively. These times coincide with the ends of periods of rapid rises in tensile strength. It is during these end periods of suture absorption that the risk of wound dehiscence and evisceration is highest. The rate of collagen formation and increase in tensile strength of the wound, in combination with the absorption rate of the suture materials, provides the parameters for activity levels the injured area can safely undertake. Abdominal binders and elastic wraps can help support the injured tissue and decrease the stress of muscle movement on the healing wound.

Maintenance of the integrity of surrounding tissue. The area surrounding the injured site must remain intact in order to assist the healing tissues. Three common insults to this surrounding tissue area are excoriation, maceration, and drying. In all instances this tissue area should be kept clean. This can be accomplished by frequent cleansing with water and/or soap. Washing is particularly advantageous in removing substances such as urine, feces, and wound exudate. If the surrounding area is macerated or excoriated, the area should be exposed frequently to drying heat for short periods. Dressings should be changed often enough to ensure that the area is kept dry and clean. Often simply exposing the area to air will produce an adequate amount of drying.

When tissues become too dry, remoisturizing can be assisted by the application of a hydrating agent. Lotions or ointments used to assist in rehydrating the tissues should not have an alcohol base because alcohol is a drying agent. Care must be taken, however, to prevent the entry of such hydrating agents into the wound, since they will only add to the debris that must be removed before healing can occur.

Evaluation criteria. Attainment of the goal of protection from further insult is evidenced when healing progresses to conclusion without incident. Inspection of the wound should reveal intact granulation tissue without breaks or bleeding. The edges of sealed wounds should be approximated, and the surrounding tissue should be clean and intact.

CONCEPT OUTLINE

I. *Conceptual definition:* Inflammation is a defensive response against cellular injury wherein the body attempts to restrict the injurious agent, neutralize it, and repair damaged tissue.

II. *Antecedent conditions*
- A. Mechanical injury
  1. Lacerations
  2. Abrasions
  3. Contusions
  4. Incisions
- B. Thermal injury
  1. Excessive temperature
  2. Electrical stimuli
  3. Ultraviolet light
  4. Radiation
- C. Chemical injury
  1. Intrinsic origin
     - a. Misplaced or improperly activated enzymes
     - b. Toxins produced by necrotic or degenerating tissues
     - c. Altered metabolism
     - d. Immune response
  2. Extrinsic origin
     - a. Chemical spills
     - b. Infectious agents
     - c. Bites or stings

III. *Behavioral definition*
- A. Objective data
  1. Local signs
     - a. Heat
     - b. Redness
     - c. Edema
     - d. Pain
     - e. Loss of function
  2. Systemic signs
     - a. Elevated temperature
     - b. Elevated WBC count
     - c. Elevated ESR
  3. Exudate characteristics
     - a. Consistency
     - b. Color
     - c. Odor
  4. Cells in tissue biopsy
  5. Culture growths
- B. Subjective data
  1. Anorexia
  2. Headache
  3. Joint ache
  4. Malaise
  5. Fatigue
  6. Pain at site of injury

IV. *Intervening variables*
- A. Agent-related variables
  1. Type of agent
  2. Virulence of agent
  3. Amount of agent
  4. Duration of agent-host encounter
  5. Extent of cellular insult
  6. Site of insult
- B. Host-related variables
  1. General health status
  2. Age
  3. Vascular competence
  4. Tissue morphology
  5. Nutritional balance
  6. Metabolic balance
  7. Hormonal balance

V. *Nursing interventions—goals*
- A. Elimination of causative agent
  1. Mechanical trauma
     - a. Extrication of agent or fragments via entry tract
     - b. Minimal manipulation of affected and adjacent tissue
     - c. Thorough cleansing of injured area and surrounding tissue
  2. Thermal trauma
     - a. Heat
       - (1) Removal of source
       - (2) Application of cold
     - b. Cold
       - (1) Immersion of affected part in water slightly warmer than body temperature
     - c. Ultraviolet light
       - (1) Limitation of exposure
       - (2) Immersion in cool bath
     - d. Electrical trauma
       - (1) Removal of source
       - (2) Assessment of cardiopulmonary status
     - e. Radiation
       - (1) Removal of source
       - (2) Monitoring of exposure
  3. Chemical trauma
     - a. External contact
       - (1) 'Copious lavage
     - b. Internal contact
       - (1) Neutralization and/or use of emetic agents
     - c. Infectious agents
       - (1) Administration of pharmaceutical agents
       - (2) Fluids increased to dilute toxins

- d. Immune response trauma
  - (1) Neutralization or suppression of inflammatory response
- B. Support of inflammatory process
  - 1. Nutritional support
    - a. Increased vitamin B intake
    - b. Increased vitamin C intake
    - c. Increased protein intake
    - d. Increased carbohydrate intake
    - e. Increased fluid intake to greater than 2000 ml/day if not contraindicated
  - 2. Meeting energy expenditures
    - a. Increased carbohydrate intake
    - b. Decrease of activities
    - c. Use of general personal hygiene measures to promote comfort and relaxation
  - 3. Reduction of temperature elevation
    - a. Use of antipyretics
    - b. Control of environmental temperature
    - c. Topical application of cold
- C. Facilitation of tissue repair
  - 1. Débridement
    - a. Cutting away of cellular debris
    - b. Use of mechanical washing action
    - c. Use of oxidizing agents
    - d. Use of dressings
  - 2. Nutritional support
    - a. Dietary supplement of vitamin C and protein
    - b. Application of heat to increase circulation
- D. Protection from further insult
  - 1. Prevention of additional contamination
    - a. Use of aseptic practices
    - b. Use of dry dressings
    - c. Use of isolation measures
  - 2. Prevention of dissemination of contaminants from injury site
    - a. Maintenance of asepsis
    - b. Use of isolation measures
    - c. Use of minimal manipulation, massage, and active movement of infected area
  - 3. Reduction of mechanical trauma
    - a. Use of dressings
    - b. Use of tensile strength and suture strength for determination of activity levels
    - c. Use of abdominal binders and elastic wraps
  - 4. Maintenance of integrity of surrounding tissue
    - a. Maintenance of cleanliness
    - b. Use of exposure or dry heat on macerated or excoriated areas
    - c. Remoisturization of dry tissues

VI. *Evaluation criteria*

- A. Subsidence of pain, swelling, and redness at site of injury
- B. Absence of growth of infectious agents in tissue and blood cultures
- C. Normal temperature, ESR, and WBC count
- D. Increased energy level
- E. Decreased anorexia, fatigue, headache, and joint ache
- F. Clean, viable tissue in open wounds
- G. Emergence of granulation tissue with progressive epithelial margination
- H. Absence of tissue separation, purulent drainage, or odor
- I. Progression from pain to soreness at injury site
- J. Greater freedom of movement of affected part
- K. Advancing tolerance for activity
- L. Intact granulation tissue
- M. Approximated wound edges
- N. Surrounding tissue clean and intact

REFERENCES

1. Beland, I. L., and Passos, J. Y.: Clinical nursing: pathophysiological and psychosocial approaches, ed. 3, New York, 1975, Macmillan Publishing Co., Inc.
2. Bickley, H. C.: Practical concepts in human disease, Baltimore, 1974, Williams & Wilkins Co.
3. Boyd, W.: A textbook of pathology: structure and function in disease, ed. 8, Philadelphia, 1970, Lea & Febiger.
4. Cohen, B. H., Lewis, L. A., and Resnik, S. S.: Wound healing: a brief review, Int. J. Dermatol. **14**:722, 1975.
5. Dingman, R. O.: Factors of clinical significance affecting wound healing, Laryngoscope **83**:1540, 1973.
6. Fingl, E., and Woodbury, D.: General principles. In Goodman, L., and Gilman, A., editors: The pharmacologic basis of therapeutics, New York, 1975, Macmillan Publishing Co., Inc.
7. Forbus, W. D.: Reaction to injury: pathology

for students of disease, Baltimore, 1943, Williams & Wilkins Co.
8. Good, R. A., and Finstad, J.: Adaptive immunity. In Frohlich, E. D., editor: Pathophysiology: altered regulatory mechanisms in disease, ed. 2, Philadelphia, 1972, J. B. Lippincott Co.
9. Groër, M. E., and Shekleton, M. E.: Basic pathopysiology: a conceptual approach, St. Louis, 1979, The C. V. Mosby Co.
10. Guyton, A. C.: Textbook of medical physiology, ed. 5, Philadelphia, 1976, W. B. Saunders Co.
11. Hersperger, J. E., and Dahl, L. M.: Electrical and chemical injuries, Critical Care Quarterly **1**:43, 1978.
12. Heughan, C., and Hunt, T. K.: Some aspects of wound healing research: a review, Can. J. Surg. **18**:118, 1975.
13. Hopps, H. C.: Principles of pathology, ed. 2, New York, 1964, Appleton-Century-Crofts.
14. Houck, J. C.: Inflammation: a quarter century of progress, J. Invest. Dermatol. **67**:124, 1976.
15. Jacoby, F. G.: Nursing care of the patient with burns, ed. 2, St. Louis, 1976, The C. V. Mosby Co.
16. Kintzel, K. C., and Lindell, D.: The immune response. In Kintzel, K. C., editor: Advanced concepts in clinical nursing, ed. 2, Philadelphia, 1977, J. B. Lippincott Co.
17. Lapp, N. L., and Juergens, J. L.: Frostbite, Mayo Clin. Proc. **40**:932, 1965.
18. Lindell, D.: Inflammation and repair: nonspecific mechanisms of immunity. In Kintzel, K. C., editor: Advanced concepts in clinical nursing, ed. 2, Philadelphia, 1977, J. B. Lippincott Co.
19. Luckmann, J., and Sorensen, K. C.: Medical-surgical nursing: a psychophysiologic approach, Philadelphia, 1974, W. B. Saunders Co.
20. McKay, D. G.: Participation of components of the blood coagulation system in the inflammatory response, Am. J. Pathol. **67**:181, 1972.
21. Nysather, J. D., Katz, A. E., and Lenth, J. L.: The immune system: development and functions, Am. J. Nurs. **76**:1614, 1976.
22. Page, A.: Inflammatory mechanisms and fever. In Frohlich, E. D., editor: Pathophysiology: altered regulatory mechanisms in disease, ed. 2, Philadelphia, 1972, J. B. Lippincott Co.
23. Pickering, R. J., and Gabrielsen, A. E.: Mechanisms involving the complement system. In Frohlich, E. D., editor: Pathophysiology: altered regulatory mechanisms in disease, ed. 2, Philadelphia, 1972, J. B. Lippincott Co.
24. Price, S. A., and Wilson, L. M.: Pathophysiology: clinical concepts of disease processes, New York, 1978, McGraw-Hill Book Co.
25. Robbins, S. L.: Pathologic basis of disease, Philadelphia, 1974, W. B. Saunders Co.
26. Robbins, S. L., and Angell, M.: Basic pathology, ed. 2, Philadelphia, 1976, W. B. Saunders Co.
27. Ryan, G. B.: Inflammation and localization of infection, Surg. Clin. North Am. **56**:831, 1976.
28. Selye, H.: The stress of life, New York, 1956, McGraw-Hill Book Co.
29. Walter, J. B.: An introduction to the principles of disease, Philadelphia, 1977, W. B. Saunders Co.

JEAN L. REESE

Chapter 11

FLUID AND ELECTROLYTE IMBALANCE

CONCEPTUAL DEFINITION

Fluid and electrolyte imbalances are disruptions in the tonicity or volume of fluid in the intravascular, interstitial, and/or intracellular compartments. Changes in the tonicity of body fluid arise from the loss or gain of either solutes or water. When a body compartment's fluid, composed of water and various solutes, becomes osmotically imbalanced, water shifts from the compartment of lower tonicity to one of higher tonicity. Abnormal hydrostatic and colloid osmotic pressures can also cause fluid imbalance in the intravascular and interstitial compartments. An excess or deficit of fluid volume in the various compartments can compromise the functioning of the circulatory, respiratory, renal, and central nervous systems.

In addition, when the concentration of specific ions is disrupted, the conduction of impulses along the cell membrane is affected. This disruption causes a range of effects on the smooth and skeletal muscle. The movement of sodium and potassium across the cell membrane is extremely important in the ability of the nerve and muscle cells to transmit electrochemical impulses along their membranes. In a normal resting state the cell membrane of the nerve fiber has potential of about −90 millivolts. This is caused by the balance of three factors: the transport of sodium out of the cell, the movement of potassium into the cell, and the large number of protein organic anions in the cell that cannot diffuse outward. The discharge, or action potential, occurs because of the huge increase in sodium permeability of the cell membrane. Sodium rushes into the cell, changing the electrical potential from negative to positive. The permeability of the cell membrane allows potassium to leave the cell, which changes the electrical potential back to negative. The active transport of sodium out of the cell and of potassium into the cell returns the cell membrane to its normal resting state.[17]

The resting state of the cell membrane is probably most influenced by the extracellular concentration of potassium. Since potassium is more highly concentrated within than outside the cell, it attempts to diffuse to the extracellular compartment. An increase or decrease in the concentration of extracellular potassium alters the cell membrane potential.

A reduction in extracellular potassium causes an increase in membrane potential, or lessened excitability of the cell membrane. This slows impulse transmission. The effects of hypopotassemia can range from muscle weakness to paralysis. This can result in striking changes in skeletal and cardiac activity. In hyperpotassemia the cell membrane potential is reduced, and the membrane becomes more reactive to stimuli.[12,27]

Anything that makes the cell membrane more permeable will usually make the membrane more excitable. In contrast, anything that decreases membrane permeability decreases excitability. It is hypothesized that there are sodium and potassium "channels" in the membrane, guarded by "gates" that open and close the channels. In the resting state of the cell membrane the gates are closed. Calcium is thought to have a role in the closure of the sodium gates. If there is a deficiency in calcium, the membrane remains very permeable to sodium ions. This results in continuous firing of the membrane. Conversely, if there is an abundance of calcium, the membrane permeability is decreased and less excitable.[17,27]

Often the effects of an abnormal concentration of a specific ion can be modified by the concentration of other ions. For instance, the ECG signs of hyperpotassemia are exaggerated by decreased serum concentrations of sodium and calcium. In contrast, increased serum concentrations of sodium and calcium reduce these signs. Other factors such as the concentration of serum proteins affect serum sodium and calcium levels.[6] The extracellular concentration of hydrogen ions is thought to affect serum potassium levels because of a reciprocal relationship. A reduction in water, or hyperosmolality, increases all ion concentrations, whereas an increase in body water, or hypo-osmolality, reduces the concentrations of all ions.

Normal dynamics

Cycling of body fluid. Although body fluid is controlled in volume and concentration in each body compartment, the hydrostatic pressure and plasma colloid pressure throughout the vascular system maintain a constant cycling of this fluid. The mechanical pressure for fluid movement comes from contraction of the cardiac muscle, which provides the hydrostatic pressure that forces plasma through the pores of the capillaries into the interstitium. This movement of fluid occurs in opposition to the pressure gradient created by the plasma colloids (oncotic pressure). The oncotic pressure gradient pulls fluid into the vascular compartment. Oncotic pressure is exerted by protein molecules, principally albumin, which cannot readily pass through the capillary pores. The hydrostatic pressure is greater than the oncotic pressure at the arterial end of the capillary bed, but it is reduced as the blood traverses the capillary bed. Water molecules are pulled from the interstitium into the venous end of the capillary bed by the oncotic pressure, which has remained constant.[18]

The concentration of proteins in the plasma far exceeds that in the interstitial fluid. The large size of the protein molecules prevents their easy exit through capillary pores into the interstitium. The concentration of proteins in the capillary filtrate is about 0.2 to 0.3 g/100 ml in contrast to the 6 to 8 g/100 ml in the plasma. Those protein molecules which do move into the interstitium are removed by the lymphatic system, which returns the protein molecules to the vascular system via the subclavian veins.[20] This reentry normally maintains the plasma colloid osmotic pressure at about 28 mm Hg. This oncotic pressure is great enough to attract the free fluid from the interstitium into the venous ends of the capillary bed and help maintain plasma volume.

Tonicity of body fluid. The sodium ion is a major factor in the maintenance of fluid volume in the vascular space and the interstitium. Unlike the albumin molecule, the sodium ion passes through the capillary walls quite freely by diffusion. Although this ion is much smaller in mass than an albumin or glucose molecule, it creates much more osmotic pressure per unit of weight.

Osmotic pressure is measured in milliosmols (mOsm), which reflects the pressure exerted by ions in a solution across a semipermeable membrane. It is not the size of the ion but the number of ions per unit of weight that determines how much water the ions attract.[15]

Sodium is the primary substance that maintains the normal plasma osmotic pressure at about 285 mOsm/L. About 95% of the cation osmols of the extracellular fluid are composed of sodium ions, which accounts for the effect of sodium. The anion osmols, principally chloride and bicarbonate, create the other half of the 285 mOsm/L of the osmotic pressure. Crystalloids such as urea, sugar, and creatinine produce only a few milliosmols of pressure in the extracellular fluid. The albumin molecule, although responsible for almost all the colloid osmotic pressure, has only negligible effect on the total plasma osmolality.[25,26] The proteins albumin and globulin contribute about 2 mOsm/L to the 285 mOsm/L of total osmotic pressure.

Normally the tonicity of fluid is uniform throughout the body's fluid compartments. The volume of fluid in the body is controlled by the intake and output of about 2000 to 3000 ml/day. The kidneys can adjust the volume and concentration of their output. However, the loss of fluid through the lungs, skin, and gastrointestinal tract remains relatively constant unless affected by disease or environmental changes.

The sodium ion concentration in the body fluid is primarily controlled by the antidiuretic hormone (ADH, vasopressin) produced in the hypothalamus. The most potent stimulus for ADH secretion is an increase in the body fluid osmolality. This means that an increase in sodium ion concentration will cause ADH to act on the renal tubules to conserve water and dilute the concentration of sodium in the body fluid. Thirst occurs with hyperosmolality. A person will usually attempt to satiate this sensation. These two mechanisms of reabsorption and ingestion add water to the body fluid.[9]

Aldosterone, a mineral corticoid secreted by the adrenal cortex, controls the reabsorption of sodium by the renal distal tubules. However, it is much less potent than ADH in affecting the concentration of sodium in the body fluid. When aldosterone concentration in the plasma increases, the rate of sodium reabsorption in the renal tubules increases, with concomitant reabsorption of chloride and other negative ions. The reabsorption of sodium by the tubules creates a strong osmotic gradient, which causes osmosis of water from the tubules into the peritubular fluid.[24] Since this leads to fluid and sodium retention in the body, it does not increase the concentration of sodium. However, this mechanism does add to the total amount of sodium ions in the body and increase the total amount of body fluid.

Aldosterone profoundly affects the concentration of potassium in body fluid because it causes the renal tubules to secrete potassium. Since almost 90% of circulating aldosterone is deactivated by passage through the liver, a decrease in the rate of portal circulation or liver metabolism can greatly increase the concentration of aldosterone in the body. The half-life of aldosterone in the body normally is 30 minutes.[24]

The fluid volume in the extracellular compartment is mediated by the atrial stretch receptors that cause reflex arterial dilation. Dilation expands the vascular area, increasing the fluid volume it can contain. An elevation in arterial pressure will increase urinary output as a result of increased glomerular filtration rate. These feedback mechanisms assist in controlling the output of fluid from the body.[4]

Interstitial compartment. Although the concentration of certain solutes in the plasma and interstitial fluid is nearly the same, the interstitial fluid has some unique properties. The interstitial space contains fluid of two different viscosities: gel and free fluid. The interstitial gel is the most abundant fluid. This gel is a mass of mucopolysaccharides in the form of coiled fibrils, which compress and restrict each other's movement. These coils provide elastic support for the cells and restrict movement of fluid through the tissues. The gel prevents the force of gravity from moving fluid to dependent body parts. In addition to the mucopolysaccharide filaments, there are collagen fiber bundles, which prevent expansion of the interstitial gel.[18]

It is theorized that the mucopolysaccharides provide optimum spacing between the cells for nutrition. Packing of the cells too tightly would not allow the outlying cells to receive nutrients, since the nutrient would not pass through one cell on its way to another. Conversely, if the cells were too far apart, nutrients would be unable to diffuse the extended distance.[18]

Another aspect of the interstitial fluid is its retention of negative pressure of about −6.3 mm Hg, which prevents accumulation of free fluid in the interstitium. This negative pressure is maintained by the plasma colloid pressure, the removal of fluid and protein molecules from the interstitium by the lymphatic vessels, and the reduction of hydrostatic pressure in the venous end of the vascular system.

Interstitial gel remains contracted. This assists in maintaining the form of the tissues. Excessive free fluid remains only in the crevices in the gel.[18] The skin clinging to the underlying structures in the axilla and the wrinkled scrotum are examples of this phenomenon. If the interstitial tissue pressure reaches zero, free fluid begins to accumulate, creating a greater distance between cells. This produces edema.

Intracellular compartment. The intracellular fluid is the last to be affected by osmotic changes in body fluids. The extracellular fluid provides a buffer between the cells and the external environment. However, the fluid in the cells is controlled by the osmolality of the extracellular fluid. Although water molecules enter and leave the cells, solutes do not pass through the cell membrane as readily. The cell does not alter the total number of ions it holds. What does change is the concentration of those ions. The composition of intracellular ions will also change to maintain electroneutrality across the cell membrane.

The cell wall, although permeable, does not stretch or increase its surface area.[7] This does not mean that the volume of the cell cannot change. A spherical container with the same surface area as an oval container holds more fluid. As the cell takes in more water, it becomes more spherical, and more space is required for expansion. Unless the cells are in a confined space such as the cranium, the surrounding tissues can usually adjust to this demand for cellular space.

Balance between compartments. Equality of osmolality, or tonicity, between the three partitions of body fluid is always sought while electroneutrality is being maintained. Although the concentration of different solutes varies considerably between the intracellular and extracellular compartments, the number of cations and anions remain the same on each side of the cell's membrane. The predominant intracellular cation is potassium. The cells also contain a large amount of negatively charged, nondiffusable protein along with anionic phosphates and magnesium cations. These substances counter the pull of the extracellular sodium and chloride. Both sodium and chloride ions are considerably fewer in number intracellularly than extracellularly. This occurs because the "sodium pump" actively removes the sodium ion from the cell. Chloride passively follows the sodium. Potassium or hydrogen and bicarbonate enter the cell in this exchange to maintain the balance of cations and anions between the two compartments.

Fluid and electrolyte imbalances are organized in the following subconcepts: isotonic, hypertonic, and hypotonic volume changes; and potassium and calcium disorders. The conceptual definition, antecedent conditions, and behavioral definition of each of these subconcepts will be discussed separately. However, the discussion of intervening variables and interventions will address the broad concept of fluid and electrolyte imbalance.

ISOTONIC VOLUME DISORDERS

Conceptual definition

In isotonic volume disorders solutes and water are gained or lost in equal ratio, with maintenance of isotonic concentrations in the extracellular fluid compartments. Expansion or contraction of the plasma and interstitial fluid results. The intracellular fluid volume is not affected because a change in tonicity is required to alter the amount of fluid in the cells.

Under normal circumstances the overingestion of fluid causes increased glomerular filtration rate and excretion of dilute urine because of the reduction in ADH secretion. The overingestion of solute or loss of water is handled by thirst and renal excretion of solute in a concentrated urine.

Antecedent conditions of isotonic volume excess

The antecedent of an isotonic extracellular fluid excess may be of exogenous or endogenous origin. Rapid intravenous administration of normal saline solution can overload the vascular system and produce a condition called hypervolemia. In this instance the rate of infusion exceeds the rate of dispersion of the fluid from the vascular system to the interstitium. When the infusion rate exceeds the rate of kidney excretion, the accumulated isotonic fluid will expand the vascular and interstitial areas.

The endogenous antecedent conditions of extracellular fluid expansion are primarily diseases that alter the function of the heart, kidneys, and liver. Congestive heart failure, whether it is caused by myocardial infarction, valvular disease, or hypertension, results in extracellular accumulation of fluid. The reduction in glomerular filtration rate caused by the lessened force of the cardiac contraction stimulates the production of ADH and aldosterone. This increases the volume of the extracellular fluid while maintaining isotonicity. The fluid is trapped in the interstitium by the increased hydrostatic pressure at the venous end of the capillary bed. This increased pressure overrides the pull of the plasma osmotic colloid pressure.

Renal failure produces retention of extracellular fluid. Reduction in the perfusion of the kidney owing to hypovolemia, vasodilation, or hypotension; disease of the kidney itself such as glomerulonephritis; and disorders such as calculi and prostatic hypertrophy that block the outflow of urine can all cause renal failure. When the kidney is not able to filter the plasma electrolytes, water and waste products are retained.

Cirrhosis of the liver causes collection of blood in the splenic venous pool, thus reducing the circulating blood volume. The kidneys compensate for this loss by retaining sodium and water. The changes in the venous hydrostatic pressure of the portal circulation operate in the same manner as those which occur in congestive heart failure. Fluid accumulates in the peritoneal cavity as well as in the interstitium of the gut. Two additional factors operate during cirrhosis to affect fluid accumulation. The decreased liver function and decreased blood flow through the liver result in longer maintenance of active aldosterone in the body. Albumin synthesis by the liver is decreased, reducing the amount of the protein available for the plasma colloid osmotic pressure. In addition, the protein concentration is diluted by the increased plasma fluid volume.

Behavioral definition of isotonic volume excess

Objective data. When the interstitial gel cannot absorb any more fluid and the negative interstitial pressure has changed to positive, free fluid begins to accumulate. External pressure on the skin is able to displace the free fluid. This produces the clinical sign of pitting edema. When pressure is removed, the indentation remains in the tissue until the displaced free fluid flows back into the area. Since this free fluid is affected by gravity, dependent parts of the body show edema first. When an upright position is maintained, edema shows initially in the feet. With the accumulation of excess fluid comes the predictable gain in body weight. As plasma accumulates in the peritoneal cavity, as is common with cirrhosis of the liver, the abdominal girth increases. This condition is called ascites.

Distension of the neck and peripheral veins and elevated central venous pressure indicate hypervolemia. Pulmonary edema may also develop, causing dyspnea, restlessness, and rales at the base of the lungs. Coughing with expectoration of pink, frothy sputum may accompany pulmonary edema. With cardiac overload, functional murmurs appear. Heart sounds are loud and snapping, and a third heart sound may occur.[5]

In an isotonic volume change, serum electrolyte concentrations usually remain in the normal range. However, the plasma protein and hematocrit levels may be low as a result of dilution. If the glomerular filtration rate is decreased, potassium concentration will increase. The specific antecedent condition may affect the kidneys' ability to remove the excess volume. Therefore the urinary output may be increased, normal, or decreased.

Subjective data. A person with increased extracellular fluid volume may feel tired, notice "puffiness" around the ankles, or complain about shoes becoming tighter. Changes in mental functioning such as irritability and forgetfulness are related to fluid volume changes interfering with oxygenation.

Antecedent conditions of isotonic volume deficit

Loss of isotonic fluid in excess of intake causes a decrease in or contraction of the extracellular fluid volume. The loss may occur via the blood vessels, kidneys, gut, or disrupted skin continuity. If the loss affects the vascular compartment first and rapidly enough, hypovolemia will occur. The fluid loss is borne by the vascular compartment, and fluid replacement from the interstitium cannot keep pace with the loss. For isotonic fluid loss to produce shock, several liters must be lost in a few hours.[26] Hemorrhage, plasma loss, acute gastric dilation, and massive diarrhea can quickly produce hypovolemia. A slow loss of extracellular fluid volume allows replacement of fluid to the vascular compartment from the interstitium. As with rapid loss, sodium and water are lost equally, resulting in minimal change in the concentration of body fluid.

Isotonic volume loss may occur when the kidney tubules lose their discriminating reabsorptive function. This occurs with such conditions as acute tubular necrosis and salt-losing nephritis and during the diuretic postoperative phase.

Diseases of the gastrointestinal tract provide several ways for the body to lose extracellular fluid: vomiting, diarrhea, fistula formation, and obstruction. Gastritis, enteritis, colitis, pseudomembranous enterocolitis, typhoid fever, cholera, and salmonellosis are examples of diseases that cause extracellular fluid loss via vomiting and/or diarrhea. A fistula caused by infection or surgical procedure that allows external drainage of gastrointestinal secretions will also produce loss of extracellular fluid volume.[6]

An obstruction in the gastrointestinal tract caused by a tumor, stricture, adhesion, incarcerated hernia, or paralytic ileus can produce sequestration of fluid. The fluid accumulated in the gastrointestinal tract is lost to the cycling fluid of the body. An extensive burn is also an avenue for loss of isotonic fluid.

Behavioral definition of isotonic volume deficit

Objective data. If several liters of isotonic fluid are lost within a few hours, shock will result. Chapter 15 discusses this concept.

Sunken cheeks, furred tongue, loss of skin turgor, and oliguria will be present with a fluid loss of about 3 L /day. The output of urine will be scanty and highly concentrated. Specific gravity of this urine may be between 1.020 and 1.040, or 1200 and 1400 mOsm/L. Since sodium is being reabsorbed as a result of aldosterone's efforts to maintain vascular volume, the urine sodium levels will decrease.[26]

If the isotonic loss is due to intestinal obstruction, abdominal girth will increase without weight loss. Initially, with an obstruction there will be increased bowel sounds from the efforts of the gut to move its contents forward. As the gut tires, bowel sounds will decrease and the gut will become silent.

A loss in weight will occur if the sodium and water leave the body. Weight loss caused by lack of caloric intake is usually limited to about 150 to 300 g/day. Weight loss greater than 300 g/day can be considered caused by fluid loss.[26]

Serum electrolytes are normal in the early course of the volume deficit, but the hematocrit level will rise in proportion to the fluid deficit. If the volume lost is pure plasma, hematocrit readings will increase 1%/100 ml of plasma loss.[26]

The continued reduction in extracellular fluid volume leads to hypotonicity, since the homeostatic mechanism of replenishing volume overrides the need to maintain tonicity. If the antecedent condition involves the gastrointestinal tract, there will probably be no fluid intake so that oxidation of body fat and protein produces water with no salts. The water is judiciously saved by the kidneys and results in hypotonicity in the extracellular fluid, which then moves into the cells. Increased intracranial pressure results from the increased volume of the cerebral cells. These signs are considered in the discussion of hypotonic volume disorders.

Subjective data. The person with isotonic volume loss will complain of thirst and a dry mouth. Complaints of lethargy and tiredness are common as hypotonicity develops.

HYPERTONIC VOLUME DISORDERS

Conceptual definition

In hypertonic volume disorders either more water than solutes have been lost or more solutes than water have been added to the body fluid. In the first instance the body fluid volume will be decreased. A decrease in body fluid will eventually occur in the second instance if it is not corrected. In each instance the hypertonicity of the extracellular compartments draws water from the cells to equalize the tonicity between compartments.

Antecedent conditions of hypertonic solute excess

Hypertonicity results when there is an excessive amount of solute such as sodium, protein, glucose, or dextrose in the plasma and interstitium. The increase in the solutes necessitates extra water so the kidneys can excrete the solute load. This water is drawn from the cells to equalize the tonicity between compartments if it is not supplied by exogenous means. The plasma volume is maintained at the expense of cell volume.

A frequent antecedent condition to this disorder is the administration of a high-protein, high-salt tube feeding without sufficient water.[13] The mistaken substitution of salt for sugar in infant formula has had dire results.[11] Persons who have an upper gastrointestinal tract hemorrhage will receive a high-protein intake from the blood. Treatment with cream or milk further adds to the body's protein load. A person with uncontrolled diabetes mellitus can develop an extremely high serum glucose level that pulls water into the vascular space. All these conditions create osmotic diuresis, which is the excretion of water by the kidney caused by the excess plasma volume. The excess plasma volume results from the hypertonicity of the plasma.

Behavioral definition of hypertonic solute excess

Objective data. A high serum sodium concentration (160 mEq/L) with a large amount of nonelectrolyte solute in the form of glucose or protein is a common finding. The plasma nonelectrolyte tonicity may be 40 mOsm/L. (The normal is about 5 to 10 mOsm/L.)[25]

A high volume of urine at a fixed osmolality of about 750 mOsm/L is an important finding when combined with serum hypertonicity. Under normal circumstances serum hypertonicity should produce a concentrated urine.[26]

Temperature may be elevated. The central nervous system is affected as in hypertonicity caused by water loss.

Subjective data. The person may express a feeling of anxiety yet be very tired. The person may also complain of thirst.

Antecedent conditions of hypertonic volume deficit

The loss of water in excess of solute occurs in three ways. The lungs normally lose about 600 to 800 ml of pure water/day through respiration. Perspiration is about one-third normal saline solution, and the kidney is able to excrete dilute urine. Increased respiration, like fever, can increase water loss by as much as threefold. Diaphoresis will cause loss of hypotonic fluid. If skin permeability is altered such as in burns, the loss of pure water is greatly increased.

Diabetes insipidus, which results in deficient ADH secretion, or a kidney that does not respond to ADH can cause fluid loss resulting in hypertonicity. An example of an unresponsive kidney occurs during the recovery phase of acute tubular necrosis. Methoxyflurane (Penthrane) anesthesia can also cause the kidneys to be refractory to ADH, which results in diuresis.[16] Lack of access to water and the inability to perceive or indicate thirst are also antecedents.

Behavioral definition of hypertonic volume deficit

Objective data. The loss of water or hypotonic fluids by the lungs or skin results in a scanty urine output with a high specific gravity. If the loss of water is a result of poor kidney function, the urine output will be high with a low specific gravity.

The serum sodium and bicarbonate levels are elevated because of the contraction of the extracellular fluid volume. The hypernatremia pulls water out of the cells. The effects of this fluid movement are particularly prominent in the central nervous system. With the movement of water out of the cells, the brain shrinks in size, and a negative pressure between it and the rigid cranium results. A depressed fontanel reflects this state in the young child. Tears in small veins of the cranium may result, producing hemorrhages that compound the fluid imbalance problem.[1,11]

Although lethargy and restlessness predominate, irritability and hyperactivity occur when the person is stimulated to respond. The irritability is evident in the young child, who often has an accompanying high-pitched cry.[1] Hallucinations, delusions, and disorientation are not uncommon. Hyperreflexia is present, representing the changes in the conductivity of the cell membrane. Signs of shock will not occur until the terminal stages, when the vascular volume can no longer be replaced by fluid from the interstitium and cells.

Subjective data. Feelings of anxiety and fear may be expressed by the person with hypertonicity and fluid volume loss. Complaints of thirst are common.

HYPOTONIC VOLUME DISORDERS

Conceptual definition

Hypotonicity results from water in excess of solutes in the extracellular fluid. Too much water (water intoxication) or nonreplacement of lost solute leads to hypotonicity. When hypotonicity occurs in the extracellular fluid compartment, water will move from the vascular space and interstitium into the cells. The cells require more area as they increase in volume. Since space is limited in the cranium, interference with central nervous system functioning occurs.

Antecedent conditions of hypotonic volume excess

Excessive ADH secretion is frequently an antecedent condition of hypotonicity with an increase in the volume of water. Psychological and/or physiological stress precipitated by fear and pain and administration of analgesics, anesthetics, and a host of other medications can cause increased ADH secretion. Drugs like cyclophosphamide (Cytoxan), morphine, meperidine hydrochloride (Demerol), amitriptyline hydrochloride (Elavil), thioridazine hydrochloride (Mellaril), and thiothixene hydrochloride (Navane) are able to stimulate ADH secretion.[16] Hypotonicity is common 12 to 36 hours after surgery, when ADH secretion is elevated and the patient is receiving hypotonic intravenous solutions. Tumors in body tissues such as oat cell of the lung can abnormally secrete ADH. Cerebral infections or trauma can stimulate ADH secretion.[15]

A gradual accumulation of water may occur in chronic caloric starvation, in which a person is not able to eat an adequate diet because of such conditions as gastrointestinal tract obstruction or long-standing cancer. Renal failure, if unrecognized, can lead to hypotonicity if fluid intake is not limited and the low urine output is not noticed.

Behavioral definition of hypotonic volume excess

Objective data. The serum sodium concentration is decreased. Every 3 mEq/L of serum sodium under normal represents 1 L of retained water in the average adults.[26] However, the usual signs of fluid retention such as edema and weight gain may be obscured. Weight gain caused by fluid retention may be offset by weight loss caused by starvation. Edema will be less obvious if the fluid gain is due to pure water, since pure water excess will be distributed to all compartments, not just extracellular ones. A unique sign of cellular volume increase is "fingerprinting." Because of the plasticity of the tissues, a fingerprint in the tissue over the sternum or tibia is retained.

Laboratory findings show a reduction in hemoglobin level because of the dilution effect. The shift of water into the red blood cells causes the mean corpuscular volume (MCV) to be increased. The hematocrit level remains unchanged because the expansion of water affects the red blood cells as well as the plasma. The serum sodium concentration is between 115 and 130 mEq/L.[25] Dilution of other plasma solutes can result in reduction of plasma tonicity to about 260 mOsm/L. Reduction of the serum sodium concentration affects the conduction of nerve impulses. Isolated muscle twitching, muscle weakness, and hyporeflexia are common signs.

The excretion of urine is decreased, and its specific gravity is low. The renal tubules are responding to increased aldosterone in an effort to retain sodium, which results in water retention as well.

As the water moves into the cerebral cells and causes increased intracranial pressure, confusion and disorientation appear. Loss of attention, incoordination, aphasia, hemiplegia, and papilledema can occur. If the movement of water is rapid or of large volume, convulsions, coma, and hypotension result.

Subjective data. The person with a low serum sodium concentration will complain of being extremely tired and loath to move. It takes much effort to engage in any physical activity. A feeling of doom or apprehension may be expressed. Abdominal cramps may be present, along with impaired sensation of taste and anorexia.[1]

Antecedent conditions of hypotonic volume deficit

Hypotonicity with fluid loss is secondary to isotonic fluid loss because there is no way to lose volumes of hypertonic fluid or solid solutes from the body.[26] The lost isotonic fluid is partially replaced with hypotonic fluid resulting from the secretion of ADH. When the water enters the vascular system, most of it will move through the interstitium into the cells. The extracellular fluid deficit persists, and the cells become swollen.

It is more important for the body to maintain volume than to maintain tonicity. Consequently, ADH saves the water that has been ingested, has been administered by intravenous solutions, or has come from oxidation of protein and fat when there has been no caloric intake.

If patients who have lost isotonic fluids are allowed to drink only water or their nasogastric tubes are repeatedly flushed with water, the concentration of serum sodium will be lowered. The same is true in the instance of diaphoresis when the fluid replacement is only water. Overzealous administration of diuretics can cause loss of sodium in excess of water, producing hypotonicity.[10,29]

Behavioral definition of hypotonic volume deficit

Objective data. The hematocrit level will be increased by the movement of water into the erythrocytes, which enlarges them, and by the movement of water out of the vascular channels to the area of higher tonicity in the tissue cells. As a result, the erythrocytes occupy more space in the reduced volume of plasma. Contraction of the vascular volume, if severe enough, can cause hypotension, rapid, low-volume pulse, and cold, clammy skin.

The signs caused by the lowered concentration of sodium and increased intracranial pressure are the same as those which occur with hypotonic volume excess.

Subjective data. The feelings experienced by the person will essentially be the same as those found with hypotonic volume excess.

POTASSIUM DISORDERS

Conceptual definition

Other ions in addition to sodium have profound effects on the excitatory properties of nerve and muscle cell membrane. Although the extracellular concentration of potassium and calcium is low, small variations in their concentrations can have a great impact on the body's functioning.

Potassium, a cation with a high intracellular concentration, has a concentration range of 3.5 to 5.0 mEq/L extracellularly. Its most important physiological functions are its effect on transmembrane potential and its role in intracellular ionic strength. In addition, potassium has specific functions in cellular metabolism, particularly in protein and glycogen synthesis.[6]

Potassium balance is controlled by intake and renal excretion. About 80% of potassium excretion depends on glomerular filtration and tubular secretion, which are the most important determinants of potassium concentration in extracellular fluid. Usually the amount of potassium ingested equals that excreted in the urine plus that excreted in the feces.[6] In cases of increased intake of potassium, increased renal excretion and increased cellular uptake of potassium, stimulated by insulin, work to maintain normal serum levels.

Antecedent conditions of hyperkalemia

Hyperkalemia is frequently caused by decreased renal excretion or a shift of potassium out of the cells because of acidosis. Renal failure, aldosterone deficiency, and the administration of potassium-sparing diuretics such as triamterene (Dyrenium) and spironolactone (Aldactone) can increase serum potassium concentration.

The release of potassium from the cells is brought about by two means. One is the destruction of the cell membrane by crushing injuries or by burns. Second, potassium ions are exchanged for the extracellular hydrogen ions when acidosis occurs.

Causes of hyperkalemia include excessive or rapid intravenous infusion of potassium chloride, large doses of penicillin G, which contains potassium ions, and rapid infusion of a large volume of bank blood.[15] A diet high in potassium coupled with normal kidney function will generally not produce hyperkalemia because of the slow absorption of potassium from the gut.[26]

Behavioral definition of hyperkalemia

Objective data. The extracellular accumulation of potassium is particularly ominous because of its effect on cardiac conductivity. Increases in extracellar potassium produce depolarization and loss of excitability of myocardial cells. If the potassium excess is severe enough, cardiac arrest in diastole will result. The ECG shows increased vertical amplitude of the T waves and atrioventricular block. As the concentration of potassium ions increases, the P waves disappear and the QRS complex spreads, with death following. The concentration of potassium at this point is about 10 to 12 mEq/L. The heart rate may be slow and regular.[15] In severe hyperkalemia flaccid muscle paralysis develops in the legs and later ascends to the trunk and arms. Diarrhea may be present because of hyperactivity of the intestines.

Subjective data. Vague muscle weakness and tingling of the hands, feet, face, and tongue are often expressed by individuals with hyperkalemia. Abdominal cramps and nausea may be other complaints.

Antecedent conditions of hypokalemia

A serum level of potassium of less than 3.0 mEq/L can result from a shift of potassium into the cells or excessive losses of total body potassium. Potassium deficit can damage cardiac and muscle cells and renal tubules.

The shift of potassium into the cell is often seen in respiratory and metabolic alkalosis. It is hypothesized that the intracellular hydrogen ion exchanges with the extracellular potassium ion to maintain the extracellular pH. Because potassium enters the cell with glucose and insulin, administration of these substances to correct diabetic acidosis will lower serum potassium concentration. Hypokalemia periodic paralysis, a rare familial disease, seems to result from unexplained movement of potassium into the cells.

Excessive losses of potassium can occur via vomiting, diarrhea, or renal excretion. Poor intake at the time of the gastrointestinal tract disturbance adds to the problem. Villous adenoma, pancreatic cholera, and abuse of enemas or laxatives can all result in large losses of potassium. As diarrheal volume increases, its concentration of potassium approaches the concentration of potassium in the plasma.[6]

Increased aldosterone secretion, such as in primary hyperaldosteronism, and excess glucocorticoid that has mineral corticoid activity can cause excess renal excretion, producing hypokalemia. Some ectopic adrenocorticotropic hormone–secreting (ACTH-secreting) tumors, adrenal cancer, and administration of ACTH cause retention of sodium and excretion of potassium. Excessive renin production such as in renal vascular hypertension or a renin-secreting tumor increases aldosterone activity, which in turn reduces the level of serum potassium.[27] Urinary loss of potassium occurs during the diuretic phase of recovery from surgery, burns, and acute renal failure. Loss of significant quantities of potassium through the skin can occur when exercising is done in a hot environment or full-thickness burns have been incurred.

The use of diuretics in the treatment of nonedematous, hypertensive individuals seems to cause hypokalemia more frequently than in edematous patients. The thiazide derivatives furosemide and ethacrynic acid can induce substantial losses of potassium. A diet consistantly low in potassium can eventually cause hypokalemia, as can a diet high in licorice.[22]

Behavioral definition of hypokalemia

Objective data. Hypokalemia is usually associated with increased membrane potential, which results in slowed transmission of impulses. Impaired neuromuscular function, ranging from weakness to paralysis, and interference with cardiac conductivity are common signs of reduced extracellular potassium. The most common types of arrhythmias produced by hypokalemia are supraventricular and ventricular ectopic beats and tachycardia, atrioventricular conduction disturbances, and ventricular fibrillation. The ECG shows low, flattened T waves, depressed ST segments, and prominent U waves.[15] The occurrence of these arrhythmias is increased if digitalis is being administered because low potassium levels accentuate the effects of digitalis.

Intestinal dilation and paralytic ileus result from the decrease in impulse conduction throughout the gut. Shallow respirations can occur because of weakened respiratory muscles. Reflexes are decreased. If the hypokalemia is chronic, polyuria can occur because of renal cell functional impairment. The renal tubules are unable to respond to ADH because of changes in chemical interactions owing to lack of potassium.[27]

CALCIUM DISORDERS

Conceptual definition

Normal calcium concentration in the plasma ranges from 4.4 to 5.4 mEq/L (9 to 11 mg/100 ml). Plasma calcium comprises ionized, nonionized, and protein-bound components. The ionized and protein-bound components contribute the greatest share. However, it is the ionized calcium that requires control within narrow limits because of its physiological influence on the threshold potential of the neuromuscular cell membrane.[27]

Calcium homeostasis is maintained by mechanisms that regulate calcium exchange between the extracellular fluid and the bone, kidney, and intestine. The major regulation comes from the parathyroid hormone (PTH) and vitamin D. These two substances cause release of calcium from the bone, enhance absorption of calcium from the intestine, and enhance reabsorption of calcium by the kidney. Calcitonin and glucocorticoid have the opposite effect. Physical stress on bone stimulates bone deposition, and the growth hormone enhances absorption of calcium from the gut. The thyroid hormone decreases intestinal absorption and enhances renal excretion of calcium. Changes in the acid-base status of the body fluid affect renal excretion of calcium. Both metabolic and respiratory acidoses increase renal excretion of calcium, whereas metabolic and respiratory alkaloses reduce it. In addition, if the concentration of plasma calcium is high, renal calcium excretion will be increased. Conversely, a low plasma calcium concentration will reduce renal excretion of calcium.[6]

Antecedent conditions of hypercalcemia

The body is not as well prepared to deal with increased concentration of calcium in the extracellular fluid as it is to deal with hypocalcemia. Hypercalcemia may stimulate thyrocalcitonin to decrease bone reabsorption. Renal excretion can aid in reducing serum calcium concentration, but often the kidney is hampered by dehydration owing to concomitant disorders. An elevation in serum calcium increases the difference in electronegativity between the resting and threshold potentials of the cell membrane. This causes the membrane to be less excitable.[27]

Metastatic tumors of bone are the most frequent causes of hypercalcemia. Destruction of the bone releases calium into the extracellular fluid. Immobilization prevents stress on bones, which causes bone loss of calcium. Excessive parathyroid activity, usually caused by a tumor of the glands, removes calcium from the bones. If severe enough, the weakened bones may fracture. A high intake of vitamin D, hyperthyroidism, milk-alkali syndrome, and acute and chronic renal failure are antecedents of hypercalcemia.

Behavioral definition of hypercalcemia

Objective data. The effects on the neuromuscular system result in generalized muscle weakness, decreased reflexes, and drowsiness. Severe hypercalcemia can result in stupor. Gastrointestinal tract effects of reduced stimulation include vomiting, constipation, and possible ileus. Renal stones may be formed from precipitation of calcium phosphate or calcium oxalate in the urine. The plasma concentration of calcium is above 5.4 mEq/L.

As with potassium imbalance, hypercalcemia can affect the cardiac muscle. Prolongation of the PR interval and atrioventricular blocks have been reported.[12]

Subjective data. The person with hypercalcemia complains of being tired and listless, having no appetite, feeling full, and/or being nauseous. Fatigue and difficulty in thinking may be expressed. Flank pain caused by nephrolithiasis and bone pain caused by loss of calcium may be reported.

Antecedent conditions of hypocalcemia

Any lowering of blood calcium concentration results in immediate action of PTH to cause reabsorption of calcium from bone to raise plasma levels. Hypocalcemia increases the negativity of the threshold potential, which decreases the difference in electronegativity between the resting and threshold potentials. This makes the cell membrane more excitable.[27]

Major antecedents for hypocalcemia are decreased parathyroid activity, vitamin D deficiency, and lack of calcum intake. Decreased PTH activity can be caused by surgical removal of the glands, thymic and immune deficiency states, and renal resistance to PTH.

Poor intestinal absorption of calcium and reduced effectiveness of PTH can be induced by vitamin D deficiency. Lack of vitamin D ingestion, no exposure to sunlight, malabsorption of vitamin D, and nutritional deficiency of calcium are factors that lower calcium plasma concentration. Hyperphosphatemia related to renal insufficiency and rapid or overcorrection of acidosis with sodium bicarbonate can reduce the serum calcium level. Transfusion with citrated blood can lower the plasma concentration of calcium.[6]

Behavioral definition of hypocalcemia

Objective data. The most profound signs of hypocalcemia are the neuromuscular reactions of tetany, muscle cramps, carpopedal spasms, laryngeal spasms, and convulsions. Emotional irritability and mild depression may also be apparent.

A plasma calcium level less than 4.4 mEq/L indicates a low concentration; however, values above the level do not rule out a low ionized calcium concentration. The plasma calcium value includes the three components, and the amount of plasma protein can alter the value. The urinary Sulkowitch test can be useful in determining the level of calcium excretion. Hypocalcemia is indicated by no precipitation of calcium oxalate in the urine. The specific changes in the ECG can be prolonged QT interval secondary to prolongation of the ST segment.[6]

Subjective data. Tingling and numbness of the hands, feet, and lips are common. The person is unable to prevent the spasms. Muscles hurt from the cramping. The person may experience fright and loss of control.

INTERVENING VARIABLES

The intervening variables apply to all types of fluid and electrolyte imbalance. The reserve of the body systems and the amount and rate of change have a profound effect on the outcome of imbalances.

Body reserve

The reserve of the body is affected by disease processes and age. Although disease processes are antecedents of fluid and electrolyte imbalance, they can also act as intervening variables. If the body has compensated for an organ that has borderline function, a stable but delicately balanced situation exists. If another disease process or an environmental event interrupts the steady-state situation, a more profound disruption will occur because of the lack of flexibility or reserve. For example, a person who has compensated heart failure may be given intravenous fluids in excess of what the heart can circulate, producing pulmonary edema. The same amount of fluid could be given to a person with normal cardiac function with negligible effects.

Chronic diseases that affect the functioning of the heart, kidneys, and lungs necessitate accurate and careful supervision of fluid therapy because of the danger of circulatory system overload or underload.

Age

The young and the elderly are particularly vulnerable to changes in fluid and electrolyte balance. The young are vulnerable because of their high metabolic rate, large surface area in relation to body mass, and distribution of body fluids. The elderly are vulnerable because of lower reserves owing to cellular changes and increased incidence of chronic disease.

A 6-month-old child's body weight is composed of almost 70% water as compared to 60% in a man. Another difference is the higher ratio of extracellular to intracellular fluid in the child. As a result, more of the child's body fluid than the adult's interfaces with the environment, gastrointestinal tract, lungs, and kidneys. There is also a greater exchange of total body fluid per day by the child than the adult.[19,28] These factors place the child in a precarious position when fluid imbalances are not treated according to the pace or amount needed by the child.

The elderly are vulnerable for different reasons. In aging, cellular activity is reduced because of decreased regional blood flow and tissue perfusion. The critical organs affected are the heart and kidneys. The heart can be spared from overexertion, whereas the kidneys have no means for reduction of work. To maintain its function, the kidney must have an unimpaired blood supply. Vascular changes and fibrotic rigidity, which increase with age, often curb the functional capacity of the kidney.[3,14] The subclinical changes in the tissues of the elderly become apparent when stress occurs. In addition, the elderly have a smaller ratio of total body water to weight than do younger people. This means that a specific amount of fluid loss will create more of a deficit in the elderly person than in a younger person. However, the average water requirement for the elderly is 25 ml/kg/day compared to 35 ml/kg/day for average adults aged 22 to 55 years in a temperate climate.[3] This decrease in requirements makes the elderly prone to overhydration.

Rate and amount of change

The rate and amount of loss or gain has a decided effect on the treatment and outcome of the imbalance. Rapid losses of body fluid come almost entirely from the extracellular fluid compartment. Signs and symptoms range from thirst and oliguria to vascular collapse, depending on the amount of fluid lost. In the adult, extracellular fluid comprises about 23% of the body weight. A 2% loss of body weight owing to fluid loss will cause thrist and oliguria. A 5% to 10% loss of body weight owing to fluid loss can result in tachycardia and postural hypotension. A 10% to 15% loss of body weight owing to fluid loss can produce stupor and shock.[6]

The loss of body fluid over a period of days rather than in a short time results in a more even volume distribution between the extracellular and intracellular compartments. As a result, the effects are less severe. Fluid from the intracellular compartment has time to move into the extracellular compartment, namely the vascular system, which prevents vascular collapse.

The gains and losses of body fluid handled easily by healthy people can have severe consequences in people with little reserve. Rapid, large changes will not be tolerated as well by a person with decreased reserve.

NURSING INTERVENTIONS—GOALS AND EVALUATION CRITERIA

The overall goal for nursing intervention is to maintain or reestablish fluid and electrolyte balance. Although monitoring the patient's condition is of prime importance in achieving these goals, nursing intervention involves more than keeping a record of fluid intake and output. The nurse must place fluid intake and output in the context of the patient situation. The nurse must have some idea of the amount, type, and rate of fluid intake and output that is required by the patient. This is not to say that the nurse will be prescribing fluid or electrolyte replacement, but the alertness of the nurse to changes in the patient's condition can often prevent imbalances or lessen the intensity of an imbalance.

Prevention or reduction of fluid overload

Patients with chronic diseases affecting the heart, lungs, or kidneys are primary candidates for overhydration. One of the goals for these patients is to prevent the accumulation of excessive fluid. These patients should receive instructions regarding the effects of sodium in the diet, the use of potassium supplements, the use of medications that affect cardiac function and water excretion, and the planning of activities. It is important for these patients to be able to recognize the following symptoms indicative of excessive fluid accumulation: increasing fatigue, weight gain without diet change, chest pains, difficulty breathing, and edema.

When the patient is available for monitoring the nurse should assess the following indicators of fluid volume excess at least daily: adventitious lung sounds; increased body weight; edema, particularly pitting edema; and decreased energy levels and mentation. Body weight should, of course, be obtained at the same time each day, after the patient has voided, and with the patient dressed in like clothing.

When the patient accumulates an excessive fluid volume, the goal is to help reduce this volume. The nurse should closely monitor the effectiveness of medications administered to increase fluid excretion. To make judgments about medication effectiveness and assist the patient in comfortably adjusting to the response, the nurse must know the expected action. For instance, when furosemide (Lasix) is given intravenously, urine output should begin to increase dramatically within 5 to 30 minutes. The patient should be informed of this usual response, and a bedpan, commode, or bathroom should be made available for the patient's use. The patient should also be informed of the necessity for accurate measurement of the output and told how to save the urine until the measurement is obtained. If the patient has a urinary catheter, the collection bag should be emptied frequently to prevent overflow. A timed urine output is often measured to obtain a time profile of the kidneys' output response. If the patient does not experience diuresis, the physician should be notified.

If the patient's condition necessitates restriction of the amount of fluid ingested, the patient should assist in planning the distribution of fluid ingestion throughout the day. The amount of fluid to be ingested at meals and between meals should be considered. Including the patient in these decisions not only helps the patient gain a better understanding of the regimen, but allows the patient to modify the plan in a way that may increase compliance with the regimen. The patient and family must, of course, understand how important it is to measure the intake and how to do so accurately.

When restricted amounts of fluid are to be administered intravenously, equipment must be used that will prevent the accidental administration of large amounts of fluid. The minidripper and the 100 ml drip chambers of Metroset equipment or an automatic infusion pump can provide this type of protection.

Behavioral criteria that indicate that fluid overload has been prevented or reduced include reduction in weight or lack of weight gain, decrease or absence of adventitious lung sounds, fading of extra heart sounds, reduction in or absence of edema, reduced incidence of fatigue, and urinary output that equals the volume of fluid intake.

Prevention of fluid deficit

Patients who have high risks for dehydration, the elderly and the young, are also the people who are usually the least able to freely obtain water for their own needs. Another group of patients who have a high risk of fluid loss are those whose fluid needs change quickly because of renal function or fluid compartmental shifts. Postoperative patients and patients recovering from acute renal failure or burns are in this group. It is essential to base intervention activities for fluid balancing on intake and output measurements that include insensible fluid losses.

When a patient is capable of oral ingestion and is not on a restricted fluid regimen, a supply of fluid should always be available. Fluid ingestion should be scheduled for high risk patients. It should not be assumed that these patients will meet their fluid needs without assistance. The patient should be included in the planning so that preferred fluids can be made available at the times the patient would be most likely to enjoy them. The elderly often ingest larger amounts of fluid most comfortably during the morning. As the day progresses, they usually ingest smaller and smaller amounts of fluid. Plans that include two thirds of the fluid ingestion goal by the noon meal take advantage of such drinking patterns.

The full range of fluid sources should be considered. Pudding, Jell-O, ice cream, soup, and Popsicles are sources of fluids that are often overlooked. If the patient is a child, the inclusion of fluid ingestion during play can assist in increasing fluid volume. Tea parties with real fluid instead of pretend tea or Popsicles with TV watching can often increase fluid ingestion.

When patients lose fluid by vomiting, an antiemetic such as prochlorperazine maleate (Compazine) may be administered intramuscularly. Although such medication will not restore appetite, it should reduce the loss of fluid by vomiting. If diarrhea is the source of fluid loss, antispasmotics such as diphenoxylate hydrochloride plus atropine (Lomotil), can be given to reduce bowel motility.

When patients receive high-protein tube feedings, enough water must be supplied to decrease the osmotic load presented to the kidneys. This prevents obligatory urine volume loss. Infants receiving prepared formula also need additional water supplements. A cue that osmotic loads are being put through the kidneys is a urinary output exceeding intake in a situation that does not normally produce diuresis.

It is of prime importance to restore the fluid volume of the patient who is dehydrated. The rate and amount of the fluid loss determine the intensity of treatment. When the fluid loss is sudden and great, parenteral fluid replacement requires the type of intravenous equipment that can deliver a large volume of fluid or blood in a short time. A Venoset with a maxidripper and a large-bore needle or catheter meets these requirements.

Behavioral criteria that evidence restoration of fluid include normal blood pressure levels, full pulse volume, filling of the peripheral veins, normal response to stimuli, improved skin turgor, wetness of the mucous membranes, and urinary output that equals fluid intake.

Maintenance of normal potassium levels

Since plasma potassium concentration is related to glomerular filtration rate, a patient who has either a high or low urine output has a risk of potassium imbalance. Supplemental potassium is often administered to a person who has high urine output from a diuretic phase of disease or from movement of potassium into the cells. When potassium is given intravenously, it must be thoroughly mixed and diluted with other fluid to avoid sudden increase in plasma concentration.[16] A potassium bolus should never be administered.

Patients who are being treated with diuretics that cause potassium loss need to increase dietary potassium ingestion. These patients should be instructed to eat foods high in potassium such as bananas, citrus fruits, apricots, dates, and lentils.[23]

If serum potassium levels remain persistently low (3.0 to 3.2 mEq/L), a liquid potassium supplement may need to be used. However, the danger in using potassium supplements is the development of hyperkalemia.[8] The patient must understand why extra potassium is needed and that tiredness, constipation, and irregular cardiac rhythm indicate that their potassium level should be checked.

Common causes for hyperkalemia are too rapid an infusion of potassium, renal failure, and massive tissue trauma. To reduce the level of potassium, a calcium salt, glucose, insulin, and sodium bicarbonate are often administered. Monitoring of ECG changes and neuroconductivity provide parameters regarding treatment effectiveness. Sodium polystyrene sulfonate (Kayexalate), a cation-exchange resin, is often used to reduce the high potassium concentrations that accompany kidney failure. Since Kayexalate can dry and harden in the colon, a laxative should accompany its oral administration.[16]

Evaluative criteria include a serum potassium level in normal limits and an ECG tracing that reflects no abnormalities attributable to altered potassium levels.

Maintenance of normal calcium levels

Serum calcium levels are important for regulation of neuromuscular excitability. The nurse must be aware of situations that have the potential to produce either an excess or depletion of calcium. Investigation of a person's dietary habits can uncover information about calcium and vitamin D excesses or deprivations. Instruction in a balanced diet and provision of alternatives for a person to have balanced meals are the preferred means of dealing with abnormal calcium levels caused by dietary habits. However, if dietary changes will not sufficiently alter the level of calcium, calcium salts may be used as supplements. The usual method of administration is oral ingestion of divided doses with meals. The patient must be informed of the purpose for this medication and be able to recognize the following cues that indicate that an adjustment in dosage is needed: muscle cramps, irritability, and tingling and numbness of extremities.

For emergency situations parenteral calcium salt preparation may be administered. The patient should be warned that a tingling sensation may be produced. Parenteral solutions of calcium chloride should never be injected into tissue because they will cause necrosis and sloughing of that tissue.

Sodium sulfate, prednisone, calcitonin, or mithramycin may be used to reduce hypercalcemia. Edetate disodium is a chelating agent that can reduce the serum calcium level very quickly. It is administered slowly in a dilute parenteral solution.

Behavioral evidence that this goal has been achieved includes general increase in muscle strength, normal reflexes, and an ECG without indications of abnormal calcium effects.

CONCEPT OUTLINE

I. *Conceptual definition:* Fluid and electrolyte imbalances are disruptions in the tonicity or volume of fluid in the intravascular, interstitial, and/or intracellular compartments.

II. *Isotonic volume disorders*
- A. Conceptual definition: An isotonic volume disorder is a state in which equal ratios of solutes and water have been lost or gained.
  - 1. Isotonic volume excess
    - a. Antecedent conditions
      - (1) Rapid intravenous administration of saline solution
      - (2) Diseases of heart, kidneys, and liver
    - b. Behavioral definition
      - (1) Edema
      - (2) Weight gain
      - (3) Increased abdominal girth (with cirrhosis)
      - (4) Pulmonary edema
      - (5) Decreased plasma protein and hematocrit levels
  - 2. Isotonic volume deficit
    - a. Antecedent conditions
      - (1) Vascular fluid loss
        - (a) Hemorrhage
        - (b) Burns
      - (2) Gastrointestinal fluid loss
        - (a) Vomiting, diarrhea
        - (b) Fistula formation
        - (c) Obstruction
        - (d) Gastric dilation
    - b. Behavioral definition
      - (1) Sunken cheek, furred tongue
      - (2) Scanty, concentrated urine if kidneys functional
      - (3) Weight loss
      - (4) Normal electrolyte concentrations at early stage
      - (5) Elevated hematocrit level
      - (6) Increased abdominal girth with obstruction
      - (7) Thirst, dry mouth
      - (8) Tiredness if hypotonicity develops

III. *Hypertonic volume disorders*
- A. Conceptual definition: A hypertonic volume disorder is a state in which more water than solutes have been lost or more solutes than water have been added to body fluids.
  - 1. Hypertonic solute excess
    - a. Antecedent conditions
      - (1) High-protein and high-salt tube feedings without sufficient water
      - (2) Upper gastrointestinal tract hemorrhage with cream or milk treatment
      - (3) High serum glucose level
    - b. Behavioral definition
      - (1) High serum sodium concentration
      - (2) High nonelectrolyte serum solute concentration
      - (3) High volume of urine at fixed osmolality
      - (4) Elevated temperature
      - (5) Signs and symptoms of cerebral hemorrhage
      - (6) Anxiety, fatigue
      - (7) Thirst
  - 2. Hypertonic volume deficit
    - a. Antecedent conditions
      - (1) Fever with increased respiration
      - (2) Diaphoresis
      - (3) ADH lack
      - (4) Kidneys unresponsive to ADH
      - (5) Unavailability of water
      - (6) Inability to perceive or indicate thirst
    - b. Behavioral definition
      - (1) Scanty, concentrated urine
      - (2) High, dilute urine output if kidneys dysfunctional
      - (3) Elevated serum sodium and bicarbonate levels
      - (4) Depressed fontanel
      - (5) High-pitched cry
      - (6) Cerebral hemorrhages
      - (7) Lethargy, restlessness
      - (8) Irritability, anxiety
      - (9) Hyperreflexia
      - (10) Thirst

IV. *Hypotonic volume disorders*
- A. Conceptual definition: A hypotonic volume disorder is a state in which water is in excess of solutes in extracellular fluid because of excess water or loss of solutes.

1. Hypotonic volume excess
   a. Antecedent conditions
      (1) Excessive ADH secretion
         (a) Stress
         (b) Drug administration
         (c) Tumor secretion
      (2) Chronic caloric starvation
   b. Behavioral definition
      (1) Decreased serum sodium level
      (2) Weight gain (may be obscured by weight loss)
      (3) Edema (fingerprinting)
      (4) Reduced hemoglobin level
      (5) Increased mean corpuscular volume
      (6) Unchanged hematocrit level
      (7) Isolated muscle twitching and weakness
      (8) Hyporeflexia
      (9) Low, dilute urine output
      (10) Confusion
      (11) Incoordination
      (12) Aphasia
      (13) Papilledema
      (14) Coma
      (15) Extreme tiredness, apprehension
      (16) Impaired taste, anorexia
2. Hypotonic volume deficit
   a. Antecedent conditions
      (1) Isotonic fluid loss
      (2) Fluid replacement with water only
      (3) Nasogastric tubes flushed with water
      (4) Overzealous administration of diuretics
   b. Behavioral definition
      (1) Elevated hematocrit level
      (2) Hypotension
      (3) Rapid, low-volume pulse
      (4) Cold, clammy skin
      (5) Decreased serum sodium concentration
      (6) Increased intracranial pressure (same as in hypotonic volume excess)

V. *Potassium disorders*
   A. Conceptual definition: A potassium disorder is a state in which serum concentration of potassium is less than 3.5 or greater than 5.0 mEq/L.
      1. Hyperkalemia
         a. Antecedent conditions
            (1) Decreased renal excretion
            (2) Release of potassium from cells
            (3) Exogenous potassium administration
         b. Behavioral definition
            (1) ECG changes
            (2) Flaccid paralysis (severe)
            (3) Diarrhea
            (4) Muscle weakness
            (5) Tingling of hands and feet
            (6) Abdominal cramps
            (7) Nausea
      2. Hypokalemia
         a. Antecedent conditions
            (1) Movement of potassium into the cells
            (2) Excessive fluid loss
               (a) Vomiting
               (b) Diarrhea
               (c) Abuse of enemas or laxatives
               (d) Excessive renal excretion
               (e) Diuretic administration
               (f) Exercise in hot environment
               (g) Full-thickness burns
         b. Behavioral definition
            (1) Weakness, paralysis
            (2) ECG changes
            (3) Intestinal changes
            (4) Intestinal dilation
            (5) Paralytic ileus
            (6) Shallow respirations

VI. *Calcium disorders*
   A. Conceptual definition: A calcium disorder is a state in which serum concentration of calcium is less than 4.4 or greater than 5.4 mEq/L (less than 9 or greater than 11 mg/100 ml).
      1. Hypercalcemia
         a. Antecedent conditions
            (1) Metastatic bone tumors
            (2) Immobilization
            (3) Excessive parathyroid and thyroid activity
            (4) High intake of vitamin D
            (5) Renal failure
         b. Behavioral definition
            (1) Muscle weakness

(2) Decreased reflexes
(3) Drowsiness
(4) Vomiting, constipation, ileus
(5) Renal stones
(6) ECG changes
(7) Listlessness, fatigue
(8) Difficulty in mentation
(9) Flank and bone pain

2. Hypocalcemia
   a. Antecedent conditions
      (1) Decreased parathyroid activity
      (2) Vitamin D deficiency
      (3) Lack of calcium intake
      (4) Renal resistance to PTH
      (5) Transfusion with citrated blood
   b. Behavioral definition
      (1) Tetany, muscle cramps, carpopedal spasms
      (2) Convulsions
      (3) Irritability
      (4) Abnormal urinary Sulkowitch test
      (5) ECG changes
      (6) Tingling and numbness of extremities and lips
      (7) Muscle aches from cramping
      (8) Fear

VII. *Intervening variables*
   A. Body reserve
   B. Age
   C. Rate and amount of change

VIII. *Nursing interventions—goals*
   A. Prevention or reduction of fluid overload
      1. Instruction regarding diet, supplements, and medication
      2. Instruction regarding cues indicating fluid accumulation
      3. Monitoring of medication effectiveness
      4. Planning of fluid ingestion schedule with patient
      5. Use of equipment that prevents accidental excessive administration
   B. Prevention of fluid deficit
      1. Identification of high risk situations
      2. Provision of accessibility of fluids
      3. Planning of fluid ingestion schedule with patient
      4. Use of sufficient water with tube feedings and formulas
      5. Use of equipment that can deliver fluid at rate needed
   C. Maintenance of normal potassium levels
      1. Identification of high risk situations
      2. Observance of urine output rate
      3. Proper mixing and administration of potassium supplements
      4. Instruction regarding potassium content of foods
      5. Instruction regarding cues that indicate potassium imbalance
   D. Maintenance of normal calcium levels
      1. Identification of high risk situations
      2. Instruction regarding cues that indicate adjustment of dosage is needed
      3. Proper administration of calcium preparations
      4. Dietary instruction regarding calcium content of foods
      5. Instruction regarding drugs that reduce serum calcium concentration

IX. *Evaluation criteria*
   A. Clearing of mentation
   B. Return of muscle strength
   C. Reduction in fatigue
   D. Return of vital signs to previous levels
   E. Balanced fluid intake and output
   F. Decreased muscle irritability
   G. Return of previous ECG pattern
   H. Return to normal levels of electrolyte concentrations

REFERENCES

1. Arieff, A. I., and Guisado, R.: Effects on the central nervous system of hypernatremic and hyponatremic states, Kidney Int. **10**:104, 1976.
2. Arieff, A. I., Guisado, R., and Lazarowitz, V. C.: Pathophysiology of hyperosmolar status. In Audreoli, T. E., Groutham, J. J., and Rector, F. C., Jr., editors: Disturbances in body fluid osmolality, Baltimore, 1977, William & Wilkins Co.
3. Behnke, A. R.: Morphologic and metabolic changes associated with aging. In Bland, J. H., editor: Clinical metabolism of body water and electrolytes, Philadelphia, 1963, W. B. Saunders Co.
4. Berne, R. M., and Levy, M. N.: Cardiovascular physiology, St. Louis, 1972, The C. V. Mosby Co.
5. Bland, J. H.: General clinical considerations in water, electrolyte and hydrogen ion metab-

olism. In Bland, J. H., editor: Clinical metabolism of body water and electrolytes, Philadelphia, 1963, W. B. Saunders Co.

6. Carroll, H. J., and Oh, M. S.: Water, electrolyte and acid-base metabolism: diagnosis and management, Philadelphia, 1978, J. B. Lippincott Co.
7. Coleman, T. G., Norman, R. A., Jr., and Manning, R. D., Jr.: Equilibrium between extracellular and intracellular fluid. In Guyton, A. C., Taylor, A. E., and Granger, H. J., editors: Circulatory physiology, vol. II, dynamics and control of the body fluids, Philadelphia, 1975, W. B. Saunders Co.
8. Cronin, R. E., and Knochel, J. P.: The consequences of potassium deficiency. In Brunner, B. M., and Stein, J. H., editors: Acid-base and potassium homeostasis: contemporary issues in nephrology, vol. 2, New York, 1978, Churchill Livingstone, Inc.
9. Crowley, A. W., Jr.: Role of thirst and vasopressin in control of body fluid osmolality and volume. In Guyton, A. C., Taylor, A. E., and Granger, H. J., editors: Circulatory physiology, vol. II, dynamics and control of the body fluids, Philadelphia, 1975, W. B. Saunders Co.
10. Fichman, M. P., Vorherr, H., Kleeman, C. R., and Telfer, N.: Diuretic induced hyponatremia, Ann. Intern. Med. **75**:853, 1971.
11. Finberg, L., Kiley, J., and Lutrell, C. N.: Mass accidental salt poisoning in infancy: a study of a hospital disaster, J.A.M.A. **184**:187, 1963.
12. Fisch, C.: Relation of electrolyte disturbances to cardiac arrhythmias, Circulation **47**:408, 1973.
13. Gault, M. H., Dixon, M. E., Doyle, M., and Cohen, W. M.: Hypernatremia, azotemia, and dehydration due to high protein tube feeding, Ann. Intern. Med. **68**:778, 1968.
14. Glick, S. M.: Preventive medicine in geriatrics, Med. Clin. North Am. **60**:1325, 1976.
15. Goldberger, E.: A primer of water, electrolyte and acid-base syndromes, ed. 5, Philadelphia, 1975, Lea & Febiger.
16. Goodman, L. S., and Gilman, A.: The pharmacological basis of therapeutics, ed. 5, New York, 1975, Macmillan Publishing Co., Inc.
17. Guyton, A. C.: Textbook of medical physiology, ed. 5, Philadelphia, 1976, W. B. Saunders Co.
18. Guyton, A. C., Taylor, A. E., and Granger, H. J.: Interstitial gel: gel pressure and effect of the gel on tissue fluid dynamics. In Guyton, A. C., Taylor, A. E., and Granger, H. J., editors: Circulatory physiology, vol. II, dynamics and control of the body fluids, Philadelphia, 1975, W. B. Saunders, Co.
19. Kerrigan, G. A.: Water and electrolyte metabolism in pediatrics. In Bland, J. H., editor: Clinical metabolism of body water and electrolytes, Philadelphia, 1963, W. B. Saunders Co.
20. Kinmonth, J. B., and Taylor, G. W.: Spontaneous rhythmic contractility in human lympatics, J. Physiol. **133**:3P, 1956.
21. Kinney, J. M., and Moore, F. D.: Surgical metabolism in metabolism of body fluids. In Bland, J. H., editor: Clinical metabolism of body water and electrolytes, Philadelphia, 1963, W. B. Saunders Co.
22. Kliger, A. S., and Hayslett, J. P.: Disorders of potassium balance. In Brenner, B. M., and Stein, J. H., editors: Acid-base and potassium homeostasis: contemporary issues in nephrology, vol. 2, New York, 1978, Churchill Livingstone, Inc.
23. Mazlen, R. G.: Nutrition and cardiovascular disease. In Halpern, S. L., editor: Quick reference to clinical nutrition, Philadelphia, 1979, J. B. Lippincott Co.
24. McCaa, C., and McCaa, R. E.: Role of aldosterone in fluid volume and electrolyte control. In Guyton, A. C., Taylor, A. E., and Granger, H. J. editors: Circulatory physiology, vol. II, dynamics and control of the body fluids, Philadelphia, 1975, W. B. Saunders Co.
25. Moore, F. D.: Fluid and electrolyte management in surgical patients: twenty-one syndromes. In Hardy, J. D., editor: Rhoads textbook of surgery: principles and practice, ed. 5, Philadelphia, 1977, J. B. Lippincott Co.
26. Pestana, C.: Fluids and electrolytes in the surgical patient, Baltimore, 1977, Williams & Wilkins Co.
27. Rose, B. D.: Clinical physiology of acid-base and electrolyte disorders, New York, 1977, McGraw-Hill Book Co.
28. Weil, W. B., Jr., and Bailie, M. D.: Fluid and electrolyte metabolism in infants and children: a unified approach, New York, 1977, Grune & Stratton.
29. Weller, J. M.: Renal disease: water and electrolyte imbalance. In Sodeman, W. A., Jr., and Sodeman, W. A., editors: Pathologic physiology: mechanisms of disease, ed. 5, Philadelphia, 1974, W. B. Saunders Co.

JEAN L. REESE

Chapter 12

ACID-BASE IMBALANCE

CONCEPTUAL DEFINITION

Acid-base imbalance is a state in which there is an excess or deficit of dissociated, or "unbuffered," hydrogen ions in the body fluids. An acid-base imbalance can affect the contractile ability of the heart, decrease peripheral vascular resistance, affect cerebral blood flow, alter the loading of oxygen onto hemoglobin or the unloading of oxygen from hemoglobin into the tissues, and alter the biochemical processes responsible for energy production and use. The maintenance of hydrogen ion concentration in a specific range is necessary for cellular function and the preservation of life.

The hydrogen ion is measured in nanoequivalents (nEq), also called microequivalents. The range of hydrogen ion concentration that is compatible with life is about 20 to 120 nEq/L. The normal range is about 35 to 45 nEq/L, with 40 nEq/L being the average. Ions other than hydrogen are measured in milliequivalents, which denotes one thousandth of a unit, whereas the nanoequivalent is one millionth of a unit. The normal concentration of hydrogen is much less than that of other ions, but it has a sixfold difference in concentration that is compatible with life. The traditional and usual method of measuring hydrogen concentration is by the pH scale. A major problem with this scale is that the measurement is inverted. That is, an increased pH value means decreased hydrogen ion concentration and vice versa. The normal pH of blood is 7.4. A pH of 6.9, which indicates an elevated concentration of hydrogen ions, and a pH of 7.7, which indicates a lowered concentration of hydrogen ions, are the extremes in which humans can survive.[35]

The body is in a state of acidosis when the pH of the blood is less than 7.35 or the concentration of hydrogen ions is greater than 45 nEq/L. A state of alkalosis exists when the pH is greater than 7.44 or the concentration of hydrogen ions is less than 35 nEq/L.

Normal dynamics

Hydrogen ions are constantly produced in huge quantities by cellular metabolism. Because the body can tolerate only a minute concentration of unbuffered, or free, hydrogen ions in its fluids, a vast chemical network exists for the sole purpose of binding hydrogen and removing it from the body. The body's chemical substances are shuffled repeatedly to accept hydrogen ions and control vacillations in their concentration. Hydrogen ions are presented to the regulatory mechanisms in an acidic form, which releases the hydrogen ions for excretion or recombination to a less offensive substance. The original carrier of the hydrogen ion returns to the body fluids as bicarbonate or water, and the cycle is repeated.

Acids, those substances which give hydrogen ions to body fluids, and bases, those substances which can accept hydrogen ions from the body metabolism, are continually added to the body's fluids. The control of hydrogen ion concentration involves three basic processes: (1) intracellular and extracellular chemical buffering,

(2) regulation of carbon dioxide concentration in the blood by changes in the alveolar ventilation rate, and (3) regulation of bicarbonate concentration in the blood by changes in renal hydrogen ion excretion.

Intracellular buffers. Hydrogen ion concentration in the cells is controlled primarily by proteins and phosphates. The many proteins in the cells act as a buffer because they can either accept or release hydrogen ions, depending on the pH of the extracellular fluid. The proteins are polyanions and easily attract the positively charged hydrogen ions.[29]

The intracellular concentration of phosphates, particularly in the red blood cells and kidney tubules, adds to the buffering power. For example, monohydrogen phosphate (HPO_4) and dihydrogen phosphate (H_2PO_4) are able to reduce the strong acid hydrogen chloride (HCl) or the strong base sodium hydroxide (NaOH) to more neutral substances, respectively.

The red blood cell contains two negatively charged substances, hemoglobin and bicarbonate. Hemoglobin carries about 95% of the carbon dioxide that is metabolized from the tissue cells, and 5% remains dissolved in the plasma. Carbon dioxide will diffuse into the red blood cell when the plasma concentration of carbon dioxide exceeds that in the erythrocyte. In the erythrocyte, carbon dioxide with the catalyzing effect of carbonic anhydrase combines with water ($CO_2 + H_2O \rightarrow H_2CO_3$). The resulting carbonic acid then dissociates into hydrogen and bicarbonate ($H_2CO_3 \rightarrow H^+ + HCO_3^-$). The free hydrogen ion attaches to the hemoglobin, and the bicarbonate attaches to the intracellular potassium. When the bicarbonate concentration in the cell exceeds that in the plasma, bicarbonate diffuses into the plasma and exchanges with negatively charged chloride from the plasma. This exchange, called the chloride shift, maintains electroneutrality, or the equal matching of cations and anions on each side of the cell membrane. The chloride attaches to the potassium in the cell and forms potassium chloride (KCl).[12,13]

When the reduced hemoglobin is oxygenated in the alveolar capillaries, it reacts with potassium bicarbonate to form carbonic acid. The carbonic acid is then reduced to carbon dioxide and water. The carbon dioxide is exhaled, and the water remains in the body fluids ($H_2CO_3 \rightarrow H_2O + CO_2$). The chloride ion returns to the plasma, and potassium bicarbonate is reformed.[12,44] (See Fig. 4.)

Intracellular buffering affects the movement of other positively charged ions, notably potassium and sodium. The law of electroneutrality requires that if an ion moves from one fluid compartment to another, it must be replaced by an ion of like charge. When hydrogen concentration is reduced extracellularly, hydrogen ions released from the intracellular anions move to the extracellular fluid. In exchange for a hydrogen ion, either a potassium or sodium ion from the extracellular fluid will move into the cell. A reduction in plasma potassium and sodium concentrations results. Conversely, if extracellular hydrogen ion concentration is high, the hydrogen ions will diffuse into the cells and cause sodium and potassium to move to the extracellular fluid.[34,39] The plasma concentration of potassium is much more vulnerable to variation with the compartmental shifts of the hydrogen ion than is the sodium concentration. This is due to its low extracellular concentration. Small shifts profoundly affect potassium concentration, whereas they have negligible effect on sodium concentration.

The concentration of hydrogen ions even varies in the cell itself. Different compartments of the cell accept hydrogen ions at different rates and have optimum concentrations of hydrogen ions for specific enzymatic actions.[4]

Extracellular buffers. There are three main extracellular buffers: phosphates, proteins, and bicarbonates. Since phosphate and protein concentrations are much lower extracellularly, their buffering effects are much less in this compartment. The bicarbonate buffer system is very effective in this compartment because it can be regulated by both the lungs and the kidneys.

The normal ratio of bicarbonate to carbonic acid in the extracellular fluid is 20:1. Changes in the concentration of one element without a similar change in the other will result in an altered pH. An increase in bicarbonate without an increase in carbonic acid concentration, or a reduction in carbonic acid without a reduction

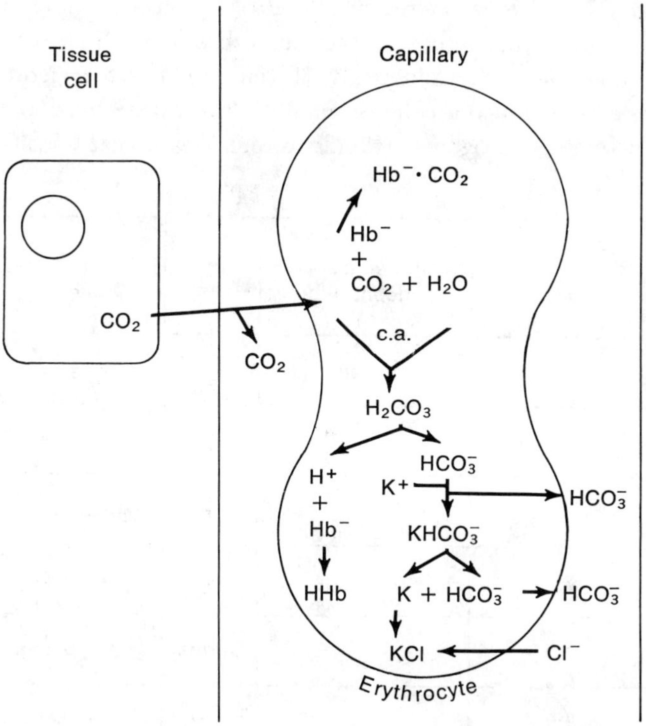

FIG. 4. Carbon dioxide blood transport and chloride shift.

in bicarbonate concentration, will cause an increase in pH. This produces a state of alkalosis. The opposite effect is an increase in carbonic acid concentration without a bicarbonate increase, or a decrease in bicarbonate without a decrease in carbonic acid, which produces a decrease in pH. This causes a state of acidosis.

When the concentrations of both bicarbonate and carbonic acid are elevated or decreased but a ratio of 20:1 is maintained, the pH remains normal. (See Fig. 5.)

Control of plasma levels of carbonic acid. Carbon dioxide is constantly produced by cellular metabolism. Minute amounts of it are dissolved in the plasma, with the bulk of it entering the red blood cells. Yet, the small amount that remains in the plasma determines the gradient that controls the entrance and exit of carbon dioxide to and from the blood. The average normal pressure of gaseous carbon dioxide ($PaCO_2$) in the arterial blood is 40 mm Hg, with a normal range of 35 to 45 mm Hg. The relationship of carbonic acid (H_2CO_3) concentration to carbon dioxide partial pressure ($PaCO_2$) is nearly equivalent, so a measurement of blood PCO_2 is like a measurement of plasma carbonic acid concentration.[43]

Removal of the carbon dioxide by ventilation controls the concentration of carbonic acid in the plasma ($H_2CO_3 \leftrightarrow H_2O + CO_2$). Hence a high $PaCO_2$ reflects hypoventilation, and a low $PaCO_2$ reflects hyperventilation. Although intracellular buffering and increased renal excretion of hydrogen ions can move the pH toward normal if ventilation is ineffective, the acid-base balance will not be restored until ventilation becomes normal. Conversely, if ventilation is too vigorous, hydrogen ions will be released from the cells to maintain the extracellular pH. The kidney will eventually retain hydrogen ions and excrete bicarbonate to offset the loss of

Bicarbonate concentration	Carbonic acid concentration	pH	Acid-base state
↑	No change	↑	Alkalosis
No change	↓	↑	Alkalosis
No change	↓	↓	Acidosis
↓	No change	↓	Acidosis
↓	↓	Normal	Compensated
↑	↑	Normal	Compensated

FIG. 5. Effect of changing ratios of bicarbonate and carbonic acid on pH.

hydrogen ions via the removal of carbonic acid from the plasma. The concentration of carbonic acid depends exclusively on the adequacy of ventilation. Any change in ventilatory efficiency will affect the pH within minutes.

Control of plasma levels of bicarbonate. Renal function has a profound effect on the pH of the plasma because the kidneys can secrete hydrogen ions into and retrieve bicarbonate ions from the glomerular filtrate. This acidification of the glomerular filtrate with ammonia production is the avenue the body uses to rid itself of "fixed" acids in contrast to the removal of the "volatile" carbonic acid by the lungs.

The level of plasma bicarbonate is controlled by the kidney. If plasma bicarbonate is increased, so are its concentration in the plasma, its filtration by the glomeruli, and its urinary excretion. When certain acid-base loads are added to the body, the kidneys stabilize the concentration of plasma bicarbonate by adjusting the excretion of either acids or bases at the same rate the load is being added. However, it takes several hours for the kidney to significantly alter the blood pH.[15]

The renal tubule cells actively secrete hydrogen ions and retain bicarbonate from dissociated carbonic acid. In the renal tubule cell, carbon dioxide, at the urging of carbonic anhydrase, combines with water to form carbonic acid. Carbonic acid then separates into a hydrogen ion, which is expelled into the lumen, and a bicarbonate ion, which moves into the peritubular capillaries. In the lumen the hydrogen ion may enter a number of different bonds. It most frequently combines with the bicarbonate ion that was freed when its partner, sodium, was reabsorbed by the tubular cell. This newly formed carbonic acid molecule is reduced to carbon dioxide and water. The carbon dioxide returns to the tubule cell, and the water is excreted. The carbon dioxide of the tubule cell then recombines with water to form

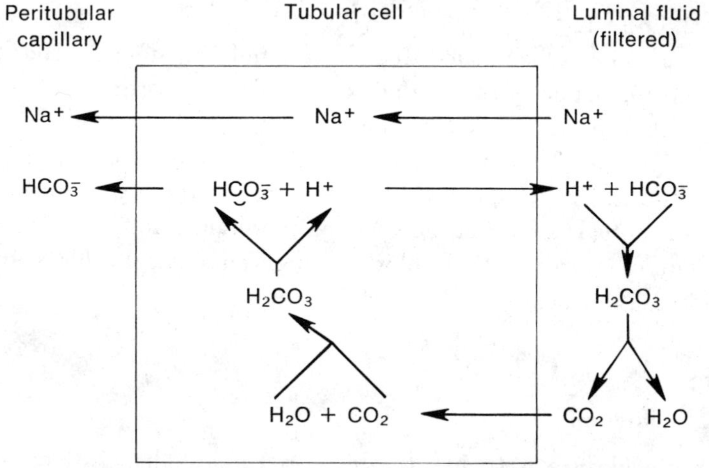

FIG. 6. Process of bicarbonate reabsorption that occurs in renal tubular cells.

carbonic acid, which again dissociates into bicarbonate and hydrogen ions. The cycle is completed when the bicarbonate ion is reabsorbed and the hydrogen ion is excreted. (See Fig. 6.) The bicarbonate ion in the glomerular filtrate is not the same one that is returned to the peritubular capillaries. It has been regenerated by the tubular cell.

Hydrogen secreted into the lumen also combines with the dibasic phosphates and with ammonia (NH_3) to form ammonium (NH_4^+).[13,39,42] The combination of hydrogen ions with these buffers in the urine prevents extreme acidification of the urine. The urinary buffers reduce the free hydrogen ion concentration so that more hydrogen ions can be secreted into the lumen by the tubules.[15] The minimum urinary pH attainable in humans is 4.5 to 5.0. The amount of acid excreted in the urine in this manner is referred to as titratable acid because it can be quantified by the amount of base that needs to be added to the urine to return the hydrogen ion concentration to 40 nEq/L, a pH of 7.4.[25]

Serum bicarbonate is measured by calculating the total carbon dioxide content, the sum of all the chemical forms in which carbon dioxide is carried in the blood (i.e., carbonic acid, dissolved carbon dioxide, and bicarbonate). To determine the bicarbonate concentration from the carbon dioxide content, the following formula is useful:

$$\text{Bicarbonate level} = CO_2 \text{ content} - (0.03 \times P_{CO_2})$$

Normal serum bicarbonate concentration ranges from 22 to 26 mEq/L.[12]

A recent addition to the determination of serum bicarbonate concentration is the calculation of base excess. The blood pH, Pa_{CO_2}, and hematocrit are used as the basis for the calculation. This measurement quantifies the total base excess or deficit. Changes in the base excess are caused by the addition or subtraction of nonvolatile acids, not by the concentrations of carbonic acid. The normal range is +2.5 to −2.5 nEq/L.[42]

In summary, the carbonic acid–bicarbonate buffer system supplies the greatest control in the regulation of pH in the extracellular compartment. There are other systems, but their impact on pH is much less.

The concept of acid-base imbalance is composed of two major subconcepts, acidosis and alkalosis. This chapter will examine each of these subconcepts separately regarding conceptual definition, antecedent conditions, and behavioral definition. The discussion of intervening variables and interventions will address the total concept of acid-base imbalance.

ACIDOSIS

Conceptual definition

A state of acidosis exists when the blood pH is less than 7.35 or the hydrogen ion concentration is greater than 45 nEq/L. An increase in hydrogen ion concentration greatly affects the delivery of oxygen to cells throughout the body. The contractile force of the heart muscle is weakened in acidosis. It appears that the overabundant hydrogen ions compete with the calcium ions in the muscle cell, reducing the number of actin-myosin interactions. The lowered pH stimulates release of stored catecholamines, which counters the depression of the cardiac muscle. Most systemic arterial vessels relax under the influence of excessive hydrogen ions. As with the cardiac muscle, the relaxation is partially checked by the sympathetic adrenal system. In contrast, cerebral vessels are affected only slightly by sympathetic adrenal factors. Acidosis tends to increase cerebral blood flow and pulmonary vascular resistance, and it is associated with venous constriction, which can cause marked movement of blood into the central circulation.[30]

An increase in extracellular hydrogen ion concentration also causes a shift to the right in the oxyhemoglobin dissociation curve. This shift increases the unloading of oxygen from hemoglobin into the tissue cells but retards the loading of oxygen onto the hemoglobin in the lung. This increases oxygen tension but lowers oxygen saturation.[30]

Antecedent conditions

An excess of extracellular hydrogen ions can occur from increased production owing to altered cellular metabolism, decreased excretion owing to impaired kidney function, or loss of alkaline fluids through the kidney or gastrointestinal tract. The clinical manifestation of these causes of excess hydrogen ion concentration is called metabolic acidosis. Respiration has a profound effect on the pH of body fluids. Although carbon dioxide removal or accumulation does not change the number of hydrogen ions in body fluids, it does intensify or reduce the buffer or response of the body. As a consequence, hypoventilation elevates the concentration of hydrogen ions.

Increased hydrogen ion production or ingestion. An excessive amount of hydrogen ions in body fluids frequently is a result of abnormal metabolism. Ketoacidosis, caused by diabetes, alcohol, or starvation, occurs because of abnormal fat metabolism. Without available carbohydrates the body turns to fats and proteins for energy. The lack of carbohydrate oxidation in diabetes mellitus causes high production of ketones from fat combustion and high phosphate and sulphate production from metabolism of body protein. The excess ketones, sulphates, and phosphates require large amounts of bicarbonate for buffering. When these acids flood the extracellular fluid, the supply of free bicarbonate is reduced.

Excessive production of lactic acid can also precipitate metabolic acidosis. Loss of blood volume, myocardial infarction, congestive heart failure, and septicemia typically require cells to use anaerobic metabolism. The end product of this metabolism is huge quantities of lactate. Lactate levels can also be increased through the ingestion of ethyl or methyl alcohol, salicylates, or ammonium chloride.[18]

Reduced excretion of hydrogen. Renal failure is probably the most common cause for the addition of hydrogen ions to the extracellular fluid. Renal failure may result from conditions such as decreased perfusion of the kidney, immune or infectious disturbances of the renal cellular structure, or mechanical blockage of the urinary tract.[8] When urine production drops below 400 to 500 ml/24 hours, the kidneys are unable to eliminate hydrogen ions and regenerate bicarbonate. The impaired tubular excretion of phosphates and/or ammonia severely restricts fixed acid excretion.[33]

Stimulation of the respiratory system by the elevated concentration of hydrogen ions is a compensatory response to metabolic acidosis. Hyperventilation lowers the $PaCO_2$, but the hydrogen ion concentration may remain elevated or within normal limits because of its excessive production.

Excessive loss of bicarbonate. Loss of bicarbonate ions from the extracellular fluid can also produce metabolic acidosis. Large amounts of bicarbonate are normally secreted into the intestine from the pancreas, the liver (bile), and the duodenal mucosa. Any disorder that interferes with the reabsorption of these basic fluids will reduce the bicarbonate concentration and lead to isotonic dehydration. Excessive loss of bicarbonate results from diarrhea, which occurs with conditions such as dysentery, food poisoning, and ulcerative colitis; from postoperative fistula formation; and from ureteral diversions such as ureteroenterostomy. Renal tubular acidosis reduces the tubular secretion of hydrogen ions. In addition, without hydrogen ion secretion the tubules are unable to regenerate bicarbonate and replenish the normal systemic bicarbonate losses.[33] The administration of chloride salts or carbonic anhydrase inhibitors also impairs this bicarbonate regeneration process.[8]

Hypoventilation. Reduced alveolar air exchange, commonly called respiratory acidosis, can be either acute or chronic. The difference between the two states is the ability of the body's mechanisms to adjust to sudden ineffective ventilation.

Hypoventilation of the alveoli can result from a malfunction in any part of the system controlling respiration. The medullary respiratory center, nervous system, bony thorax, respiratory muscles, negative pleural pressure, lung parenchyma, and airways can all be affected to produce inadequate air exchange.

Inhibitions of the medullary respiratory center by cerebral infarct, tumor, or drugs (specifically opiates, sedatives, and anesthetics) and interruption of nerve impulses to respiratory muscles such as in motor nerve diseases (e.g., Guillain-Barré syndrome, tick paralysis, and tetanus) can result in accumulation of carbon dioxide in the blood (acute hypercapnia). Defects in nerve transmission from myasthenia gravis and poliomyelitis can produce hypoventilation.[3] Severe hypo- or hyperkalemia can also paralyze the respiratory muscles by affecting neuromuscular excitability. Respiratory muscle fatigue can decrease the rate and depth of respiration.

Acute respiratory acidosis is most often produced by airway obstruction. Mucous plugs caused by ineffective coughing, bronchoconstriction such as in asthma, trauma to the upper airway resulting in edema and bleeding, the tongue falling backward in the unconscious person, and the aspiration of food or foreign objects are all examples of airway obstructions.

Inflammation of the upper respiratory tract in infants and young children can rapidly produce obstruction. Such conditions as acute epiglottitis or subglottic edema after extubation can obstruct air flow in young children easily.[43] Acute ventilatory failure may be superimposed on existing conditions, particularly those involving the cardiopulmonary system. Hypercapnea is frequently found with cardiac arrest and often is superimposed on chronic respiratory failure.

The most common cause of chronic respiratory acidosis is airway obstruction from bronchitis and emphysema. These diseases and their variations are collectively called chronic obstructive lung disease. Cigarette smoking and air pollution are major factors in the development of the obstructive process. The obstructive process increases airflow resistance on expiration, leading to overinflation and lessened efficiency of air exchange. Loss of alveolar surface area results in wasted ventilation because less inhaled oxygen exchanges with the blood. There are areas in the lung that have insufficient oxygen to exchange with the blood, so hypoxemia is produced. Extreme obesity such as in the pickwickian syndrome, ankylosing spondylitis, and kyphoscoliosis can reduce thoracic cage expansion.[16]

Behavioral definition

Objective data. The objective data present during metabolic acidosis depend on the antecedent condition. However, the bicarbonate ion concentration is always reduced. The concentrations of sodium and chloride are often altered. These ions comprise the bulk of the electrolytes in the extracellular fluid. The concentration of the cation sodium normally exceeds the concentration of the anions chloride and bicarbonate by about 15 mEq/L. The 15 mEq/L are unmeasured anions that arise principally from the negative charge on the plasma proteins.[8] The difference between the measured cation and anion concentrations is referred to as the anion gap. Determination of the anion gap is helpful in the initial search for the cause of metabolic acidosis. Either the anion gap is increased or it remains within normal limits in conditions causing metabolic acidosis. The anion gap is increased if hydrogen ions accumulate with any anion other than chloride.

The concentration of bicarbonate can be reduced and replaced by the addition of unmeasured anions such as ketones, lactate, or other organic anions. For example, if the serum sodium concentration is 140 mEq/L, the chloride, 103 mEq/L, and the bicarbonate, 10 mEq/L, there is an anion gap of 27 mEq/L. With an anion gap of this amount it is known that other, unmeasured anions are being added to the extracellular fluid. Conversely, if there is a loss of bicarbonate and the chloride is its replacement, a normal anion gap results because chloride takes the place left by the reduced bicarbonate.

Generally, loss of alkaline fluid causes the kidney to maintain fluid volume by conserving sodium. Chloride will also be conserved because it follows the sodium ion. Metabolic acidosis with this picture is called hyperchloremic acidosis because the serum concentration of chloride is increased. One example of a hyperchloremic picture would be a serum sodium concentration at 140 mEq/L, bicarbonate at 10 mEq/L, and chloride at 118 mEq/L. This results in an anion gap of 12 mEq/L, which, although in normal limits, presents an increased chloride concentration.

When metabolic acidosis is caused by the addition of hydrogen ions or organic acids to the plasma, the anion gap increases. Values such as an elevated level of serum glucose, blood urea nitrogen, serum creatinine, or serum ketones may provide clues to the cause of the acidosis. Glycosuria and ketonuria also indicate the source of excessive organic anions.

When base-loss acidosis is present, the pH does not drop below 7.25. Although compensatory hyperventilation may not be obvious, the $Pa{CO_2}$ may still be reduced.[32] Plasma sodium concentration decreases, plasma potassium may increase, and chloride is retained to take the place of the lost bicarbonate. There is no increase in unmeasured anions such as ketones, lactate, and other organic anions.

In acute metabolic acidosis deep breathing or hyperventilation is usually quite evident. The $Pa{CO_2}$ is reduced, since the body attempts to retard the falling pH through ventilation. As the level of acidosis increases, mental confusion and decreased responsiveness to stimuli may occur.

The signs present during respiratory acidosis depend on the rapidity of the onset. The person, if not sedated, will become restless and extremely dyspneic and may not be able to verbalize what is wrong. The person may appear panic-stricken and disoriented. If the airway blockage is in the upper respiratory tract, intercostal retraction on inspiration may be apparent, along with inspiratory stridor. Since the adequacy of alveolar ventilation is reflected directly by the $Pa{CO_2}$, the partial pressure of carbon dioxide may rise as high as 70 to 120 mm Hg.[32] A high $Pa{CO_2}$ with a reduction in pH indicates acute ventilatory failure.

In acute hypercapnia the plasma hydrogen ion concentration is elevated by about 0.77 nEq/L for each 1 mm Hg increase in $Pa{CO_2}$, provided this is the only disruption in the acid-base balance.[2] This relationship is linear, so hydrogen ion concentration can be computed from the $Pa{CO_2}$. A $Pa{CO_2}$ greater than 46 mm Hg is indicative of respiratory acidosis.

The bicarbonate concentration will rise only about 3 mEq/L even if the $Pa{CO_2}$ rises to 80 mm Hg.[2] This slight increase is a result of hydrogen being removed by the nonbicarbonate buffers in the extracellular fluid and not because the kidneys are saving bicarbonate.

The extracellular bicarbonate buffer system, which reacts almost instantaneously to the addition of noncarbonic acids, cannot reduce the carbonic acid concentration. Combination of the hydrogen ion with bicarbonate merely regenerates carbonic acid. This buffering is ineffective in maintaining a range of hydrogen ion concentration compatible with life when ventilation is deficient. The only correction for acute hypercapnia is adequate ventilation.[42]

Since acute hypercapnia causes vasodilation, the cerebral blood flow may be affected, producing increased intracranial pressure with papilledema. The extremities may also be warm.[21]

Neurological signs and symptoms generally are more conspicuous in acute respiratory acidosis than in acute metabolic acidosis. The explanation for this may lie in the ability of carbon dioxide to equilibrate with the cerebrospinal fluid rapidly, whereas bicarbonate seems to be retarded in passing the blood-brain barrier. The resulting higher hydrogen ion concentration in the cerebrospinal fluid may reduce cerebral cell functioning.[39] This effect in combination with accompanying hypoxemia precipitates mental confusion and, eventually, stupor, coma, and death.

Serum potassium levels are elevated as a result of potassium being exchanged when hydrogen ions move into the cells. As potassium plasma concentration rises, ventricular fibrillation may occur.[10]

Chronic respiratory acidosis, or chronic hypercapnia, shows slightly different signs because the slow onset of hypoventilation has allowed compensatory action by the kidneys. To move the pH toward normal, the kidneys excrete hydrogen ions and retain bicarbonate ions. This is evidenced by the leveling off of the increase in hydrogen ion concentration after hypercapnia has been present for 2 or 3 days.

Renal regeneration of bicarbonate in uncomplicated chronic respiratory acidosis raises the plasma bicarbonate level about 3.5 mEq/L for every 10 mm Hg increment in the Pa_{CO_2}.[41] If someone with chronic respiratory acidosis had a Pa_{CO_2} of 70 mm Hg, the bicarbonate level would be roughly 35 mEq/L, an elevation of 10.5 mEq/L from normal. The blood pH in this person would not be as low as is usual in acute respiratory acidosis with the same Pa_{CO_2}. The renal compensation that can occur in the chronic situation might keep the pH near 7.35, whereas the pH in the acute situation without the effects of renal compensation would probably be about 7.22. In chronic respiratory acidosis the hydrogen ion concentration is increased by 0.32 nEq/L for every 1 mm Hg increase in Pa_{CO_2} rather than by 0.77 nEq/L (the increase that occurs in acute hypercapnea).[41]

When acidosis is precipitated by chronic obstructive lung disease, the Pa_{CO_2} is generally about 50 to 60 mm Hg, with bicarbonate levels ranging from 35 to 50 mEq/L. If the Pa_{CO_2} exceeds 70 mm Hg, papilledema, asterixis, and coughing may result.[26] High levels of Pa_{CO_2} are tolerated better if there is no hypoxemia or severe or acute change in pH.[28]

To maintain electroneutrality across cell membranes during conditions of acidosis, the negatively charged chloride ion is excreted and the negatively charged bicarbonate ion is retained. This lowers the plasma concentration of chloride. The increased urinary chloride excretion is associated with an elevated excretion of ammonium.[6] Serum chloride levels are reduced to about 75 to 90 mEq/L.[32]

If chronic obstructive lung disease is the cause of chronic hypercapnia, the following may be present: decreased forced expiratory volume, cyanotic or pinkish skin, rounded shoulder posture with use of accessory muscles to breathe, hyperresonance to percussion, distant breath sounds, sneezing with forced expiration, coughing, and sputum production. The intercostal spaces may bulge on expiration. Shortness of breath is obvious on exertion and may be present when the person is resting. Increased heart rate and rapid ventilatory rate are present.[43]

Subjective data. The acidotic person often complains of weakness, lethargy, and nausea. However, these symptoms may be caused by electrolyte changes or the antecedent condition rather than by the elevated hydrogen ion concentration.

Persons with respiratory acidosis will also experience feelings that accompany hypoxia. The person may complain of shortness of breath or difficulty breathing and resultant anxiety. Headache, blurred vision, fatigue, loss of memory, and difficulty concentrating may also be experienced.

ALKALOSIS

Conceptual definition

A state of alkalosis exists when the blood pH is greater than 7.44 or the hydrogen ion concentration is less than 35 nEq/L. A reduction in hydrogen ion concentration causes peripheral vascular relaxation, an effect that is opposed by the sympathetic adrenal system. The cerebral blood flow decreases owing to vascular constriction caused by an acute fall in $PaCO_2$. The $PaCO_2$ determines the pH of the cerebral tissue in short-term acid-base imbalances.[30]

Alkalosis shifts the oxyhemoglobin dissociation curve to the left, which causes increased loading of oxygen onto hemoglobin in the lung, but the oxygen is not released as readily from the hemoglobin into the tissues. The saturation of the blood increases, but the PaO_2 is decreased.[30]

Enzymatic activity of the cells is sensitive to the levels of pH. A reduction in hydrogen ion concentration enhances the aerobic production of lactate and pyruvate and decreases the normal hepatic use of lactate. It is interesting that the metabolic effects of alkalosis and hypoxia are often analogous, although the conditions act on the enzymatic activities in a different way.[36]

Antecedent conditions

Alkalosis results from a loss of hydrogen ions, an excess of bicarbonate ions, or hyperventilation. The first two causes produce that condition which is clinically labeled metabolic alkalosis, and the last produces respiratory alkalosis.

Excessive loss of hydrogen. Extracellular hydrogen ion concentration can be reduced three ways: (1) loss of gastric secretions, which are high in hydrochloric acid, by vomiting or nasogastric suction; (2) hydrogen loss caused by mineralocorticoid excess, diuretics, or hypoparathyroidism; and (3) hydrogen ion movement into the cells caused by hypokalemia. Hypokalemia can either produce or contribute to metabolic alkalosis by its reciprocal relationship with hydrogen ions. Reduced plasma concentration of potassium causes potassium ions to leave the cell and be replaced by hydrogen ions from the extracellular fluid. This movement of hydrogen ions into the cell reduces the concentration of hydrogen in the plasma, thereby producing metabolic alkalosis.

Aldosterone stimulates the renal secretion of hydrogen and potassium as well as the reabsorption of sodium ions. Excessive secretion of aldosterone causes loss of hydrogen ions with concomitant retention of sodium bicarbonate. It is interesting that excessive ingestion of licorice can produce alkalosis because of that substance's mineralocorticoid-like activity.[7]

The loss of hydrogen ions from the stomach results in a net gain of bicarbonate; a loss of potassium, which causes a hydrogen ion shift into the cells; and a contraction of the extracellular fluid volume.

Excess of bicarbonate. Extracellular bicarbonate excess results from overingestion or enhanced conservation of bicarbonate by the kidney. Ingestion of large doses of sodium or calcium bicarbonate, massive blood transfusions, and the milk/antacid treatment for gastrointestinal ulcers can elevate extracellular bicarbonate concentration.

In persons with normal renal function the ingestion of sodium or calcium bicarbonate will produce only a small increase in plasma bicarbonate concentration.[39] Excessive use of milk and an antacid in the treatment of a peptic ulcer can produce the milk-alkali syndrome. Bicarbonate can be added to the vascular system through the transfusion of eight or more units of bank blood because the citrate used for anticoagulation of the blood is metabolized into bicarbonate.[27]

Sodium bicarbonate is most often given for treatment of lactic acidosis and ketoacidosis. Excessive accumulation of extracellular bicarbonate can occur when the restoration of perfusion or vigorous administration of insulin coupled with rapidly administered bicarbonate reduces the production of hydrogen ions. Since the kidney primed to save bicarbonate, it cannot adjust to the sudden load of bicarbonate, and alkalosis results because of the overtreatment for acidosis.

The kidney conserves bicarbonate when the arterial volume is decreased.[23] Loss of effective circulating volume of blood caused by actual fluid loss from the body, sequestration of fluid in the intestine, failure of the heart, or cirrhosis of the liver will stimulate the kidney to conserve sodium, which carries with it water and bicarbonate. The need for sodium conservation and defense of fluid volume supercedes the body's need for acid-base or potassium equilibrium.[3,11,17]

Hyperventilation. Hypocapnia (reduced $PaCO_2$) results from hyperventilation stimulated by physical and/or psychological factors. The physical impetus generally is initiated by hypoxemia or acidosis. Hypoxemia can be caused by abnormal lung conditions such as interstitial pulmonary disease, emboli, or atelectasis. Congestive heart failure, right-to-left cardiac shunts, anemia, and living in high altitudes can all lead to hypoxemia with coexisting hyperventilation.[45] Lactic acidosis or ketoacidosis lowers the blood pH, which stimulates ventilation as a compensatory mechanism.

Anxiety caused by emotional stress or central nervous system disorders can produce respiratory alkalosis. In these cases the PaO_2 is normal and not a stimulus. Cerebral vascular accidents, meningitis, brain tumors, and head trauma are examples of central nervous system causation. Drugs such as salicylates and epinephrine can stimulate respiration, as can liver disease, fever, and gram-negative septicemia. Even the normal condition of pregnancy produces a slight respiratory alkalosis. Mechanical ventilatory support systems can produce respiratory alkalosis when improperly adjusted.[20]

Behavioral definition

Objective data. Metabolic alkalosis is characterized by a low hydrogen ion concentration in the blood (elevated pH) and/or an increased plasma bicarbonate concentration with a compensatory increase in the $PaCO_2$. The body attempts to impede the extreme swing in the pH by slowing the loss of hydrogen ions by retaining carbonic acid through hypoventilation. Generally, $PaCO_2$ increases 0.6 to 0.7 mm Hg for every 1.0 mEq/L increment in the plasma bicarbonate concentration.[39] There are limits to the effectiveness of respiratory compensation because hypoventilation reduces the PaO_2, which in turn stimulates ventilation. Many patients with metabolic alkalosis maintain a normal $PaCO_2$. If respiratory compensation does occur, $PaCO_2$ usually remains less than 55 mm Hg.[3] A formula for estimating how much a bicarbonate increase should affect $PaCO_2$ follows[39]:

$$PaCO_2 \text{ (mm Hg)} = 0.9 \times HCO_3 \text{ (mEq/L)} \pm 5$$

Manifestations of metabolic alkalosis are less pronounced than those which occur with respiratory alkalosis because of its slower rate of development. Signs of neuromuscular irritability and tetany are most frequent. Periods of mental confusion, belligerence, and being "unreasonable" may be followed by drowsiness and coma as the alkalosis progresses.

Respiratory alkalosis is characterized by a low $PaCO_2$, an elevated pH, and a variable reduction in the plasma concentration of bicarbonate. In uncomplicated respiratory alkalosis, for each 10 mm Hg decrease in the $PaCO_2$ the bicarbonate concentration drops about 2 to 3 mEq/L as a result of the intracellular buffers giving up hydrogen ions in the acute hypocapneic situation.[1] With renal compensation in chronic hypocapnia the bicarbonate concentration will drop about 5 mEq/L for each 10 mm Hg decrease in $PaCO_2$. In this instance the kidneys have responded to reduce the conservation of bicarbonate or the secretion of hydrogen ions. This action prevents a profound change in the pH. Serum potassium concentration is generally reduced because the potassium takes the place of hydrogen in the cell.

In rapidly developing respiratory alkalosis irritability of the central and peripheral nervous systems produces profound signs. Altered levels of consciousness, increased deep tendon reflexes, sweating, cramps, and carpopedal spasms occur.[6] These signs usually occur when the pH rises to 7.54 or higher.[19] Although sometimes hyperventilation may be interspersed with periods of apnea, the person may still remain in a state of alkalosis.[40]

Subjective data. Weakness, cramps, and postural dizziness may be caused by the hypovolemia and hypokalemia that accompany alkalosis. Paresthesia and light-headedness tend to occur less often during metabolic alkalosis than during respiratory alkalosis, possibly because of the slow speed at which the bicarbonate compound crosses the blood-brain barrier. The slower rate of onset results in a slower change in the cerebrospinal fluid pH.[31] However, light-headedness and tingling and numbness of lips and extremities are common complaints in respiratory alkalosis.[40] An increase in membrane excitability and a decrease in cerebral blood flow are thought to be the reasons for these abnormalities.[9] A sense of panic, palpation, and chest pain may also occur when the Pa_{CO_2} drops.[12]

INTERVENING VARIABLES

The major intervening variables that alter the course of acid-base imbalance are the rate, severity, and extent of the antecedent conditions and the person's compensatory mechanisms and age.

Rate, severity, and extent of antecedent conditions

A fast rate of onset is particularly ominous because of the lack of time for the body to make adjustments. In the instance of acute hypoventilation the continued high metabolic production and diffusion rate of carbon dioxide can profoundly reduce the blood pH before the kidney or other buffer systems are able to respond. This is also true of episodes of hyperventilation that are not interrupted by unconsciousness. For instance, if a hydrogen load is presented to the body fluids, the extracellular buffering by bicarbonate is immediate, the respiratory buffering by decreasing Pa_{CO_2} takes minutes to hours, the intracellular buffering takes 2 to 4 hours, and increased renal excretion of hydrogen takes hours to days.[39] The kidneys and other buffers can match the rate only of gradually changing respiratory or metabolic disorders to maintain the blood pH within limits compatible with life.

The severity and extent of insult may be so overwhelming that compensatory mechanisms are unable to offset the imbalance. Although the rate of the insult may precipitate severe imbalance before external assistance can be employed, the severity and extent of changes in the cell structures determine the long-term impact on the body. For example, a person who develops acute tubular necrosis from hypoperfusion may have a severe functional disability for a short time. After perfusion is reestablished, the kidneys can function fully if there is no residual damage. On the other hand, a person may gradually lose kidney function because of repeated renal infections that destroy renal structures. Even though the change is gradual, the amount of structural damage can become so great that the kidney permanently loses its ability to regulate the excretion of acids and bases.

The severity and extent of the insult may be lessened or intensified by other events. For example, air pollutants, respiratory infections, or states of anxiety can easily upset a delicately balanced chronic respiratory state by reducing the amount of gaseous exchange or increasing the need for oxygen.[5] A decrease in bicarbonate concentration because of losses brought about by diarrhea or a reduction in regeneration caused by renal inflammation will intensify an existing acidosis.

The level of an acidotic state may be lessened by the loss of gastric fluid through vomiting or nasogastric suction. The ingestion of large amounts of bicarbonate by the person with respiratory acidosis may modify the pH. However, this would not affect the $Pa{CO_2}$. Metabolic alkalosis can be reduced by diarrhea or heightened by hyperventilation. Respiratory alkalosis can be intensified by gastric losses of hydrochloric acid or by the addition of bicarbonate to the body.

Compensatory mechanisms

The reserve of the compensatory systems greatly affects the severity of acid-base imbalances. If the buffer system is not depleted and the lungs and kidneys have the ability to respond unconditionally, an acid-base disorder can be better tolerated. In contrast, the inability of the compensatory systems to respond will intensify the imbalance. For instance, if the respiratory reserve is decreased and metabolic acidosis develops, the adjustment of the pH by the lungs will be hampered. Another example is a renal system that is unable to increase the regeneration of bicarbonate to offset acidosis caused by an impaired respiratory system. Often deficiencies in a compensatory system are not apparent until the system is stressed.

Age

The body's risk of functional and structural cell damage increases with age because of increased exposure to disease processes and other stressors. The elderly, when confronted with a new assault on the body, may develop a more severe clinical picture, require more rigorous treatment, and have longer convalescence as compared to younger adults with the same degree of assault.

The young child has a smaller reserve than an adult because of the relatively larger amount of surface area in relation to body mass. Because of the child's increased metabolic rate, fluid turnover is more rapid and the child is more prone to dehydration.

The relative size of organ structures to body space is often larger in the child than in the adult. For example, the size of the swollen tongue and epiglottis presents more danger of airway occlusion in a child than in the adult. The infant's oxygen requirement per kilogram of body weight is $1^1/_2$ times that of an adult, and the infant has little ability to increase tidal volume because of lung expansion constrictions. The large heart, the intestines pressing upward on the diaphragm, and flexible thoracic cage inhibit large increases in gas exchange.[43] Acid-base imbalance can occur more easily in an infant because of decreased bicarbonate and buffer activity.

NURSING INTERVENTIONS—GOALS AND EVALUATION CRITERIA

Nursing intervention operates in three major areas: (1) prevention, (2) education, and (3) monitoring for changes. To intervene, the nurse must recognize which situations place the patient at a high risk, what the patient needs to know to prevent an acute state or to maintain a balanced chronic state, and what cues indicate important changes in a patient's condition.

Maintenance of normal or compensated ventilation and kidney function

Acid-base imbalance can be prevented initially, or the imbalance can be maintained as a steady-state compensation. In the latter instance nursing intervention would be aimed toward preventing occurrences that would interrupt the steady state.

The nursing goal of maintaining normal ventilation is of prime importance. Interventions for this goal are discussed under the concept of hypoxia (Chapter 13). Identification of patients who are prone to ventilatory changes is essential. Patients who have depressed levels of consciousness, conditions that necessitate horizontal positioning, a reluctance to breathe deeply or cough, mechanical breathing assistance, a disease process that can rapidly affect neuromuscular control, or a high level of anxiety are vulnerable to acute changes in ventilation.

A person with a depressed level of consciousness needs to be positioned on the side so that the tongue does not fall back and occlude the upper airway. The use of artificial airways and removal of secretions by suctioning help secure airway patency. Aspiration is also a primary danger in these individuals. Oral administration of food or fluid to a semiconscious person invites aspiration. If a feeding tube is required, the placement of the tube must be checked prior to feeding, and the amount and rate of the feeding must be adjusted to avoid regurgitation and possible aspiration.

Positioning the patient during oral intake is of vital importance. Having the patient sit upright with the head slightly forward reduces the danger of aspiration. If the patient's head cannot be elevated, a side-lying eating position is better than a supine one. Even though a patient may not be in a high risk group, an airway occlusion can still occur because of food particles. The nurse needs to be able to perform the Heimlich maneuver in such instances.

Deep breathing and coughing reduce the occurrence of mucous plugs and pooling of secretions in the lungs.[38] Patients who have had thoracic or abdominal surgery frequently reluctant to inhale deply. A regular and consistant routine of turning, coughing, and deep breathing needs to be carried out for any patient who does not periodically breathe deeply. Humidification "loosens" secretions for easier removal.

If the change in ventilation is due to anxiety, the nurse must gain the person's cooperation. Using a calm and quiet but firm approach, the nurse can have the person hold his or her breath to allow enough carbon dioxide to accumulate to avoid neuromuscular irritability and unconsciousness. Generally, self-induced respiratory alkalosis aborts itself. The person who hyperventilates loses consciousness, and the body adjusts the $Paco_2$ by hypoventilating. However, the signs of neuromuscular irritability may occur either before or after the period of unconsciousness. These manifestations are frightening, and an explanation regarding the cause of the symptoms needs to be given to the person to allay more anxiety.

To maintain the compensatory steady state, nursing techniques should be performed in such a way as to prevent events that could cause an acute situation. For instance, it is essential that sterile technique be used during suctioning to avoid a superimposed pulmonary infection in the person who already has compromised breathing because of chronic obstructive lung disease. Likewise, the person who has decreased renal reserve is at great risk with an indwelling catheter if sterile technique is not followed when the drainage equipment is handled.

Behavior that indicates prevention of imbalance is the maintenance of the blood pH, $Paco_2$, and Pao_2 within normal or compensated limits.

Increase of use of maintenance or prevention techniques

Education of the patient includes (1) prevention and (2) maintenance of optimal function in chronic states. One of the prime areas for teaching prevention of acid-base imbalances relates to cigarette smoking. Since smoking is highly correlated with the development of obstructive lung disease, the individual needs to be aware of the hazards of this habit. The nurse can influence the individual's decision not to smoke.

When a patient has a chronic disease, the educational goal is to teach the patient how to maintain an optimal level of adjustment through the use of compensatory mechanisms.[5] When the patient has a chronic respiratory disease, the patient and/or significant others should be taught how to manipulate breathing equipment competently and confidently, to perform coughing and breathing techniques correctly, and to follow a plan of conditioning exercises. Chapter 13 discusses the techniques more extensively.

In all attempts to teach a patient, the individual's emotional and physical needs must be considered. Education about breathing techniques is of prime importance in helping reduce patient anxiety.[22,24]

Patients who have arteriosclerosis, diabetes mellitus, or chronic renal failure should receive instruction about the diet, medications, and daily living habits necessary for the avoidance of acidosis. Instruction regarding the signs and symptoms that indicate the need for medical assistance should be included. Self-monitoring such as urine testing by the person with diabetes or pulse taking by the person with cardiac disease should be taught. This should facilitate the patient's monitoring for changes in body functioning. Persons with chronic disease need to receive information that will allow them to maximize their independence and maintain the quality of their life.

When hyperventilation is a recurring response to stress, the person may be taught relaxation techniques to alleviate anxious episodes. The relaxation techniques should, of course, only be taught when the person is able to focus on the technique, not during an acute episode.[37]

The person who chronically ingests excessive milk and alkaline antacids for relief of peptic ulcer pain can develop metabolic alkalosis. The patient should be informed of the hazards of such treatment, and other forms of treatment should be investigated.

The criterion indicative that education has successfully prevented or reduced acid-base imbalance is maintenance of a compensated state or of normal blood pH, $PaCO_2$, and PaO_2.

Identification of change in acid-base balance

The cues regarding change in acid-base imbalances arise from changes in ventilation, urinary output, specific type of electrolytes gained or lost by the fluid compartments, and the disruption in normal metabolic functions.

Observing and responding to pertinent cues is the beginning of any nursing intervention. Being able to assist in adjusting the rate of medical treatment in relation to the cues is a prime nursing function. For instance, if there is a loss of isotonic fluids, the goal of nursing intervention is to pace intravenous fluid administration with the losses without creating hypervolemia. The cues for managing fluid infusion rate would be changes in blood pressure, pulse rate, lung sounds, mentation of the patient, and urinary output.

If the situation is an emergency such as in hypoperfusion owing to cardiac arrest, the goal is to maintain oxygenation of the blood, maintain tissue perfusion, and control the wide swing in the pH. The nurse must be able to initiate and maintain the cardiopulmonary resuscitation procedure and monitor the intravenous administration of specific drugs such as sodium bicarbonate.

In the case of acidosis caused by diabetes, glucose solutions, insulin, and potassium must be given at a rate that will prevent sudden shifts in electrolytes while normalizing the pH. The nurse's role is to monitor the rate of infusion and be alert to signs and symptoms that indicate too rapid a change. A particularly important sign is the occurrence of cardiac arrhythmias. Pulse and ECG recordings provide signs of electrolyte maintenance.

Adjustment of pH in patients with chronic renal failure with dialysis techniques must also proceed at a rate that will not cause rapid shifts in electrolytes and water between compartments, which would result in cerebral edema. A change in mental functioning, difficulty speaking, and weakness of the extremities are indications of possible increased intracranial pressure.

It is necessary for the nurse to recognize when a patient cannot breathe without mechanical assistance or needs increased concentration of oxygen in the air that is exchanged. Restlessness, dyspnea, or a frightened appearance may indicate lack of oxygen. Once the machine and/or oxygen is in operation, monitoring of arterial blood gas levels and observation of the patient's response are necessary to determine the efficiency of ventilation.

Criteria indicative of successful treatment include clearing of mentation, return to previous cardiac rhythm, increased muscle strength, reduction in muscle spasms, reduction in fatigue, normal or compensated Pa_{CO_2}, normal or compensated bicarbonate levels, normal potassium concentrations, a pH within normal range, maintenance of normal blood pressure, and balanced fluid intake and output.

CONCEPT OUTLINE

I. *Conceptual definition:* An acid-base imbalance is a state in which there is an excess or deficit of dissociated, or "unbuffered," hydrogen ions in the body fluids.

II. Acidosis
   - A. *Conceptual definition:* Acidosis is a state in which the hydrogen ion concentration in the blood is greater than 45 nEq/L or the blood pH is less than 7.35.
   - B. *Antecedent conditions*
     1. Increased hydrogen ion production or ingestion
        - a. Abnormal metabolism
          - (1) Ketoacidosis
          - (2) Lactic acidosis
        - b. Ingestion
          - (1) Alcohol
          - (2) Salicyclates
          - (3) Ammonium chloride
     2. Reduced excretion of hydrogen
        - a. Renal failure
     3. Excessive loss of bicarbonate
        - a. Diarrhea
        - b. Gastrointestinal fistula formation
        - c. Ureteral diversions
        - d. Renal tubular acidosis
     4. Hypoventilation (chronic and acute)
        - a. Neuromuscular interference
          - (1) Cerebral infarct or brain tumor
          - (2) Gullain-Barré syndrome
          - (3) Tick paralysis
          - (4) Tetanus
          - (5) Potassium imbalance
          - (6) Myasthenia gravis
          - (7) Poliomyelitis
        - b. Airway obstruction
          - (1) Mucous plugs
          - (2) Foreign objects, food, or tongue
          - (3) Bronchoconstriction
          - (4) Inflammation
          - (5) Chronic obstructive lung disease
        - c. Impediments to thoracic cage expansion
          - (1) Ankylosing spondylitis

(2) Kyphoscoliosis
(3) Extreme obesity

C. *Behavioral definition*
1. Objective data
a. Metabolic acidosis
(1) Bicarbonate level reduction
(2) Variable anion gap
(3) Hyperventilation
(4) Abnormalities in serum levels of glucose, ketones, chloride, and potassium
(5) Reduced total base excess
b. Respiratory acidosis
(1) Variable bicarbonate level elevation
(2) Elevated $PaCO_2$
(3) Depression of pH variable
2. Subjective data
a. Weakness
b. Lethargy
c. Mentation changes

III. Alkalosis

A. *Conceptual definition:* Alkalosis is a state in which the hydrogen ion concentration in the blood is less than 35 nEq/L or the blood pH is greater than 7.44.

B. *Antecedent conditions*
1. Excessive loss of hydrogen
a. Loss of gastric secretions
b. Renal loss
c. Movement into cells
2. Excess of bicarbonate caused by overingestion or administration
a. Antacids
b. Sodium or calcium bicarbonate
c. Blood bank transfusions
3. Hyperventilation
a. Physical causes
(1) Acidemia
(2) Hypoxia
(3) Central nervous system abnormalities
(4) Drugs
(5) Mechanical ventilatory support
b. Psychological cause
(1) Anxiety

C. *Behavioral definition*
1. Objective data
a. Metabolic alkalosis
(1) Elevated blood pH
(2) Elevated serum bicarbonate level
(3) Normal or increased $PaCO_2$
b. Respiratory alkalosis
(1) Low $PaCO_2$
(2) Elevated blood pH
(3) Variable reduction in serum bicarbonate level
(4) Reduced serum potassium level
(5) Irritability of central and peripheral nervous systems
i. Hyperreflexia
ii. Carpopedal spasms
iii. Cramps
2. Subjective data
a. Weakness
b. Paresthesia
(1) Tingling
(2) Numbness
c. Sense of panic

IV. *Intervening variables*

A. Rate of onset
B. Severity and extent of antecedent conditions
C. Compensatory mechanisms
D. Age

V. *Nursing interventions—goals*

A. Maintenance of normal or compensated ventilation and kidney function
1. Positioning
2. Deep breathing and coughing routine
3. Mechanical breathing assistance
4. Use of artificial airways
5. Removal of secretions
6. Humidification of secretions
7. Correct placement of feeding tubes
8. Adjustment of feeding rate and amount to patient's capacity
9. Use of Heimlich maneuver
10. Use of explanations and calm approach to reduce anxiety
11. Use of aseptic techniques with ventilation and renal drainage equipment

B. Increase of use of maintenance or prevention techniques
1. Patient and family education
a. Abstention from smoking
b. Use of breathing equipment
c. Breathing exercises
d. Relaxation techniques
e. Diet
f. Medications
g. Self-monitoring techniques

C. Monitoring of indications of change in acid-base balance
   1. Ventilation patterns
   2. Balance of fluid intake and output
   3. Cardiac rhythm
   4. Muscle strength
   5. Mental activity
   6. Arterial blood gas levels
   7. Electrolyte blood levels
   8. Blood pH

VI. *Evaluation criteria*
   A. Clearing of mentation
   B. Return to previous cardiac rhythm
   C. Increased muscle strength
   D. Reduction in muscle spasm
   E. Reduction in fatigue
   F. Normal blood pressure
   G. Balanced fluid intake and output
   H. Return to normal or compensated levels of $PaCO_2$, serum bicarbonate and potassium levels, and blood pH

REFERENCES

1. Arbus, G. S., Herbert, L. A., Levesque, P. R., Etsten, B. E., and Schwartz, W. B.: Characterization and clinical application of the "significance band" for acute respiratory alkalosis, N. Engl. J. Med. **280**:117, 1969.
2. Brackett, N. C., Jr., Cohen, J. J.. and Schwartz, W. B.: Carbon dioxide titration curve of normal man: effect of increasing degrees of acute hypercapnia on acid-base equilibrium, N. Engl. J. Med. **272**:6, 1965.
3. Carrol, H. J., and Oh, M. S.: Water, electrolyte and acid-base metabolism: diagnosis and management, Philadelphia, 1978, J. B. Lippincott Co.
4. Carter, N. W.: Intracellular pH, Kidney Int. **1**:341, 1972.
5. Cherniack, R. M., and Lertzman, M. M.: Management of patients with chronic airflow obstruction, Med. Clin. North Am. **61**:1219, 1977.
6. Cohen, J. J., and Madias, N. E.: Acid-base disorders of respiratory origin. In Brenner, B. M., and Stein, J. H., editors: Acid-base and potassium homeostasis: contemporary issues in nephrology, New York, 1978, Churchill Livingstone, Inc.
7. Conn, J. W., Rouner, D. R., and Cohen, E. L.: Licorice-induced pseudoaldosteronism, J.A.M.A. **205**:492, 1968.
8. Emmett, M., and Narins, R. G.: The clinical use of the anion gap, Medicine **56**:38, 1977.
9. Fencl, V., Vale, J. R., and Broch, J. A.: Respiration and cerebral blood flow in metabolic acidosis and alkalosis in humans, J. Appl. Physiol. **27**:67, 1969.
10. Foulds, H. P. S., Kendel, D., and de Mowbray, R. R.: Changes in serum potassium level and in pH of arterial blood in respiratory acidosis, Lancet **1**:405, 1958.
11. Garella, S., Chang, B. S., and Kahn, S. I.: Dilution acidosis and contraction alkalosis: review of a concept, Kidney Int. **8**:279, 1975.
12. Goldberger, E.: A primer of water, electrolyte and acid-base syndromes, ed. 5, Philadelphia, 1975, Lea & Febiger.
13. Guyton, A. C.: Textbook of medical physiology, ed. 5, Philadelphia, 1976, W. B. Saunders Co.
14. Heineman, H. O.: Metabolic alkalosis in patients with hypercalcemia, Metabolism **14**:1137, 1965.
15. Hills, A. G.: Acid-base balance: chemistry physiology, pathophysiology, Baltimore, 1973, William & Wilkins Co.
16. Holley, H. S., Milic-Emili, J., Becklake, M. R., and Bates, D. V.: Regional distribution of pulmonary ventilation and perfusion in obesity, J. Clin. Invest. **46**:475, 1967.
17. Kassirer, J. P., and Schwartz, W. B.: The response of normal man to selective depletion of hydrochloric acid, Am. J. Med. **40**:10, 1966.
18. Kelman, A. S.: Lactic acidosis. In Brenner, B. M., and Stein, J. H., editors: Acid-base and potassium homeostasis: contemporary issues in nephrology, New York, 1978, Churchill Livingstone, Inc.
19. Kilburn, K. H.: Neurological manifestations of respiratory failure, Arch. Intern. Med. **116**:409, 1965.
20. Kilburn, K. H.: Shock, seizures and coma with alkalosis during mechanical ventilation, Ann. Intern. Med. **65**:977, 1966.
21. Kontos, H. A., Richardson, D. W., and Patterson, J. L., Jr.: Vasodilator effect of hypercapnic acidosis on human forearm blood vessels, Am. J. Physiol. **215**:1403, 1968.
22. Koss, J. A., and Christoph, C.: Oxygen therapy and other respiratory therapy in acute respiratory failure, Critical Care Quarterly **1**:53, 1979.
23. Kurtzman, N. A., White, M. G., and Rogers, P. W.: Pathophysiology of metabolic alkalosis, Arch. Intern. Med. **131**:702, 1973.
24. Lagerson, J.: Pulmonary rehabilitation, Critical Care Quarterly **1**:75, 1979.

25. Lennon, E. J.: Body buffering mechanisms. In Frohlick, E. D., editor: Pathophysiology: altered regulatory mechanisms, ed. 3, Philadelphia, 1976, J. B. Lippincott Co.
26. Levinsky, N. G.: Acidosis and alkalosis. In Thorn, G. W., Wintrobe, M. M., Adams, R. D., Bennett, I. L., Braunwald, E., Isselbacher, K. J., and Petersdorf, R. G., editors: Harrison's principles of internal medicine, ed. 8, St. Louis, 1977, McGraw-Hill Book Co.
27. Litwin, M., Smith, L., and Moore, F. D.: Metabolic alkalosis following massive transfusion, Surgery **45**:805, 1959.
28. Martin, L.: Respiratory failure, Med. Clin. North Am. **61**:1369, 1977.
29. Masoro, E. J., and Siegel, P. D.: Acid-base regulation: its physiology and pathophysiology, Philadelphia, 1971, W. B. Saunders Co.
30. Mitchell, J. H., Wildenthal, K., and Johnson, R. L., Jr.: The effects of acid-base disturbances on cardiovascular and pulmonary function, Kidney Int. **1**:375, 1972.
31. Mitchell, R. A., Carmen, C. T., Severinghaus, J. W., Richardson, B. W., Singer, M. M., and Shnider, S.: Stability of cerebrospinal fluid pH in chronic acid-base disturbances in blood, J. Appl. Physiol. **20**:443, 1965.
32. Moore, F. D.: Fluid and electrolyte management in surgical patients. In Hardy, J. D., editor: Rhoad's textbook of surgery: principles and practice, ed. 5, Philadelphia, 1977, J. B. Lippincott Co.
33. Narins, R. G.: Renal acidosis. In Brenner, B. M., and Stein, J. H., editors: Acid-base and potassium homeostasis: contemporary issues in nephrology, New York, 1978, Churchill Livingstone, Inc.
34. O'Connor, G., and Kunace, R. T.: Renal transport of hydrogen and potassium. In Brenner, B. M., and Stein, J. H., editors: Acid-base and potassium homeostasis: contemporary issues in nephrology, vol. 2, New York, 1978, Churchill Livingstone, Inc.
35. Pestana, C.: Fluids and electrolytes in the surgical patient, Baltimore, 1977, Williams & Wilkins Co.
36. Relman, A. S.: Metabolic consequences of acid-base disorders, Kidney Int. **1**:347, 1972.
37. Richter, J. M., and Sloan, R.: A relaxation technique, Am. J. Nurs. **11**:1960, 1979.
38. Risser, N. L.: Preoperative and postoperative care to prevent pulmonary complications, Heart Lung **9**:57, 1980.
39. Rose, B. D.: Clinical physiology of acid-base and electrolyte disorders, St. Louis, 1977, McGraw-Hill Book Co.
40. Saltzman, H., Heyman, A., and Sieker, H. A.: Correlation of clinical and physiological manifestations of sustained hyperventilation, N. Engl. J. Med. **268**:1431, 1963.
41. Schwartz, W. B., Brackett, N. C., and Cohen, J. J.: The response of extracellular hydrogen ion concentration to graded degrees of chronic hypercapnia: the physiologic limits of the defense of pH, J. Clin. Invest. **44**:291, 1965.
42. Shapiro, B. A.: Clinical applications of blood gases, Chicago, 1973, Year Book Medical Publishers, Inc.
43. Shapiro, B. A., Harrison, R. A., and Trout, C. A,: Clinical application of respiratory care, Chicago, 1975, Year Book Medical Publishers, Inc.
44. Slonim, N. B., and Hamilton, L. H.: Respiratory physiology, ed. 3, St. Louis, 1976, The C. V. Mosby Co.
45. Wasserman, K., Whipp, B. J., and Castagna, J.: Cardiodynamic hyperpnea: hyperpnea secondary to cardiac output increase, J. Appl. Physiol. **36**:457, 1974.

RITA A. FARREN FRANTZ

Chapter 13

HYPOXIA

CONCEPTUAL DEFINITION

An inadequate supply of oxygen or the inability of the body to use the oxygen that is present will alter cellular function and structure and will disrupt oxygen-dependent metabolism. Whenever the availability of oxygen is diminished or the cellular demand for oxygen exceeds the ability of the body's systems to deliver it, a state of hypoxia occurs. As the impingement of a hypoxic state increases, an identifiable pattern of biochemical disarray and intracellular dysfunction occurs, which may ultimately culminate in cell death.

Initially, hypoxia impairs oxidative phosphorylation and produces a dysfunction of the cell's energy-releasing systems. This produces a depletion in the cell's adenosine triphosphate (ATP) reserves. Although the deletion in ATP reserves with hypoxia is well documented, the source of breakdown in the cell's energy-producing systems has not yet been verified. On the basis of a study of liver autolysis, it has been suggested that hypoxia initially produces a loss of respiratory cofactors that the cell requires to carry on the Krebs cycle.[2] It also has been proposed that hypoxia injures mitochondrial membranes through release of extramitochondrial lipolytic enzymes.[5] However, Vogt and Farger[9] found that mitochondria in hypoxic renal tubular cells with rapidly depleted ATP reserves still retained the ability to carry out oxidative phosphorylation. They contend that other, as yet unidentified, mechanisms cause the depleted ATP reserves.

Regardless of the source, the dissipation of ATP reserves as a result of hypoxia leads to reduced energy availability for the cell's sodium pump function.[4] As a result, sodium is not extruded from the intracellular fluid in adequate amounts to maintain normal cellular osmolarity. The increased intracellular concentration of sodium causes water, which passively follows sodium, to enter the cell in rising amounts. This produces a phenomenon called cellular swelling, accompanied by swelling of the mitochondria and endoplasmic reticulum. In an attempt to compensate for the reduced levels of ATP, the cell activates glycolytic reactions that produce small amounts of ATP in the absence of a sufficient amount of oxygen. This anaerobic production of ATP can extend cellular life for a few minutes when oxygen is unavailable.[3]

However, the end products of these glycolytic reactions are pyruvic acid and hydrogen ions, which react with each other and form lactic acid. This lowers the intracellular pH and disrupts cell membrane integrity. Increased cell membrane permeability permits an influx of sodium and calcium. The increasing levels of intracellular sodium further burden the sodium pump, and the calcium disrupts links in the oxidative phosphorylation process. In addition to shifting the osmotic balance of the cell, the increased cell membrane permeability allows intracellular enzymes to diffuse into the intercellular fluid and ultimately into the bloodstream. The movement of these enzymes into the blood indicates significant levels of cell injury and cell death.

Three of these enzymes that can be isolated by quantitative analysis are aspartate transaminase (AST),* isoenzymes of lactic dehydrogenase (LDH), and creatine phosphokinase (CPK). These enzymes are found in varying degrees in a majority of the body tissues. The cells of the lung, pancreas, liver, and heart contain high concentrations of AST and LDH. The enzyme CPK is found only in cells of the heart, brain, and skeletal muscles. In addition to these enzymes, large amounts of potassium escape from damaged cells, resulting in a state of serum hyperkalemia.

As oxygen deprivation continues, the cell becomes less and less able to restore its energy supply. Intracellular disorganization becomes increasingly rapid. Ultimately the nucleus shrinks, impairing deoxyribonucleic acid (DNA) and ribonucleic acid (RNA) synthesis. Finally the lysosomes rupture, releasing their catalases, which digest the cell components and completely destroy the cell. Initial cytoplasmic changes in response to oxygen insufficiency are reversible, but nuclear changes indicate irreversible cell injury.[7]

If the hypoxic state is accompanied by interference in the elimination of carbon dioxide, it is possible that the carbon dioxide tension (Pa_{CO_2}) will rise above the level of 50 mm Hg. Retained carbon dioxide will combine with water in the plasma to form carbonic acid. The hypoxic state then begins to disrupt the body's acid-base balance. The increased hydrogen ions begin depressing the body's pH below 7.35. As hypoxia persists and cellular metabolism is disrupted, lactic acid spills into the bloodstream, further depressing the body's pH. Generally the kidneys compensate for the rising level of carbon dioxide by retaining the buffer, bicarbonate, in an attempt to maintain a normal 20:1 ratio of bicarbonate to carbonic acid. These acid-base changes, which often accompany hypoxia, frequently result in a low serum chloride level. This reflects the ion exchange that occurs when the kidneys excrete chloride ions, which are negatively charged, in exchange for bicarbonate ions, also negatively charged.

ANTECEDENT CONDITIONS

When there is an adequate supply of environmental oxygen, three types of physiological deficiencies can precipitate hypoxia. Pulmonary failure, inadequate oxygen transport, and ineffective cellular use of available oxygen will all interrupt the process of oxygenation.

Pulmonary failure

Hypoxia owing to pulmonary failure results either from failure to inspire an adequate volume of air for exchange or from failure to diffuse the air adequately

*Aspartate transaminase (AST) is now international standard nomenclature for what was formerly called glutamic oxaloacetic transaminase (GOT).

across the alveolocapillary membrane. Ventilatory failure can occur as a result of airway obstruction, restricted movement of the thoracic cavity, or depression of the respiratory center.

Aspiration of foreign bodies, bronchospasm, or the presence of tenacious mucus can produce partial or complete obstruction of the airflow. Chronic bronchitis, emphysema, and asthma are examples of conditions in which these types of obstructions occur.

Restricted movement of the thoracic cavity occurs with pneumothorax or pleural effusion when the air or fluid in the pleural space presses on the lung, impeding the flow of air. Conditions such as extreme obesity, pregnancy, and ascites restrict thoracic movement by impinging on the downward movement of the diaphragm. Impaired function of respiratory muscles, which occurs with neuromuscular disorders such as muscular dystrophy and myasthenia gravis, results in hypoventilation and reduced volume of inspired oxygen. Hypoventilation also occurs when the individual voluntarily immobilizes the respiratory muscles. This is common in patients with pleurisy and in postoperative patients who use voluntary splinting of high abdominal and thoracic incisions to cope with postsurgical pain.

Brain stem injury or drug-induced depression of the respiratory center will reduce the volume of inspired air through depression of respiratory stimulation. Central nervous system depressants such as narcotics (morphine sulphate, codeine) and sedatives (barbiturates) and excessive ingestion of alcohol commonly depress the respiratory rate. Muscle relaxants such as curare, often administered in conjunction with anesthesthetics, relax the diaphragm and other respiratory muscles so that ventilation is depressed.

Regardless of the precipitating factor, the ultimate effect of ventilatory failure is an increase in the $Paco_2$ and a decrease in the Po_2. Because of the affinity of hemoglobin for oxygen, manifestations of ventilatory failure result primarily from the elevated $Paco_2$. The effects of low Po_2 levels appear only in the late stages of ventilatory failure.

The second major source of pulmonary failure is impaired diffusion of oxygen across the alveolocapillary membrane. When excessive mucus accumulation occurs, as happens with pulmonary infections, diffusion across the membrane is impeded. This also occurs when the surface area is reduced by alveoli destruction, as occurs in emphysema and severe chronic bronchitis. Obstruction of pulmonary circulation with an embolus or distention of the pulmonary capillaries with edema also interferes with alveolar-arterial gas exchange. In all cases of impaired alveolocapillary diffusion the major effect is reduced exchange of oxygen. In these instances accumulation of carbon dioxide is prevented by hyperventilation in the remaining portion of the lung.[1]

Inadequate oxygen transport

Hypoxia owing to inadequate transport and delivery of oxygen can arise from failure of the heart pump, hypovolemia, loss of vascular tone, or decreased oxygen-carrying capacity of the blood.

Inadequacy of the heart as a pump is the most common cause of hypoxia in industrialized nations.[7] This "pump failure" can be produced by congenital anomalies that cause blood to flow through abnormal pathways in the heart, thereby reducing the volume of oxygenated blood pumped to systemic circulation. Conditions that compromise the contractility of the myocardium such as myocardial infarction decrease cardiac output. Valvular disorders contribute to pump failure by limiting the forward flow of blood, thereby reducing output by the ventricles. Cardiac arrhythmias diminish output through weak, ineffective contractions. Regardless of the underlying cause, any condition that compromises the effectiveness of the heart will result in reduced amounts of oxygenated blood being delivered to the cells.

Defects in the vascular system also can cause ineffective transport and delivery of oxygen. When the volume of circulating blood is reduced such as occurs with acute hemorrhage, venous return to the heart is diminished, ultimately resulting in decreased cardiac output of oxygenated blood. The ability of the vascular system to deliver oxygen-enriched blood is also hindered by the loss of tone in the arterial walls. Such a decrease in elasticity, which characterizes the generalized atherosclerotic process, impedes the flow of blood to the tissues.

Inadequate levels of the oxygen-carrying components in the blood impose limitations on oxygen delivery. This may take the form of reduced hemoglobin levels, which render the red blood cells incapable of transporting a full complement of oxygen. Correspondingly, a depressed red blood cell (RBC) level arising from such factors as nutritional deficiency, malabsorption, and increased red blood cell destruction decreases the amount of oxygen carried by a given volume of blood. The end result of any limitation on the vascular system's ability to deliver oxygen is cellular hypoxia.

Excessive tissue demands for oxygen such as occurs with thyroid disorders and extreme exercise can produce manifestations of hypoxia owing to inability of the body's transport system to keep pace with oxygen use in the tissues. Such oxygen deficiency can also occur when an individual experiences extreme stress, increasing the metabolic rate beyond the capability of the body to deliver the needed oxygen.

Ineffective cellular use of oxygen

Ineffective tissue oxygenation or oxygen use is a third major source of hypoxia. Effective diffusion of oxygen to body tissues can be impeded by tissue edema. Although adequate amounts of oxygen are delivered to the tissues, the edema interferes with the absorption of oxygen. Poisoning of cellular enzymes with such substances as carbon monoxide, arsenic, and formaldehyde renders the enzymes incapable of catalyzing chemical reactions crucial to maintenance of cellular respiration. Breakdown of this vital function results in cellular hypoxia.

BEHAVIORAL DEFINITION

Although the initial effects of hypoxia occur at the cellular level, eventually the whole body systemically responds to the effects of oxygen insufficiency. Objective signs of this systemic response are most obvious in the neurological, respiratory, and cardiovascular systems.

Objective data

The earliest alteration in bodily function that occurs in response to hypoxia is disrupted neurological function. Initially, hypoxia decreases night vision. Even a slight decrease in oxygen saturation of the arterial blood depresses the normal function of the rods in the retina.[3] As hypoxia intensifies, neurological function is further compromised. Drowsiness and lassitude begin to appear. The low tolerance of the cerebral cortex for hypoxia manifests itself with a decrease in the ability to make judgments, to remember, and to carry out discrete motor movements. If hypoxia continues, the end result is coma with decreasing respiratory center activity. The respiratory center no longer responds to stimulation by the chemoreceptors, and ultimately respirations cease.

Before this point of respiratory depression is reached, the respiratory system responds to falling oxygen levels by increasing the rate of respiration without increasing its depth. When the arterial oxygen saturation drops below 93%, chemoreceptors in the respiratory center stimulate an increase in the rate of pulmonary ventilation.[3] If the state of hypoxia persists or accelerates, respirations may become difficult and labored, resulting in a condition called dyspnea. The dyspneic patient attempts to promote gaseous exchange by using the accessory muscles of respiration, including the scalenus, sternocleidomastoid, trapezius, and latissimus dorsi. Contraction of these muscle groups increases upper airway pressure in an attempt to open constricted air passages. However, in actuality, use of these muscles aggrates air hunger by decreasing the elasticity of the lung tissue and increasing the resistance to air flow. In addition, it increases the need for tissue oxygenation because of the increased metabolic demand.

Specific respiratory characteristics often give clues to the particular antecedent that produced the oxygen deficiency. Bradypnea, or oligopnea, a slow respiratory rate, occurs as a result of depression of the respiratory center or ineffective action of the respiratory muscles. Orthopnea is the need to have the head elevated to breathe effectively. Orthopnea occurs when fluid accumulates in the pulmonary tissues. Its severity is commonly measured in terms of the number of pillows required behind the head to relieve the breathing difficulty, such as two-pillow orthopnea. Cheyne-Stokes respirations are distinguished by periods of apnea, absence of respirations, lasting from 30 seconds to 3 minutes interposed with a single deep respiration. Such a pattern of respirations is associated with pump failure that delays transport of blood to and from the brain. As a result of the delayed circulation, carbon dioxide accumulates in the blood during the apneic period until it ultimately reaches a critical level. This causes the chemoreceptors in the respiratory center to initiate a deep breath, which lowers the carbon dioxide level. In a few seconds the oxygenated pulmonary blood reaches the respiratory center and inhibits respirations. Thus Cheyne-Stokes breathing is characterized by a pattern of periodic waxing and waning of respiration.

Examination of the thorax can provide additional clues to the antecedent condition and indications of the severity and location of the problem. Uneven expansion of the chest wall indicates a lack of airflow in the underlying lung tissue. Hyperresonance found on percussion of the chest walls indicates overinflated alveoli such as with emphysema. Dullness indicates fluid-filled or consolidated lung tissue. Decreased breath sounds on auscultation indicate either reduced air flow in underlying lung tissue or overinflation of lung tissue. Expiratory wheezing suggests air is being forced through constricted bronchioles such as with bronchospasms. Air being driven through a partially closed glottis such as occurs with a partially obstructed larynx or tracheal spasms produces the harsh sound of stridor. Rales are associated with fluid secretions in the alveoli. The gurgling and harmonic sounds characteristic of rhonchi result from the movement of air over fluid and mucus in the airways.

Cough is associated with hypoxia when airway patency is compromised by an obstruction. Certain characteristics of the cough suggest the source of the obstruction. A cough of "foghorn" quality accompanied by expiratory wheezing when the person lies on the affected side indicates a localized bronchial obstruction. Diffuse airway obstruction produces a weak, ineffective cough in which secretions are raised only with extreme effort. Mucus accumulation associated with obstructive lung disease precipitates a persistent, productive cough that is usually most severe when the person assumes an upright position.

Airway patency is often reduced by secretions that impede ventilation. Characteristics of these secretions provide additional insight into the source of hypoxia. Chronic obstructive lung disease is marked by thick, tenacious sputum. Edema that impedes exchange at the alveolocapilary level causes large amounts of pink, frothy sputum to be produced. When hypoxia is precipitated by destruction of pulmonary tissue such as with tuberculosis and carcinoma, the secretions frequently contain frank blood. Yellow- or greenish-tinged, thick and odoriferous sputum indicates an infection such as pneumonia.

Like the respiratory system, the cardiovascular system responds to decreased oxygen availability by attempting to compensate for the inadequacy. One of the earliest cardiovascular signs is tachycardia, aimed at increasing the rate of oxygen transport to the body tissues. Tachycardia is frequently accompanied by a slight rise in blood pressure, indicative of sympathetic nervous system activity that causes vasoconstriction and increased peripheral resistance. Cardiac auscultation may reveal the presence of arrhythmias or murmurs, which reduce cardiac output and diminish the quantity of oxygenated blood pumped to tissues.

In oxygen deficiency an excessive concentration of deoxygenated hemoglobin circulates in the capillaries. Deoxygenated hemoglobin is characterized by an intense dark blue color, which is reflected through the skin as cyanosis. This sign of hypoxia may vary owing to a number of factors.[3] The intensity of cyanosis depends on the concentration of deoxygenated hemoglobin, regardless of the concentration of oxygenated hemoglobin. The intense dark blue color of deoxygenated blood overpowers the weak red color of oxygenated blood, causing the blue color to be reflected through the skin. Generally, cyanosis is evident when the arterial blood contains greater than 5 g/100 ml of deoxygenated hemoglobin. Consequently, in conditions such as polycythemia, which raises the amount of hemoglobin in the blood, cyanosis is common. Therefore hypoxia accompanied by cyanosis in an anemic person is much more critical than in a person with polycythemia.

The rate of blood flow through the skin and the skin thickness may affect the intensity of cyanosis. If blood flow through the capillaries of the skin is slowed markedly such as occurs with exposure to extreme cold, metabolism of the skin cells further extracts oxygen from the blood. This increases the concentration of deoxygenated hemoglobin and intensifies the cyanosis. Decreased skin thickness enhances the degree of cyanosis. The intense blue color appears more readily on individuals with very thin skin such as newborns and in very vascular areas such as nail beds and lips. Since pigmentation of the skin also affects cyanosis, the color of the mucous membranes often offers a more reliable index than does that of the skin.

In addition to these objective systemic signs, a number of laboratory tests can provide more definitive measures of the impact of hypoxia on cellular function. Among the most commonly used procedures are blood studies, including arterial blood gas, serum enzyme, and electrolyte levels and a complete blood count (CBC).

The arterial blood gas levels provide the best indication of pulmonary ventilation, diffusion effectiveness, and cellular metabolism. The most obvious arterial blood gas indicator of hypoxia is a decreased $Pa{O_2}$. A rise above the normal $Pa{O_2}$ usually indicates hyperventilation or the administration of oxygen under pressure. Increased $Pa{CO_2}$ indicates insufficient ventilation, whereas a decreased level indicates hyperventilation. Variation in $Pa{O_2}$ and $Pa{CO_2}$ is one method for the body to maintain the pH in its normal range. The particular combinations of $Pa{O_2}$, $Pa{CO_2}$, and pH give information as to the status of the buffer systems and clues about the cause of the disruptions.

When reduced oxygen capacity of the blood is the antecedent of hypoxia, the CBC should exhibit decreases in the number of red blood cells, the amount of hemoglobin (Hb), and/or the hematocrit (Hct). However, in the individual who is compensating for long-standing hypoxia not precipitated by reduced oxygen-carrying capacity, this pattern may be reversed. In such instances the kidneys produce large quantities of erythropoietin, which stimulates red blood cell production by the bone marrow. As a result, long-term hypoxia is characterized by elevated RBC, Hb, and Hct levels.

When the antecedent to hypoxia involves a pulmonary infection, the CBC will document the presence of inflammation by an elevation in the white blood cell (WBC) count and the erythrocyte sedimentation rate (ESR). Elevations in the levels of serum potassium and of the intracellular enzymes LDH, AST, and CPK provide an indication of the level of cellular damage precipitated by the hypoxic condition. A depression of the blood pH below 7.35 during a hypoxic state and/or elevated serum chloride level suggests a shift in acid-base balance.

Further definition of the parameters of an individual's oxygen insufficiency is obtained from tests of pulmonary function. Taken in total, these tests reflect the adequacy of air movement to and from the respiratory membrane. Among the most significant findings associated with hypoxia are reduced vital capacity and decreased maximal breathing capacity. In cases of airway obstruction, hypoxia will be further defined by decreased vital capacity and depressed measures of forced expiratory volume and maximal midexpiratory flow. In conjunction with arterial blood gas levels, pulmonary function tests reflect the adequacy of (1) air movement to and from the alevoli, (2) diffusion across the alveolocapillary membrane, (3) transport and delivery of oxygen and carbon dioxide between the lungs and body tissues, and (4) cellular use of oxygen.

Bacteriological studies are important indicators of the extent to which infection is fostering hypoxia. Sputum analysis and nose and throat cultures are sources of data that can identify the causative organism.

Direct visualization of the cardiopulmonary structures provides additional objective evidence of hypoxia. Through such techniques as x-ray studies, bronchoscopy, angiography, and isotope scanning structural irregularities relating to the hypoxia can be identified. ECGs can identify arrhythmias that cause or result from hypoxia.

Subjective data

Hypoxia produces other, more generalized effects on the body. Because of its effects on cellular metabolism, hypoxia reduces the work capacity of the muscles. The lack of oxygen needed for muscles to perform their work becomes evident in descriptions of fatigue or weakness even with minimal exertion. Frequently this is accompanied by reports of increasing effort being required to carry out routine tasks or inability to perform activities that previously were done with no difficulty.

The hypoxic individual may relate episodes of breathlessness or feeling out of breath. When questioned, the individual may recount situations that were avoided because of the fear that they would cause fatigue or breathlessness. Anorexia often develops because the person lacks the strength to eat or fears that eating will aggravate breathlessness.

With severe hypoxia the fear of not being able to get one's breath fosters anxiety, which, when not relieved, can reach panic proportions. The individual's whole being is consumed with the activity of breathing. Such fear increases metabolic demands and oxygen requirements, intensifying the breathing difficulty. When hypoxia is less severe, the individual often employs defense mechanisms to deal with anxiety. Isolation techniques may be employed to avoid activities that require muscular exertion and the expenditure of energy. To deal with doubt and insecurity about the lack of strength, the individual may attempt to control the environment through compulsive rituals and obsessions. Such defense mechanisms enable the individual to conserve energy and preserve self-image.

INTERVENING VARIABLES

The effects of hypoxia on the human organism are in large part a function of the antecedent condition. However, certain other factors influence the degree to which hypoxia affects the organism. A common denominator of these variables is their impact on the metabolic rate. With an increase in metabolic rate, oxygen consumption rises to meet increased energy demands. This intensifies the state of hypoxia. Conversely, a drop in metabolic rate reduces the demand for oxygen and decreases the intensity of hypoxia manifestations.

Foremost among these intervening variables is exercise. Maximal muscle exercise involving the entire body can increase the metabolic rate to 2000% of normal.[3] Such an increase in metabolic rate dramatically raises oxygen consumption and correspondingly intensifies the hypoxia. The intensity of hypoxia also varies with age and sex. The newborn child's metabolic rate in relation to body surface area is almost two times that of an elderly person.[3] Thus young children are less tolerant of hypoxia than are the elderly. However, the older individual has less reserves to cope with hypoxia. Decreased elastic recoil of the lungs, increased chest wall rigidity, and reduced physical power accompany the aging process. These physical changes increase residual volume of the lungs and decrease the vital capacity, causing a depression in the alveolocapillary diffusion. This imposes restrictions on the elderly individual's capability to compensate for reduced oxygen levels. Sex hormones also influence oxygen use. A man's metabolic rate is 10% to 15% higher than a woman's.[3] As a result, hypoxia of the same degree will be felt more intensely by the man.

Stress or anxiety can significantly influence the individual's oxygen requirements. The secretion of epinephrine, which accompanies anxiety, often increases the metabolic rate of the body as much as 100% above normal.[3] This heightened metabolic rate exaggerates oxygen demands and aggravates hypoxia.

Variations in the level of the thyroid hormone, thyroxine, alter the metabolic rate and consequently modify the impact of hypoxia on the body. Maximal secretion of thyroxine can increase the metabolic rate to as much as 100% above normal. Absence of thyroxine reduces the metabolic rate to 50% of normal.[3] Thus the manifestations of hypoxia can be intensified or subdued by the presence of a thyroid disorder.

Body temperature is closely tied to metabolic rate. An increase in body temperature, regardless of the cause, generates a heightened metabolic rate. This puts an additional burden on the body to supply oxygen to cells and exaggerates the hypoxia. A lowered body temperature such as occurs with hypothermia reduces metabolic demands and decreases the potential for hypoxia.

Ultimately, by influencing the metabolic rate, these variables intensify or diminish the effects of inadequate oxygen.

NURSING INTERVENTIONS—GOALS AND EVALUATION CRITERIA

The general goal of nursing interventions in hypoxic states is to increase tissue oxygenation to a level that will meet oxygen demands. This broad goal can be attained through the achievement of the following five specific goals of nursing care: (1) maintenance of airway patency, (2) provision of maximized ventilation, (3) increase of oxygen transport, (4) reduction of tissue oxygen demands, and (5) reduction of incidence or risk of infection.

Maintenance of airway patency

Airway patency is so crucial to the management or reduction of hypoxia that if it is not maintained, efforts toward the achievement of the other goals are useless. Therefore it is essential that initial efforts at promoting tissue oxygenation be directed at determining whether there is a patent airway for ventilation.

If relaxation of the tongue is causing upper airway obstruction, the tongue can be lifted from the posterior pharyngeal wall by placing a finger behind each ramus and moving the mandible forward. An oropharyngeal airway may be inserted to maintain the tongue in the forward position. Lower airway obstruction, generally resulting from accumulated secretions or bronchospasms that block free movement of oxygen and carbon dioxide, is most effectively cleared by productive cough initiated by the patient. To increase the cough's productivity, the patient should be instructed to inhale deeply and then try to force all the air out of the lungs with an explosive cough using the abdominal muscles. When the small, distal airways are obstructed, the most effective coughing consists of a deep inspiration followed by three consecutive coughs aimed at emptying the lungs of all air with each cough. This process is most effective when carried out while sitting up.[8]

When the patient is unable to initiate efforts to clear the airways of secretions, mechanical suction may be needed to maintain a patent airway. Insertion of a sterile catheter through a nostril past the pharynx and into the trachea induces a cough by laryngotracheal irritation. Suction can then aspirate the secretions produced by the cough. When secretions are especially tenacious, 5 to 10 ml of sterile normal saline solution or a dilution of sterile normal saline solution and a mucolytic agent may be instilled through the catheter to liquify the secretions and facilitate removal.

Frequent changing of position will allow gravity to increase the evacuation of secretions by facilitating their movement to larger, more central airways, where they can be more easily removed by coughing or suction. Movement of secretions is enhanced further by postural drainage, which uses gravity to drain secretions from the lung periphery to the more central areas of the tracheobronchial tree, from which it can be expelled more effectively. When accompanied by percussion, postural drainage can result in the evacuation of copious amounts of thick, tenacious sputum.

Although the specific pharmacological agents used to maintain airway patency vary, the following groups of medications are commonly used to help achieve this goal. Antihistamines are used to reduce the edema of the tracheobronchial airways that occurs in allergic reactions. Among the more commonly used antihistamines are diphenhydramine hydrochloride (Benadryl), chlorpheniramine maleate (Chlor-Trimeton), and brompheniramine maleate (Dimetane). Adrenocorticoids, anti-inflammatory agents, can also enhance air movement by decreasing inflammatory edema of the bronchial walls. Prednisone is a frequently used agent in this group. Since corticoids decrease the body's inflammatory response, the hypoxic patient receiving them has an increased susceptibility to infection, and additional precautions must be taken to protect this patient from the added hypoxic burden of respiratory infections.

Bronchodilators used to relieve bronchial spasms are primarily of two types. One type is adrenergic agents such as isoproterenol (Isuprel) hydrochloride and epinephrine hydrochloride (Adrenalin), and the other type is theophylline compounds, particularly aminophylline. Both groups of medications act directly on the bronchial smooth muscle to relieve bronchospasms.

Antitussives and expectorants, two types of cough preparations, affect airway clearing. Antitussive agents are used to inhibit the cough reflex in the cough center and are available in many forms, the most familiar being codeine (methylmorphine). Because of the helpful airway-clearing action of a cough, antitussive agents should be used only when the patient's level of fatigue requires a period of uninterrupted rest. Expectorants are used to facilitate movement of secretions. A commonly used preparation is saturated solution of potassium iodide (SSKI), which acts by liquifying mucus so it can be expelled more easily by coughing. Tyloxapol (Alevaire) and ethasulfate (Tergemist), both mucolytic detergents, are used for the same reason. Glyceryl guaiacolate enhances the flow of secretions from the airways be decreasing viscosity. Regardless of the expectorant used, the patient should avoid taking fluids, food, or other medications after ingestion of the expectorant, since washing of the expectorant from the pharyngeal mucosa interferes with its effect.

Behaviors that can be used to evaluate the achievement of the goal of maintaining airway patency include clearly audible breath sounds and a decrease in adventitious lung sounds. If a cough has been present, the initial signs of effectiveness would include increased productivity of the cough. Then, as the antecedent condition diminishes, the secretions that have obstructed the airway should become less viscous, decrease in volume, and return to a normal mucoid white color. As the cough becomes less productive, it should also decrease in frequency. Other behaviors indicative of relief of the hypoxic state also relate to increased tissue oxygenation; they will be considered in the following discussions. However, if airway obstruction is the only antecedent to the hypoxic state, all the behaviors outlined in the following discussions should occur at the achievement of airway patency.

Provision of maximized ventilation

Although the maintenance of a patent airway is essential to the avoidance of hypoxia, that alone may not be sufficient to restore optimum tissue oxygenation. In addition, interventions may have to be directed at maximizing ventilatory efforts. Breathing can usually be facilitated by positioning the patient with head and chest elevated. This position allows for unrestricted movement of the respiratory muscles during ventilation. Positioning the shoulders slightly back when the person is sitting increases the area for downward movement of the diaphragm and thus enhances diaphragmatic breathing. Reducing the gravitational weight of the arms also allows for greater expansion of the chest wall. The head should not flex forward, since this increases resistance to airflow in the upper airways. A pillow placed lengthwise behind the back and head should prevent this flexion. When severe dyspnea is present, the patient often breathes easier while sleeping if positioned sitting with head and arms leaning over a padded overbed table.

Ventilatory efforts can be enhanced further by deep breathing exercises aimed at helping the patient use the diaphragm and abdominal muscles for more efficient ventilation. Deep breathing increases lung expansion and equalizes the distribution of air in the alveolar sacs. In addition, it decreases intrapleural pressure, which, in turn, stimulates blood flow to the lungs. To obtain maximum diffusion of oxygen from deep breathing, the tracheobronchial tree should be cleared of secretions by suction or by a patient-initiated productive cough before the beginning of the exercises. While lying flat on a firm surface, the patient should breathe deeply through the nose, feeling a rise in the abdomen during inhalation. This is followed by a slow, easy exhalation through pursed lips, accompanied by tightening of the abdominal muscles. This exerts pressure on the diaphragm and forces air out of the lungs. Depending on the severity of the hypoxia, this maneuver should be repeated 5 to 10 times every 1 to 2 hours. Once adept at deep breathing in the supine position, the patient should be helped to develop this pattern of breathing in sitting, standing, and both lateral positions. The ultimate goal for the patient with chronic ventilatory failure or impaired alveolocapillary diffusion is incorporation of this controlled diaphragmatic breathing in the unconscious breathing pattern.

If secretions retained in the tracheobronchial tree precipitate or aggravate hypoxia, deep breathing exercises may be used as an adjunct to deep coughing to clear the airway of obstruction. The deep inspiratory breaths can increase the tidal volume as much as threefold, providing additional air during expiration to force out accumulated secretions.[8] Deep breathing may be induced by the use of blow gloves or blow bottles. Deep breaths may also be stimulated by rebreathing devices that stimulate the respiratory center by increasing carbon dioxide levels.

Respiratory stimulants such as caffeine, sodium benzoate, and carbon dioxide gas, which affect the central nervous system, may be used to intensify the activity of the respiratory center in the medulla. Also, with narcotic- or barbiturate-induced respiratory failure, nalorphine (Nalline) hydrochloride and levallorphan tartrate (Lorfan), narcotic antagonists, may be used to counteract respiratory depression.

Specific behavioral outcomes to evaluate the effectiveness of ventilatory efforts include decreased pulse and blood pressure, reduced respiratory rate, and increased ease of breathing. The increased ease in breathing should be accompanied by a decrease in anxiety behavior as demonstrated by muscle relaxation. As the ability to eliminate carbon dioxide improves, arterial blood gas levels should become more normal. Dropping of the $Paco_2$ should be accompanied by pH shifts toward or above 7.35. Serum chloride levels should return to normal as acid-base balance is regained. Pulmonary function tests should indicate increases in tidal volume, vital capacity, and forced expiratory flow. As these pulmonary functions improve, there should be a gradual increase in exercise tolerance, and the patient should be able to pursue more intense activity for longer periods.

Increase of oxygen transport

Although positioning and deep breathing exercises greatly improve oxygenation, oxygen therapy is often instituted when the manifestations of hypoxia are marked. The aim of oxygen therapy is to maximize the oxygen-carrying capacity of the arterial blood so that a Pao_2 of approximately 100 to 150 mm Hg can be achieved, given a normal hemoglobin level.[6]

Special precautions are required in patients with a history of long-term ventilatory insufficiency whose stimulus to breathe arises from the reduced Pao_2. In these patients special oxygen delivery devices such as a Venturi mask are employed to regulate the oxygen concentration. The goal of this oxygen therapy is to attain a PaO_2 of approximately 80 mm Hg. This is sufficient to provide relief of hypoxia manifestations in these patients without destroying their ventilation stimulus.[6]

When hypoxia is produced by ineffective respiratory muscle action or by increased airway resistance, oxygen therapy can be augmented by mechanical respirators. Intermittent positive pressure breathing devices modify the character of respirations by providing oxygen or an air-oxygen mixture under increased pressure to the bronchi at a set rate. This increases tidal volume and promotes a more uniform distribution of gases at the alveolocapillary membrane. Intermittent positive pressure breathing devices further enhance oxygenation by forcing gas beyond accumulated secretions, thus producing an airway-clearing cough.

To counteract the drying effects of oxygen and promote removal of secretions, administered oxygen should always be humidified.

When a decreased oxygen-carrying capacity of the blood produces hypoxia, dietary supplements such as folic acid, vitamin B_{12}, iron, and protein may be administered to enhance the production of red blood cells and hemoglobin. When hypoxia results from pump failure, oxygen transport may be enhanced by the direct action of cardiotonic preparations such as digitalis and antiarrhythmic drugs on the myocardium. The aim is that myocardial contractions become more efficient and regular, with resultant improved tissue oxygenation.

Behavioral indicators of increased oxygen transport to body tissues include a return to normal of the pulse, blood pressure, and respiratory rates. These indicators also accompany increased ventilation. Skin color should improve from cyanotic or pallor to pink. As more oxygen reaches the neurons of the central nervous system, levels of awareness and concentration ability should increase, visual acuity should improve, and headaches should decrease. Enhanced oxygen transport can also be documented by improved Hb, Hct, RBC, and PaO_2 levels as well as electrocardiographic tracings indicative of more synchronized electrical conduction in the cardiac muscles.

Reduction of tissue oxygen demands

Efforts to promote tissue oxygenation must be accompanied by interventions directed at decreasing the tissues' oxygen demands. To this end the patient's activity level must be planned to balance the ability of the body's systems to deliver oxygen to tissues. Because of the effects of hypoxia on cellular metabolism, the patient deprived of oxygen fatigues easily. Nursing care must be organized to allow the patient periods of uninterrupted rest. Activities such as bathing, positioning, and eating should be carried out in ways that require the least expenditure of patient energy. Sequencing and clustering of activities should be planned with the aim of energy conservation. Small rest pauses may be required during activities such as bathing. Small, frequent feedings might counteract the fatigue and shortness of breath the patient may experience with the normal three large meals each day. Gas-forming foods should be avoided because of the upward pressure they exert on the diaphragm, which can reduce maximal excursion. Planned rest periods before meals may increase the patient's appetite.

Hypoxic fatigue may so limit the patient's activity level that passive activity such as range of motion exercises may be needed to reduce the risk of complication from physical immobilization. Since excessive heat or cold will increase the metabolism, the room temperature should be maintained at a level comfortable for the patient.

Because of the effects of anxiety and fear on hypoxia, efforts should be made to provide for psychological comfort and well-being. The presence of a nurse can reassure the severely dyspneic patient who is extremely frightened. Anticipation of the patient's needs and prompt answering of the call light convey the nonverbal message that the staff knows about and can be trusted to attend to the patient's needs. Careful explanation of procedures and tests helps to reduce the fear of the unknown and to return cognitive control to the patient. The patient's psychological comfort and well-being, and ultimately oxygen demands, can be greatly affected by the nurse's ability to recognize the patient's psychological response to hypoxia, to preserve the patient's identity, and to provide the patient with avenues of control.

Behavioral indications that tissue demands have been reduced include an increase in the number of activities in which the patient can engage without becoming overly fatigued. An increase in nutrients ingested and increased appetite provide additional evidence of successful management of oxygen demands.

Relaxed patterns of breathing, general muscle relaxation, and more relaxed conversation patterns all indicate increased psychological comfort.

Reduction in incidence or risk of infection

Because of the hypoxic patient's increased susceptibility to infection, special safeguards are required to prevent infection and keep the environment safe. Efforts should be made to protect the patient from exposure to individuals with known infections, particularly those involving the respiratory tract. All equipment used for oxygen therapy should be properly sterilized and changed every 24 hours to prevent transmission of infection through contaminated equipment. Good hand-washing technique is a must in all aspects of patient care.

A variety of antimicrobial agents, including tetracycline, penicillin, and cephalosporin antibiotics, are used to treat pulmonary infections.

Hydration is especially significant when the hypoxia is accompanied by tenacious secretions or fever. Increased fluid intake is needed to reduce the tenacity of the secretions and prevent dehydration. In the absence of cardiovascular and renal limitations, fluids should be forced up to 4000 ml/day. Clear liquid are preferable to fluids such as milk that coat the oral pharynx and make it more difficult to expectorate secretions.

The hypoxic patient requires special attention to oral and nasal hygiene. When the hypoxia is accompanied by secretions, the mouth becomes coated with mucus, which harbors microorganisms and reduces the patient's appetite. To reduce microorganisms and make food more palatable, oral hygiene should be carried out every 3 to 4 hours, including before each meal.

A mixture of four parts mouthwash and one part hydrogen peroxide will facilitate débridement of mucus from the oral mucosa. In addition, teeth or dentures should be thoroughly cleaned with a toothbrush. The nasal passage also require special attention to keep them patent and moist. The patient should be provided with tissues and an emesis basin to blow mucus from the nasal pharynx or to expectorate mucus that drains into the oral pharynx from the sinuses. If the patient cannot carry this out independently, the nurse should check the patency of the nasal airways frequently with a nasal speculum. Dried secretions can be cleansed away with a moist applicator. This should be followed by an application of a lubricant such as glycerin or petroleum jelly to moisten dried mucous membranes. To further prevent drying of the mucous membranes, the patient's room should be well ventilated and free of pollutants. Smoking by the patient and others should be strongly discouraged. Of course, when oxygen therapy is used, smoking must be prohibited. Humidification of the room air by a bedside humidifier may also help reduce membrane drying.

A daily bath helps decrease bacterial growth on the skin. Lotions should be substituted for powders during back rubs to avoid the danger of the patient inhaling the powder. Men should be shaved daily, particularly when receiving oxygen by mask or expectorating copious secretions. In these situations the beard could serve as a reservoir for the growth of microorganisms. Electric razors should be used with caution to avoid inhalation of hair particles.

Useful criteria in the determination of the effectiveness with which infections are being reduced include the character of the oropharyngeal mucous membranes. A hydrated, intact mucous membrane is an indication that portals of entry are minimal. Maintenance of a normal WBC count, ESR, and temperature is a further indication that the body is not involved in an inflammatory response.

CONCEPT OUTLINE

I. *Conceptual definition:* Hypoxia is a state wherein oxygen-dependent cellular metabolism is disrupted as a result of either diminished availability of oxygen or cellular demand for oxygen that exceeds ability of body's systems to deliver it.

II. *Antecedent conditions*
  A. Pulmonary failure
    1. Failure to inspire an adequate volume of air
      a. Obstructed airway
      b. Restricted movement of the thoracic cavity
      c. Depression of the respiratory center
    2. Impaired diffusion across alveolocapillary membrane
      a. Excessive mucus accumulation
      b. Alveoli destruction
      c. Obstruction of pulmonary circulation
      d. Edema of lung tissue

B. Inadequate oxygen transport
  1. Failure of heart pump
    a. Congenital anomalies
    b. Decreased myocardial contractility
    c. Valvular disorders
    d. Cardiac arrhythmias
  2. Defects in vascular system
    a. Reduced volume of circulating blood
    b. Decreased levels of oxygen-carrying components
C. Excessive tissue demands for oxygen
  1. Decreased metabolism
  2. Physical exertion
D. Ineffective cellular use of oxygen
  1. Tissue edema
  2. Inhibition of cellular enzymes

III. *Behavioral definition*
A. Objective data
  1. Neurological changes
    a. Decreased night vision
    b. Restlessness
    c. Drowsiness and lassitude
    d. Decreased ability to make judgments, remember, and carry out discrete motor movements
    e. Coma
    f. Cessation of respiration
  2. Respiratory changes
    a. Increased respiratory rate
    b. Dyspnea and air hunger
    c. Altered pattern of respiration
    d. Uneven chest wall expansion
    e. Abnormal percussion sounds
    f. Abnormal breath sounds
    g. Adventitious lung sounds
    h. Cough
    i. Sputum production
    j. Elevated or reduced $Paco_2$
    k. Reduced PaO_2
    l. Decreased serum chloride level
    m. Radiological changes in thoracic cavity structure and tissue density
    n. Bacterial culture growths
    o. Elevated WBC count
    p. Abnormal pulmonary function tests
  3. Cardiovascular changes
    a. Tachycardia
    b. Slight rise in blood pressure
    c. Arrhythmias or murmurs
    d. Cyanosis
    e. Abnormal ECG
    f. Decreased Hb, Hct, and RBC levels
    g. Increased CPK, LDH, and aspartate (AST) levels
B. Subjective data
  1. Fatigue
  2. Breathlessness
  3. Anorexia
  4. Restless feelings or fears

IV. *Intervening variables*
A. Activity level
B. Age
C. Sex
D. Stress level and tolerance
E. Thyroid hormone activity
F. Body temperature
G. Anxiety

V. *Nursing interventions—goals*
A. Maintenance of airway patency
  1. Manual opening of upper airway
  2. Patient-initiated cough
  3. Suctioning
  4. Positioning
  5. Pharmacological agents
    a. Bronchodilators
    b. Antihistamines
    c. Anti-inflammatory agents
    d. Antitussives
    e. Expectorants
B. Provision of maximized ventilation
  1. Positioning for maximum movement of respiratory muscles
  2. Deep breathing exercises
  3. Pharmacological agents
    a. Respiratory stimulants
    b. Narcotic antagonists
    c. Carbon dioxide
C. Increase of oxygen transport
  1. Oxygen therapy
  2. Mechanical ventilation
  3. Dietary supplements
    a. Folic acid
    b. Vitamin B_{12}
    c. Iron
    d. Protein
  4. Pharmacological agents
    a. Cardiotonic preparations
    b. Antiarrhythmic drugs
D. Reduction of tissue oxygen demands
  1. Activity level balanced with oxygen availability
  2. Maintenance of comfortable room temperature

3. Development of trust relationship to reduce anxiety
   a. Prompt answering of call light
   b. Explanation of procedures and tests
   c. Provision of benchmarks of progress

E. Reduction of incidence or risk of infection
   1. Prevention or reduction of exposure to individuals with infections
   2. Hand washing by personnel
   3. Fluid intake increased to 4000 ml/day
   4. Oral and nasal hygiene every 3 to 4 hours, particularly before meals
   5. Daily bath
   6. Discouragement of smoking by patient and others in environment
   7. Room air humidification
   8. Antimicrobial agents

VI. *Evaluation criteria*
   A. Neurological changes
      1. Improved visual acuity
      2. Increased ability to concentrate
      3. Decreased incidence of headaches
      4. Increased level of awareness
   B. Respiratory changes
      1. Decreased respiratory rate
      2. Increased ease of breathing
      3. Less adventitious lung sounds
      4. Return of normal breath sounds
      5. Return of secretions to more mucoid, white color
   C. Cardiovascular changes
      1. Normal pulse rate and blood pressure
      2. Increased force and regularity of heartbeat
      3. Normal color of skin and mucous membranes
      4. Normal CPK, LDH, AST, Hb, Hct, and RBC levels
   D. Other changes
      1. Increased muscle relaxation
      2. Increased relaxed conversation patterns
      3. Increased exercise tolerance
      4. Expansion of social interaction
      5. Reduced fatigue
      6. Increased appetite and ingestion of nutrients

REFERENCES

1. Comroe, J. H.: The lung: clinical physiology and pulmonary function tests, ed. 2, Chicago, 1962, Year Book Medical Publishers, Inc.
2. Gallagher, C. H., Judah, J. D., and Rees, K. R.: Enzyme changes during liver autolysis, J. Pathol. Bacteriol. **72**:247, 1956.
3. Guyton, A. C.: Textbook of medical physiology, Philadelphia, 1976, W. B. Saunders Co.
4. Majno, G., LaGattuta, M., and Thompson, T. E.: Death and necrosis: chemical, physical, and morphologic changes in rat liver, Virchows Arch. [Pathol. Anat.] **333**:421, 1960.
5. Ozawa, K., Seta, K., Araki, H., and Handa, H.: The effect of ischemia on mitochondrial metabolism, J. Biochem. (Tokyo) **61**:512, 1967.
6. Phipps, W. J., and Barker, W. L.: Respiratory insufficiency and failure. In Meltzer, L. E., Abdellah, F. G., and Kitchell, J. R., editors: Concepts and practices of intensive care for nurse specialists, Philadelphia, 1969, The Charles Press.
7. Robbins, S. L., and Angell, M.: Basic pathology, ed. 2, Philadelphia, 1969, W. B. Saunders Co.
8. Secor, J.: Patient care in respiratory problems, Philadelphia, 1969, W. B. Saunders Co.
9. Vogt, M., Farber, E.: On the molecular pathology of ischemic renal cell death, Am. J. Pathol. **53**:1, 1968.
10. Walter, J. B.: An introduction to the principles of disease, Philadelphia, 1977, W. B. Saunders Co.

LAURA K. HART

Chapter 14

ISCHEMIA

CONCEPTUAL DEFINITION

Ischemia is a state of reduced or absent blood perfusion of tissues. It often refers both to varying degrees of blood perfusion deficiency and to conditions that involve varying extents of body function. The term is used to refer to local, compartmental, regional, and systemic reductions in or cessation of circulatory flow. This chapter will not address the dynamics of the systemic concept of ischemic shock; such a discussion can be found in Chapter 15. The concept of ischemia discussed here will be limited to the reduction of local or compartmental circulatory flow, ranging from slight impairment to complete cessation.

Normal cell metabolism depends on the receipt of oxygen and nutrients and the removal of metabolic waste products. When reduction in blood perfusion of tissues interferes with the exchange of these substances, the function and energy metabolism of the cells are affected.[41,51]

Cells oxidize carbohydrate and/or lipid fuels to generate chemical energy in the form of adenosine triphosate (ATP). This process of oxidizing substrates and conserving energy in the form of ATP is called oxidative phosphorylation. When abundant oxygen and substrates are available, most cells convert this high-energy phosphate group to creatine phosphate, which acts as a reservoir for the high-energy phosphate bond.

Glucose and its storage form, glycogen, are the only substrates the cells are capable of using for an energy source in both the presence and absence of oxygen. The conversion of one molecule of glucose to pyruvate yields two molecules of ATP. This occurs whether the conversion is accomplished aerobically or anaerobically. Anaerobic metabolism is unable to progress beyond this initial conversion. However, under aerobic metabolism, pyruvate can continue to be converted and burned via the Krebs cycle and the electron transport chain, yielding 36 more molecules of ATP.[24] During anaerobic metabolism the ATP yield from a glucose molecule is approximately 18 times less than that produced by aerobic pathways.[74]

When blood flow to a tissue is restricted, the availability of oxygen and substrates regulates the rate of the oxidative phosphorylation process.[59] During states of hypoxia the creatine phosphate stores are depleted and the concentrations of the metabolic end products of this conversion, adenosine phosphate (ADP), adenosine monophosphate (AMP), and inorganic phosphate, increase.[5,7] The end product of the anaerobic glucose conversion, lactic acid, is also increased.

Anaerobic metabolism of glucose can continue as long as glucose remains available as a substrate. When blood perfusion is totally occluded, the endogenous glycogen is the only fuel available for energy generation. Since intracellular triglyceride stores cannot be metabolized anaerobically when glycogen tissue stores are depleted, ATP production stops owing to the lack of available anaerobic substrate. As a result of this impaired energy production, the cell's ion transport ability is reduced and its parenchymal function is restricted.[74]

As energy production decreases, ions that require active transport to move through the cell membrane begin having their movement governed by the concentration gradient. Among the substances that require active transport for movement are sodium, potassium, calcium, iron, hydrogen, chloride, iodide, urate ions, and several sugars and amino acids. As the energy available for active transport is reduced, sodium and calcium begin moving into the cell, and potassium and magnesium move out. These changes in ion concentrations are accompanied by cellular swelling.[48-51,73]

In addition to reducing energy production, anaerobic metabolism produces the waste product lactic acid, which reduces the cell's pH.[25,48,79] A lowered pH can trigger the release and activation of lysosomal enzymes, resulting in disruption of the mitochondrial and plasma membranes. These catabolic enzymes are able to digest cell components. As cell membranes are broken, intracellular enzymes such as lactic dehydrogenase (LDH), aspartate transaminase (AST),* and creatine phosphokinase (CPK) leak through the damaged membranes.

Tissues can tolerate being perfused with blood with very low oxygen content much longer than they can tolerate the hypoxia that accompanies lack of blood perfusion.[32,37,38] It appears that this difference relates to the tissue acidosis caused by the accumulation of lactic acid.[30] Ischemia seems to be a self-perpetuating mechanism in which ischemically induced edema generates more ischemia. Cellular swelling produces pressure, which further impairs circulation, precipitating a vicious circle that can result in cell death.[18]

The ability of tissue to survive and recover from ischemia depends on how long the tissue's cells can withstand ischemic insult and on the extent to which nutritive blood flow to the cells can be reestablished. The reaction of the microcirculation to ischemic injury is critical to the tissue's ability to repair ischemic damage. When ischemic capillaries are injured to the point that they lose their integrity, leaky capillary membranes and ischemic tissues become susceptible to further injury from the increased tissue edema that may accompany reperfusion.[54,55,59] In addition to such tissue edema, a no-reflow phenomenon has been observed during the reperfusion of many ischemic tissues.[2] The hyperemic response that occurs after long-term ischemia does not reperfuse tissues equally.[40,47] Postischemic endothelial swelling and blebs have been held partially responsible for the poor initiation of recirculation.[8,14,17,28]

Functional disturbances such as hemoconcentration, increased blood viscosity, white blood cell stickiness, and thrombus formation have also been suggested as the cause of reduced reperfusion of microvessels. However, most investigators conclude than these changes cannot completely explain the no-reflow phenomenon. It has been advanced that the blood is altered as it returns to the ischemic tissues.

---

*Aspartate transaminase (AST) is now the international standard nomenclature for what was formerly called glutamic oxaloacetic transaminase (GOT).

Hemoconcentration and secondarily increased viscosity occur.[61] In addition, the rapid deoxygenation of the red blood cells in combination with the low pH environment decreases red blood cell deformability.[42] Thus it appears that the low pH of the ischemic tissue is the primary variable that impedes reflow.[61,79]

ANTECEDENT CONDITIONS

When ischemia is defined as a reduction in or absence of local or compartmental tissue perfusion that initiates and limits anaerobic metabolism, the conditions that can singularly initate this phenomenon are limited. Local ischemia is most commonly initiated by the interaction of a number of antecedents. The major factors that influence how adequately blood flow meets metabolic needs include the effectiveness of the cardiac pump, the patency of the vessels, the volume and viscosity of the blood, and the level of the cells' metabolic demand.

When ischemia is limited to the perspective of a local phenomenon, only factors that affect the patency of the vessels or the level of local metabolism can singularly initiate this concept. When failure in the cardiac pump or reduced blood volume reaches a level that singularly initiates local tissue ischemia, the systemic condition of ischemic shock is usually also precipitated. In such situations shock rather than local ischemia would be the priority problem. Discussion of such antecedents is found in Chapter 15.

Reduced vessel patency

Conditions that affect the patency of vessels are of four types: (1) pathological conditions of the cardiovascular system that reduce or obstruct the vessel lumens, (2) conditions that precipitate severe reflexive vasoconstriction, (3) extracorporeal mechanical pressure on the blood vessels, and (4) intracorporeal mechanical pressure on the blood vessels.

Restriction or obstruction of vessel lumens. The patency of blood vessels, arterial and venous, can be affected by changes in vessel elasticity and competency as well as by changes in blood viscosity that precipitate the development of thrombi and emboli.

Arteriosclerosis refers to a group of pathological processes that cause thickening and loss of elasticity of arterial walls. These processes may precipitate the formation of focal intimal plaques (atheromata), calcification of the media of muscular arteries, and/or proliferative fibromuscular or endothelial thickening of the walls of small arteries and arterioles.[60] These arteriosclerotic processes cause thickening and induration of arterial walls. The deposit of calcium in the arterial walls reduces the vessels' elasticity and prevents the vessels from dilating to accommodate the increased volume of blood demanded by increased metabolic needs. When these disease processes cause intimal degeneration and/or plaque formation, tears, roughening, ulceration, and clot formation on the arterial lining occur. Clots, or thombi, can occur anywhere in the cardiovascular system. A thrombus is a mass containing red blood cells, granular leukocytes, and platelets bound together by fibrin.[32]

A thrombus may partially or completely close the lumen of the affected vessel, increasing resistance to the flow and changing the flow from laminar to turbulent. Turbulent flow requires more energy or pressure to maintain the delivery of a given volume of blood. Turbulent flow also increases the risk of thromboembolism, a detached intravascular fragment of a thrombus that is carried in the blood to a site distant from its point of origin.[60] Such fragments become lodged in vessels that are too small to permit passage. This usually causes complete or partial occlusion of the vessel, precipitating another instance of ischemia. The large and small pulmonary arteries are the most common and the most lethal sites of emboli. However, these emboli are usually of venous origin. The brain, lower extremities, spleen, and kidneys are the most frequent sites of arterial emboli.[60]

The majority of arterial thrombi develop as a result of arteriosclerotic processes. However, other causes of arteritis such as syphilis, bacterial endocarditis, lupus erythematosus, and other debilitating illnesses may also precipitate thrombus formation. In these situations hypercoagulability of the blood may assist thrombus initiation.

In the slower moving venous blood flow, thrombus formation appears to be affected by blood stasis. However, stasis of the blood alone is not able to induce thrombosis. Usually two or more of the following prediposing factors must be present to initiate thrombus formation: vascular changes, stasis, and hypercoagulability. The contribution of the condition of the venous wall to the formation of thrombi is not well understood.[60]

Phlebothrombosis occurs predominately (90%) in the lower extremities.[32] Two of the major factors that precipitate stasis in these limbs are incompetent valves and reduced or absent skeletal muscle activity. Trauma to or inflammation near the veins may break or roughen the endothelial lining of the veins, providing a clotting nidus. However, a normal flow rate, which confines formed elements to the central column of the blood and sweeps off wandering platelets, significantly prevents or limits thrombosis. The dilution, removal, and inhibition of activated procoagulants also protect against thrombogenesis and nidus enlargement.[60]

A high risk of venous thrombosis is associated with the third trimester of pregnancy and the postdelivery period, when fibrinogen, clotting factors, and the number and adhesiveness of platelets increase.[72] High risk also accompanies congestive heart failure; varicositis of the lower legs; severe burns; major trauma; fractures, particularly of long bones; upper abdominal and pelvic surgery; disseminated cancer; and prolonged bed rest or part immobilization.[26,67,68] Hypercoagulability and flow stasis appear to be the dominant influences in these conditions.

When a thrombus does form, the underlying vessel tissue responds to it as a foreign body, with an inflammatory response. The process of thrombus organization and canalization most commonly follows the inflammatory reaction as the body attempts to repair tissue and, at least in part, reestablish blood flow.

Thromboangiitis obliterans (Buerger's disease) is an arterial and venous pathological condition characterized by segmental thrombi and acute and chronic inflammation. These processes often obliterate flow and lead to gangrene. The arteries initially become involved, with accompanying veins and adjacent nerves secondarily affected. A striking feature of this disease is that it occurs almost exclusively in men and tobacco smokers.[60]

Reflexive vasoconstriction. The peripheral vascular beds most susceptible to vasospastic disorders are characterized by a high degree of sympathetic regulation as well as by regulation by and response to locally circulating vasoactive substances such as histamine, prostaglandins, polypeptides, and catecholamines.[52] Vasospastic disorders that precipitate local ischemia are of two types: (1) primarily vasospastic disorders and (2) diseases in which vasospasm is associated with other systemic, regional, or local disorders.

The most common vasospastic disorder is Raynaud's disease. This disease is characterized by episodic, symmetrical vasoconstriction of the small arteries and arterioles of the extremities. The vasospasms of Raynaud's disease may be so severe and prolonged that ulcerations and frank gangrene of the affected parts may be precipitated. These vasospasms are particularly aggravated by exposure to cold.

Raynaud's phenomenon, unlike Raynaud's disease, is a syndrome of arterial insufficiency caused by organic arterial occlusions. Persons with this phenomenon may also present the sequential blanching, cyanosis, and rubor characteristic of the vasospasms of Raynaud's disease.[52]

Another major secondary vasospastic condition results from cold injury or frostbite. The mechanisms that precipitate cell injury in this disorder appear to include cell freezing, vasospasm, microcirculatory stasis, endothelial swelling, and changes in the physical state of the ground substances.[13,34]

Extracorporeal mechanical pressure. External pressure is one of the primary antecedents of local ischemic tissue destruction. The extent of destruction resulting from external pressure depends on (1) the presence of a bony prominence close beneath the skin, (2) the thickness and morphology of the padding tissue between the bone and skin, (3) the duration of the pressure, and (4) the integrity of the skin.[56]

One of the major factors that affects the type of tissue destruction that occurs from external pressure is the manner in which pressure is distributed in heterogeneous, semisolid cutaneous and muscle tissue. When tissues are compressed between two unequal surfaces such as a mattress and a bony prominence, the greatest amount of compression occurs immediately beneath the compression surfaces. In addition, the greatest amount of tissue deformation occurs adjacent to the smaller of the two surfaces. The force of the compression diminishes as the distance from the opposing forces increases, and the area affected by the force increases as the distance from the smaller surface increases. The tissue adjacent to the impinging surfaces is subjected to increased tension rather than to compression.[33,44] This tension is greatest when the impinging surface is angular or pointed and when the pressure forces are not only vertical but shearing.[15,16,23,44] When a shearing force is exerted against muscle tissue, the blood vessels in the tissue are stretched at their anchoring points in the deep fascia. This may explain the multiple thrombi of small vessels that frequently accompany decubitus ulcers. In addition, shearing forces produce extensive tissue dissection or cleavage in the plane of the greatest concentration of force. This area of undermined tissue extends circumferentially about the point of pressure at the level of the deep superficial fascia.[15,58]

The prime factors that produce tissue pathology by external pressure are the magnitude of the applied force per unit of surface and the duration of the pressure.[44] However, the extent of muscle degeneration is also affected by whether the muscle is stretched and by its content of mitochrondria.[27]

The malleability of the opposing surfaces also modifies the magnitude of the pressure exerted on any given point. The more pliable the support, the greater the area of surface contact. This pliability reduces the force exerted on any single unit of surface.[44] When the body is in a recumbent position, only about $^1/_5$ of the body's surface is available for weight bearing.[33] If the pressure exerted on the recumbent body were evenly distributed over the body's surface, each square inch would receive less than $^1/_3$ pound of pressure. When a person is recumbent in an ordinary hospital bed, the weight of the body falls heavily on certain parts, with the combined area of these points being very small. The points that receive the greatest stress are those in which the bone skeleton approaches the skin. When the body is recumbent, these bony points include the occiput, scapulae, sacrum, spinous processes, trochanters, heels, and ankles. The knees and toes can also receive pressure from the bedclothes.[57]

The tissue ischemia that results from prolonged low extracorporeal pressure can lead to irreversible cellular changes, which ultimately progress to necrosis and ulceration. High pressure, exerted even for short periods, reduces or stops the capillary flow. In addition, venous thrombosis can occur in the larger vessels, so when the pressure is relieved, ischemia prevails owing to the large-vessel involvement.[40] The development of ischemic ulcers is one of the major problems confronting a person whose mobility is impaired. The debilitated person may fail to reposition body parts because of lack of strength, reduced neurological control, or impaired sensation. When a person does not experience the sensation of pressure, areas of the body may be subjected to excessive pressure for prolonged periods. The distribution of such pressure depends on the person's functional status. Trochanteric and sacral ulcers are most prevalent in patients who must maintain recumbent positions, whereas ulcers over the ischial tuberosities are found in those who are able to maintain sitting positions.

Intracorporeal mechanical pressure. Intracorporeal pressure on blood vessels is a common concomitant of (1) exudate and collagen formation associated with the inflammatory process, (2) intracavity or extracellular fluid accumulation such as edema and ascites, and (3) rapid cellular proliferation such as that associated with tumor growth and pregnancy. Intracorporeal pressure precipitates ischemia by direct pressure on adjacent vessels. The extent of such ischemia relates to the specific site or vessels involved. For example, intracorporeal pressure in the peritoneal cavity that results from conditions such as ascites, pregnancy, or tumor growth usually affects the abdominal veins, interfering with circulatory return from the lower extremities.

Chronic inflammatory processes apply pressure on vessels in a different manner. Chronic inflammation differs from the acute response by its emphasis on fibroblastic proliferation rather than exudate production. For this reason chronic inflammation is often characterized by extensive scarring. The production of collagen and its shrinkage produce fibrous scars that may deform repaired tissues and compress vessels. An example of this process is the adhesions that may occur after abdominal surgery. The bowel may be narrowed and the vessels slowly strangled by shrinking, fibrous, adhesive scarring. Another example of shrinkage pressure is exhibited by the collagen formation that accompanies arthritis. The collagen fibers deposited in the joints often form rings around the capillaries and compress them when the fibrin shrinks during inactive periods, pinching off the circulation as if a knot were being tied by the fibrils.[60]

Increased metabolic demand

Cellular functions depend on the circulatory system for the delivery of the necessary substances for metabolic activity. Therefore the adequacy of local and compartmental tissue perfusion is influenced not only by the amount of blood delivered to the tissue but also by the metabolic demands of the tissue. When hypermetabolic states create a situation in which there is a relative oxygen deficiency, vasodilation of the part normally occurs to restore adequate tissue perfusion. Cerebral and coronary vessels are particularly sensitive to tissue perfusion deficiencies. Excess carbon dioxide precipitates cerebral vasodilation, whereas lack of oxygen causes coronary vasodilation. However, when vessels are unable to or limited in ability to dilate and/or when the cardiac pump is unable to increase flow volume, ischemia can be precipitated by increased metabolic demand.

It is also possible for demands of hypermetabolic states to surpass the ability of a competent cardiac pump to increase perfusion or the ability of the vessels to dilate. For example, it has been noted that the changes in tissue lactate, phosphocreatine, and ATP levels that are induced by 90 minutes of tourniquet ischemia of an extremity are less than those which occur during heavy exercise.[25]

It has been suggested that in conditions of peripheral arterial insufficiency the muscles' energy metabolism and oxygen consumption become adapted to reduced supplies of nutrients.[36] The most pronounced increases in metabolic capacities observed have been in mitochondrial enzyme activity.[6] However, when physical exercise increases the cells' metabolic demands, the balance between oxygen supply and consumption is markedly disturbed. It has been noted in patients with occlusive arteriosclerosis that muscle PaO_2 and $PaCO_2$ remained normal when the extremities were at rest. However, with exercise the blood flow to the parts reduced abruptly, muscle PaO_2 decreased, and carbon dioxide accumulated.[36]

The redistribution of the body's blood flow to meet extraordinary demands for increased perfusion may precipitate ischemia in the body parts from which the blood has been shunted. For example, during heavy exercise the blood has been shunted. For example, during heavy exercise the blood flow to skeletal and coronary muscles is increased dramatically, whereas skin, kidney, and splanchnic circulation is reduced. Since the heart and brain functions depend on aerobic metabolism, peripheral circulation is often reduced when cardiac output is limited.

BEHAVIORAL DEFINITION

The signs and symptoms indicative of local or compartmental ischemia evolve from reductions in the cells' energy production, increase in anaerobic products, structural changes in the affected tissue, and decreases in vascular patency.

Objective data

Loss of function. Among the earliest indications of local ischemia is a reduction in the parenchymal function of the tissue. Weakness in or absence of contractility of striated muscle generally precedes structural changes.[41] For example, in patients with ischemic lower extremities, signs of disuse such as muscle atrophy are often present in the buttocks, thighs, and legs.

Altered levels of awareness to the point of unconsciousness quickly follow brain ischemia. Even short, transient ischemic attacks may interrupt consciousness and motor function. Reduction in excretions or secretions from affected organs also occurs. An ischemic kidney excretes less urine or no urine. Since the ischemic bowels' absorption ability is reduced, patients with this problem may exhibit apparently unexplained abdominal distention and/or forceful diarrhea, which is positive for occult blood in about 75% of the cases.[4] When the skin is affected, it becomes dry because oil glands reduce secretions, and the nails become dry, hard, and brittle. Although hair is often lost, this is not a reliable indicator of reduced perfusion. However, reduced or absent perspiration is such a reliable indicator that the continuance of foot sweating is an indication that peripheral arterial insufficiency is not present.[11]

Changes in tissue structure. Local ischemic problems of the skin and striated muscle offer the assessment advantage of direct visability of color, size, and tissue firmness changes.

One of the first indications that extracorporeal pressure has precipitated ischemia in endothelial cells is the occurrence of hyperemia immediately following the release of pressure. Since the extent and duration of the hyperemic flare are proportional to the needs of the tissue, this phenomenon provides an indication of the degree of tissue insult. The more deeply red the tissue and the more prolonged the coloring, the greater has been the ischemic insult.[20,33,41,43] When both endothelial and underlying striated muscle experience ischemia, structural deterioration occurs first in the muscle. The edematous condition of the fibrils, and progressive vacuolization, and the granular, albuminous, and fatty degeneration are evidenced by changes in the firmness of the muscle tissue. The consistency of the tissue changes from firm to soft and then mushy, possibly progressing to a jelly liquid feel as lysosomal enzymes become active. Such tissue changes undermine and extend circumferentially about the base of the cutaneous hyperemic tissue. As ischemia progresses, the color of the cutaneous tissue begins to fade until blanched. Accompanying this color change, the skin takes on a stretched, tight, shiny appearance as the endothelial cells become edematous. The central portion of the underlying muscle may be deep, hyperemic, dark red, or the color may change to black as underlying clotting and necrosis occur. The cutaneous involvement usually has a hyperemic demarcation. If necrosis progresses, the cells will begin to slough. Such ulceration can progress to the depth of the underlying bone structure.

Indications of the amount of structural change occurring in ischemic tissues that cannot be observed directly include increased serum enzyme levels, nonspecific indices of tissue necrosis, and inflammation.

Two nonspecific indicators of ischemic injury and necrosis are the systemic indicators of inflammation: leukocytosis and an elevated erythrocyte sedimentation rate (ESR). Leukocytosis appears within a few hours after the onset of an infarct, reaches levels of 12,000 to 15,000, and persists for up to 7 days. The higher the white blood cell count, the more severe the tissue damage. The ESR rises more slowly, usually peaking within a week, and remains elevated for several weeks.[81]

The intracellular enzymes AST, LDH, and CPK are liberated from cells when lysosomal activity precipitates membrane leakiness. AST and CPK blood levels will rise and fall rapidly after cell membrane injury. These enzyme levels usually return to normal within 3 days after injury. AST is liberated from damaged cardiac and skeletal muscle, liver, kidney, and lung tissue, and red blood cells. CPK is present in significant concentrations only in the heart, skeletal muscle, and brain.

LDH levels begin rising after injury, peak in 3 to 4 days, and return to normal in approximately 2 weeks. There are five common LDH isoenzymes, and tissues differ with respect to the specific preponderant LDH isoenzyme. For example, LDH_1 predominates in the cardiac muscle, whereas the more slowly migrating LDH components predominate in liver tissue and skeletal muscle.[81]

One of the major hindrances to the treatment of ischemic bowel is the difficulty of differentiating the diagnosis before intestinal gangrene develops. However, it has been found that inorganic phosphate levels in the blood and peritoneal fluid rise when the mucosa of the gut begins to slough. This occurs early during an ischemic episode, when the intestinal muscle is still viable.[71]

The probability of internal ischemic organs ulcerating or rupturing during the initial phases of an ischemic event is slight. However, as necrosis occurs and tissue begins to degenerate, the possibility of ulceration and rupture increases. An example is the muscle weakness that can occur in an ischemic portion of the heart. As the dead muscle becomes thinner, the degree of systolic stretch becomes greater. In situations of severe injury this can progress until the heart ruptures, causing rapid development of cardiac tamponade.[24]

Reduced vascular patency. Reduced strength in or absence of a normally palpable pulse is a reliable indicator of reduced patency. However, in an obese or muscular person the popliteal pulse is often difficult to feel. The variability in the location of the dorsalis pedis pulse also reduces the reliability of meaning of its absence. In conditions of peripheral arterial insufficiency the arterial walls may feel firm, hard, tortuous, and calcified on palpation.

The color of the skin after exercise or when position is changed also provides indications of the state of patency. Of course, if the normal pigmentation of the skin is dark, color changes are less reliable indicators of perfusion deficiencies. Distal pallor accompanied by coolness of the skin is characteristic of reduced arterial patency. When an afflicted extremity is raised above the heart, the skin will blanch because arterial flow is further reduced by the effects of gravity. When the peripheral vessels are so damaged that they are no longer able to constrict, the skin takes on a reddish-blue color called rubor. The hallmarks of lower extremity ischemia are pallor on elevation, increased venous filling time, and dependent rubor. Venous filling time is determined by having the patient elevate the legs and exercise the toes. Then the patient should sit up with the feet in a dependent position. The venous filling time is determined by how quickly color returns to the extremity. When veins are competent, this should take less than 15 seconds.[11] When incompetent veins are present, distal swelling and cyanosis also characterize the reduced venous outflow. The increased hydrostatic pressure in the capillaries prevents reabsorption of fluid from the tissue and promotes edema. Fluid first accumulates in the most distal areas such as over the toes, in and above the instep, and at the ankle. As venous incompetency progresses, edema moves up the leg. As the permeability of the vessel walls increases, red blood cells move into surrounding tissue, disintegrate, and deposit hemosiderin. The distribution of this pigment, which stains the tissue brown, is usually limited to the distal third of the lower extremities.[60]

Another sign that vessel patency or competence has been reduced is a slowing of the body's rate of healing. Cuts, bruises, or burns are slow to heal and frequently become infected. Even small injuries heal slowly and may reopen with slight additional trauma to the site.

A number of diagnostic tests can more specifically delineate vessel patency. Angiography uses contrast dye and x-ray films to obtain an image of the vascular tree. An oscillometer can be used to measure alterations in pulse volume. A Doppler ultrasound flow detector can be used to follow flow sounds in the vessels, determine points of occlusion, and map collateral circulation.

Subjective data

Pain. Although ischemia frequently causes pain, the mechanism by which pain is initiated has not yet been determined. One possible cause is the large amount of lactic acid that accumulates as a result of anaerobic metabolism. However, other chemical agents released from the ischemic cells, such as histamine and bradykinin, may also stimulate the pain.[24] The pain initiated by the accumulation of these substances can be sharp and intolerable. The intensity and distribution of the pain are related to the extent and duration of the ischemia and to the nerve pathways that transmit messages from the site. For example, the pain of angina pectoris and myocardial infarction have approximately the same distribution, over the chest, up the neck, and down the arms. However, the infarct pain is more prolonged and has an intolerable, crushing, viselike character.

Ischemia of the lower extremities can precipitate intermittent claudication and rest pain. Intermittent claudication is characterized by cramping, tightness, weakness, numbness, and/or tiredness; it occurs with exercise and is relieved by resting. The site of the pain depends on the level of arterial occlusion. The most common site is the calf muscle, but this pain may also occur in the hips, thighs, and buttocks if the occlusion is in the aortoiliac area. The distance the person can walk before pain occurrence depends on the speed of walking and the surface gradient.[12]

Rest pain, which rarely extends above the foot, indicates the presence of a series of arterial blocks. The pain, caused by nerve ischemia, is worse at night. It often occurs during sleep, when the extremity is no longer dependent and peripheral circulation is reduced. The pain has a persistent character with peaks of intensity that may be relieved by placing the legs in a dependent position and exercising the muscles of the extremity.

The character of the pain or discomfort produced by venous incompetence is also influenced by the presence of edematous pressure. The characteristic heavy, dull, diffuse aches, muscle cramps, and fatigue can often be relieved by elevation of the leg to assist venous outflow.

Diminished function. Ischemic neuropathy may occur when reductions in circulatory flow persist. Numbness and tingling may be experienced. In addition, diminished sensitivity to temperature, pressure, and mechanical trauma may occur. When asked how they cut, bruised, or burned themselves, patients may say that they do not know. Usually the patients are not aware of the injury until they see the injured site.

Fatigue is another symptom of loss of function. It can accompany the early phase of cardiac, kidney, liver, and bowel ischemia. In the latter three instances the fatigue often relates to reduction in the body's ability to eliminate toxins and/or metabolic wastes.

INTERVENING VARIABLES

A number of host and environmental factors not only influence vessel patency and general metabolic levels but also affect the ability of the tissue to survive reduced perfusion.

Host factors

Host factors such as age, sex, and race influence a person's risk of acquiring an antecedent pathological condition that precipitates ischemia. Once the pathological condition occurs, these variables do not necessarily affect the level of its impact. However, the metabolic balance and nutritional status of the host as well as the characteristics of the affected tissues do modify the impact of the ischemic insult.

Nutritional status and metabolic balance. The metabolic dysfunction of diabetes mellitus decreases cellular ability to survive ischemic insult because of the cells' reduced ability to efficiently metabolize the substrates necessary for cellular energy production. In addition, diabetics have a predisposition and low resistance to infection. The metabolic demands of the inflammatory response and healing process in a diabetic, whose blood flow is already compromised, may exceed the ability of the vascular system to meet perfusion demands. The incidence of necrosis is high for diabetics when both local ischemia and infection are present.[12] The diabetic is also disadvantaged by the common presence of neuropathy, which reduces sensitivity to pressure sensations as well as awareness of tissue trauma.

Any condition that increases the body's general metabolic rate also increases demand on circulatory flow. An example is the metabolic effect of body temperature elevation or the healing process. Almost any illness or injury, whether it is only a mild infection or a fracture, is accompanied by a negative nitrogen, phosphorus, sulfur, and calcium balance. This is evidenced by loss of weight and wasting of tissues. The more severe the illness, the more pronounced the result. These negative balances peak about 2 to 8 days after the illness onset and often do not return to normal for several months.[40] As these imbalances occur, increases in interstitial fluid (edema) also occur. Edema directly reduces the diffusion of oxygen, nutrients, and wastes to and from the capillaries and cells by increasing the distance between these structures. Anemia would, of course, further restrict the tissue access to oxygen.

When the cells are nutritionally depleted, even minimal pressure of short duration can precipitate necrosis and ischemic ulceration. In addition, tissues that are dehydrated, dry, and inelastic require little shearing force to damage their fragile cells.[57]

Tissue type and location. It has been noted that muscle tissue is more susceptible to ischemic injury than is the dermal, epidermal, and even fatty tissue.[9,22,33] Studies of the pathogenesis of ischemic ulcers have found striated muscles degenerating and becoming infiltrated long before any dermal changes appear.[22,33] Although striated muscles begin degenerating rapidly after 2 hours of no-flow ischemia, the cells of the skin exhibit little damage even after 8 hours of ischemia.[80] Two reasons have been advanced to explain this difference in sensitivity. The first possibility is that the epidermis is able to use surface oxygen. This explanation is supported by the fact that the hair follicles are the first structures of the skin to have their activity inhibited, and these follicles depend entirely on oxygen supplied by the underlying capillary circulation. The second possible reason is that muscle tissue exhibits the no-reflow phenomenon, whereas the skin does not. After release of pressure certain areas of the muscle remain temporarily or permanently incapable of resuming blood flow. However, the skin, which has no true parenchymal cells, does not exhibit the same cellular swelling, and reflow is quickly resumed.[80]

Lung tissue has also demonstrated the ability to use surface oxygen during periods of no-flow ischemia. Lung tissue has been found to tolerate at least 5 hours of ischemia without significant damage as long as lung ventilation is present.[54]

The mitochondrial changes that occur in striated muscles are similar to those noted in ischemic myocardium. However, in myocardial muscle, mitochondrial swelling and structural disorganization are present after only 40 to 60 minutes of ischemia. This more rapid alteration is probably due to the myocardial cells' greater dependence on aerobic metabolism.[65] In addition, irreversible alterations occur more rapidly in myocardial cells than in striated muscles. Irreversible changes have been reported to occur in less that 1 hour, whereas irreversible changes do not often occur in striated muscle until approximately 4 hours after ischemia has been initiated.[3]

Total cessation of brain perfusion results in depletion of brain oxygen stores[69] and unconsciousness[62] within 10 seconds. Glucose and glycogen stores are depleted, and anaerobic metabolism stops within 4 minutes after flow cessation.[69] All energy-requiring reactions stop within about 5 minutes.[53,69] These rapid changes indicate the dependence of brain tissue on aerobic metabolism and the inability of brain tissue to store glucose or oxygen.

In addition to dependence on aerobic metabolism and ability to store glucose and oxygen, the energy needs of the parenchymal cells also influence the quickness of the occurrence of irreversible changes. For example, renal cortical cells can experience irreversible ischemic injury in about 1 hour,[18,39] whereas the peristalsis of the bowel will continue for about 6 to 8 hours after onset of ischemia.[71]

Environmental factors

Smoking, cold, and emotional stress can accentuate ischemia by increasing vasoconstriction. Other environmental factors such as heat, humidity, and acids affect the survival of ischemic tissue by affecting tissue integrity.

Vasoconstrictors. Emotional stress can excite the sympathetic system and precipitate vasoconstriction through the sympathetic alarm reaction. Sympathetic vasoconstriction fibers are distributed to all segments of the circulation. However, the distribution of these fibers in the brain, heart, and skeletal muscles is rather poor. The kidney, gut, spleen, and skin have many more of the fibers, so the effects of sympathetic vasoconstriction are more pronounced in these tissues.

The body's response to cold is both a central sympathetic response directed by the hypothalamic thermostat and a local vascular response governed by peripheral receptors. The vascular changes precipitated by emotional stress and cold exposure in persons who have vasospastic disorders can be so sudden and severe that the viability of the involved digits becomes questionable.

The mechanisms by which smoking influences circulatory flow have often been disputed. However, the amount of nicotine absorbed from two cigarettes has been shown to decrease blood flow to the skin of the foot by so much as 40%.[52] Abstention from smoking also appears vital to the control of Buerger's disease.

Altered tissue integrity. When the body is exposed to a warm, humid environment, the skin can become soft and moist, increasing the risk of maceration. This occurs particularly in skin areas where the process of evaporation has been restricted. For example, plastic bed covers, which restrict air flow, can produce a wet environment first by stimulating the sweat response and then by restricting the evaporation process. In addition to softening the skin, wet bedclothes also cause considerable friction to contacting body surfaces.

Skin that has been soiled by urine, feces, or other acidic excretions can lose antibacterial properties and become excoriated by the acids. Any skin trauma, no matter how slight, can open a portal of entry, precipitate an infection, and accelerate the effects of local ischemia.

NURSING INTERVENTIONS—GOALS AND EVALUATION CRITERIA

The primary goals of nursing intervention for local or compartmental tissue ischemia are (1) increase of arterial blood flow and venous return, (2) reduction of metabolic demands, and (3) relief of ischemic pain.

Increase of arterial blood flow and venous return

The subgoals that can assist in increasing the flow of the blood through the circulatory system include (1) facilitation of effects of gravity, (2) increase of structural support of vessels, (3) reduction of external compression, (4) reduction of internal obstructions, (5) vasodilation, and (6) inhibition of vasoconstriction.

Facilitation of effects of gravity. Gravity exerts a downward pull on vascular flow, moving blood to the most dependent (lower than the heart) body parts. The position of the body that will facilitate the flow of blood by gravity depends on whether the flow deficiency is of arterial or venous origin. If arterial insufficiency exists in the lower extremities, gravity will improve flow when the legs are placed in a dependent position. When venous incompetence is present, the legs must be elevated to take advantage of the downward pull of gravity. Prolonged periods of standing or sitting with the legs dependent should be avoided when venous deficiency is present.

Increase of structural support of vessels. When the body is upright, approximately 600 to 700 ml of blood is added to the volume of the lower extremities. It appears that the action of the muscle pumps in the calves and thighs is the primary factors that offsets this increase in lower limb blood volume.[70] The deep veins, which contain the bulk of the venous blood in the lower extremities, have thin walls that contain a minimum of smooth muscle. These vessels are sparsely innervated and derive their structural support from the surrounding skeletal muscles.[46] When skeletal muscles contract, they compress the veins and assist the action of the intrinsic valves by exerting a pumplike action on the venous flow. The activity of walking can increase the venous pressure in the calf to 100 mm Hg during the compression phase.[78]

A program of moderate exercise and rest can balance the advantages of the structural support of muscle contraction to both venous and arterial circulation against the disadvantage of increasing metabolic demands by activity.

The structural support afforded the veins by muscle exercise can be augmented by elastic bandages or elastic stockings, which exert an even, external pressure from the toes to the thighs. Other mechanical and anatomical methods that can be used to help maintain adequate venous circulation in the immobilized patient are discussed in Chapter 5. Chapter 5 also discusses a number of active and passive exercises for patients who are not ambulatory.

An exercise that combines the use of gravity and active muscle movement to facilitate arterial and venous flow is the Buerger-Allen routine. The exercise consists of three phases. First the person assumes a recumbent supine position. The legs are elevated for 30 seconds to 3 minutes, until the legs blanch. The person then sits up, putting the legs in a dependent position with the feet resting on the floor. The feet are then flexed, extended, abducted, and adducted as far as possible. The toes are also flexed, extended, abducted, and adducted. Both the feet and toes should be exercised for about 3 minutes, until the feet become pink. After this the person lies down for 5 minutes with legs horizontal and covered to keep them warm. If the legs become blue or painful when in the dependent position, the person should stop, lie down, and elevate the legs until the color fades and the pain subsides. The legs should then be placed in the horizontal position for 5 minutes. The number of times these exercises are performed during a day depends on the severity of the ischemic problem.

Manual massage of tissue facilitates increased blood flow through two actions. Massage motions alternately apply pressure to the underlying vessels, facilitating the forward movement of blood and lymph. This activity increases circulation in both the deep veins and the arterioles and capillaries of the area.[63,75] In addition, gentle, stroking massage motions facilitate reflexive vasodilation by stimulating the vasomotor nerves of the blood vessels. Deeper massage pressure, particularly over bony structures, appears to release acetylcholine and histamine into the massaged tissue, further stimulating vasodilation.[66,76,77] It has been found that after removal of flow obstruction, ischemic muscles are able to perform twice as much work after a minute of massage than without the massage.[75]

The use of manual massage of tissue with ischemia that was precipitated by external pressure, in conjunction with the release of the pressure, greatly facilitates the tissue's recovery. When the position of the immobilized patient is changed, the tissue over the bony prominences that received the greatest amount of force should be massaged.

Reduction of external compression. The most effective way to prevent detrimental effects of pressure ischemia is to relieve the pressure before cellular changes have occurred. The critical time interval during which pathological changes occur in both normal and denervated skeletal muscle following subjection to pressure is between 1 and 2 hours. Persons who are unable to move themselves should alternately be turned from side to back to side at least every 2 hours day and night.[41] Very obese or very debilitated patients may need to be turned hourly.[35,57] The use of modified Fowler's positions for the bedridden patient who is unable to move or is insensitive to pressure should be restricted. These positions exert shearing force on the sacral areas.

Persons who have reduced sensitivity to pressure should develop a routine of altering their position at least hourly. When the sitting position must be used, the arms should be used to push the body up off the surface on which it is resting. This relieves the pressure completely for a few minutes and allows for alteration in pressure distribution when sitting is resumed.

The external pressure exerted on the body can be reduced by altering the nature of the opposing surface. The surface should be kept clean and smooth so that angled surfaces do not come in contact with the skin. Sheets should be kept free of such things as wrinkles and crumbs. Increasing the pliability of the contacted surface also assists in reducing pressure by distributing it over a larger amount of the body's surface and thereby reducing the intensity of the pressure on any one point. Pillows used to support the extremities help to mitigate pressure effects. Water beds can effectively conform to the body's contours. Foam-filled, water-filled, and viscoelastic gel cushions significantly reduce the pressure exerted on the ischial areas when the person is sitting.[12] Bed cradles and foot boards are useful devices to help relieve the pressure of the bedclothes on the knees and ankles. However, none of the available aids to redistribute pressure can replace the benefits of changing the position of the body so that pressure is completely removed from ischemic sites.

Reduction of internal obstructions. When a person experiences an arterial or venous thrombosis, activity or massage of the affected part could facilitate detachment of a thromboembolus. Bed rest and restricted movement of the affected part are indicated until the tail of the thrombus becomes firmly attached to the vessel wall. If the thrombus is venous, the affected part should be elevated about 6 inches above the heart level to facilitate blood flow and reduce the risk of new thrombi. Increasing the blood flow from the area should also reduce edematous pressure in the area. Once the threat of embolism is over, active exercise and/or ambulation should be used to promote venous return. Warm packs continually applied to the area can assist in reducing the obstruction by facilitating resolution of the inflammation as well as relieving vasospasm at the site.[45]

Anticoagulant therapy is used to prevent intravascular thrombosis by decreasing blood coagulability. Anticoagulant drugs have no direct effect on a blood clot that has already formed. Rather, these drugs are used prophylactically to prevent clot formation. The body can then deal with the obstruction by means of canalization, resolution, and/or formation of collateral circulation.

The most commonly used anticoagulants are parenterally administered heparin and orally administered coumarin derivatives. Heparin prevents coagulation by increasing the blood's clotting time. This is done by interfering with the formation of thrombin, preventing the conversion of fibrinogen to fibrin, and preventing platelets from releasing thromboplastin. The oral anticoagulants primarily decrease prothrombin activity. Because of the differences in action, the usefulness of coumarin derivatives is limited primarily to venous thromboembolic disorders.

Heparin has the advantage of almost immediate effect after intravenous administration, whereas coumarin derivatives require at least 18 hours to elevate prothrombin time (PT) to therapeutic levels.[21] Disadvantages of heparin are that it is expensive and requires parenteral administration. Intramuscular administration of heparin is usually avoided owing to frequent, painful hematoma formation at the injection site.

The dosage of anticoagulants should be monitored by laboratory tests. Heparin can be monitored by the whole blood–clotting time (Lee White time). The therapeutic clotting time is two to three times the normal 5 to 10 minutes. The whole blood activated partial thromboplastin time (PTT) provides a more accurate measure. The PTT should be kept at twice the normal level. The most widely used method to control oral anticoagulants is the PT. Since this measure varies with technique and laboratory conditions, therapeutic levels are kept between 2 and $2\frac{1}{2}$ times that of the control.[21]

Patients taking anticoagulants should continually be monitored for signs of bleeding. The epithelial membranes are the usual sites of the first signs of increased bleeding tendency. Hematuria, epistaxis, ecchymosis, and bleeding gums are common early signs. In addition, patients with wounds often have increased bleeding or hematoma formation in the wound area. The effects of heparin are reduced within 3 to 4 hours after administration; this is an advantage if bleeding occurs. Oral anticoagulants may sustain their actions for 24 to 72 hours after administration is discontinued.

Two other substances, streptokinase and low-molecular-weight dextran, have also been used to assist in reducing thrombus obstructions. However, both drugs are still considered experimental regarding their internal coagulation effects. Streptokinase is an enzyme that breaks down fibrin. It has proven effective in topical application, but tests of internal effectiveness are still inconclusive. Low-molecular-weight dextran (dextran 70 and dextran 40) coats the vascular endothelium and blood elements, reducing the contact and aggregation factors that trigger coagulation.[21]

A few other medications are used in situations that have a high risk of arterial thrombosis. Drugs such as aspirin, dipyridamole, and prostaglandins, although still experimental in this use, appear to control platelet aggregation, thereby reducing thrombosis.

Vasodilation. According to the vasodilator theory of local blood flow regulation, the metabolic substances produced during ischemia (lactic acid, adenosine, adenosine phosphate compounds, histamine, potassium and hydrogen ions, and carbon dioxide) diffuse back to the precapillary sphincters, metarterioles, and arterioles to cause dilation. These dilation efforts can be augmented by local application of or exposure to heat. The skin temperature receptors transmit impulses both to the spinal cord and the hypothalamus. When the local cord reflexes are stimulated by heat, both local vasodilation and mild sweating are initiated. The sweating initiates still another vasodilation mechanism. The sweat gland releases bradykinin, which diffuses into surrounding tissue and causes further vasodilation. In addition to the local reflex action to heat application, heat applied to the abdomen also causes reflexive dilation of the arteries of the lower extremities.[24]

When the temperature of the cells is increased, the rate of enzyme activity increases, as does the metabolism of the tissue. Therefore the use of heat to achieve vasodilation must be governed by the effect that an increase in the metabolic demands of the tissues will have on the ischemia level. When the ischemia is caused by intracorporeal vascular deficiencies, application of heat directly to the ischemic area should be avoided because of the body's inability to respond to the increased metabolic demand. In addition, the decreased sensitivity of such ischemic tissues to temperature may allow a person to be burned without realizing it. Therefore patients with peripheral vascular disorders should not use hot water bottles, heating pads, or hot soaks to increase circulation to the extremities. However, the application of heat to the abdomen can effect vasodilation of the extremities without metabolic and neurological risks.

When tissues can tolerate mild elevations in metabolic demands, heat application can facilitate the recovery from ischemic insult. This is particularly effective with cutaneous and striated muscle ischemia caused by external pressure. After the pressure has been removed, intermittent application of heat can facilitate cell recovery. Often dry heat from a light source is used to avoid the possible macerating effects of moist heat.

The use of vasodilator medications to relieve the ischemia of peripheral vascular deficiency has been fairly ineffective. None of the available peripheral vasodilators has demonstrated a greater dilation effect than that caused by the ischemic vasodilator substances present in the tissues. To date, there has been no significant evidence that vasodilators improve the activity capacity of ischemic muscles.[1,10,21] In addition, no known drug decreases cerebrovascular resistance as much as ischemically precipitated increased $PaCO_2$.[21] Although vasodilator drugs have demonstrated vasodilation on normal vasculature of resting parts, the arteries must be capable of dilating for these agents to be effective. Therefore these drugs are of little benefit to patients whose pathological condition has reduced this ability.

The oldest and still most useful regional vasodilator drugs are the nitrites. The basic action of these drugs is to relax smooth muscle. Although all smooth muscle is affected, there is a difference in the effect on the vascular smooth muscle of different tissue beds. Amyl nitrate and nitroglycerin are most commonly used for their rapid effect on the resistance of the coronary circulation, particularly in the large coronary arteries and conducting vessels during anginal attacks.[21] Slower, yet long-acting, nitrates such as pentaerythritol tetranitrate (Peritrate) and isosorbide dinitrate (Isordil) are used prophylactically to prevent anginal attack. However, tolerance to their action may be developed in a few weeks, limiting their usefulness in the management of this ischemic problem. Nitroglycerin is now also being used in a paste form applied topically to the sternal area to provide a sustained effect over 4- to 6-hour periods.

Inhibition of vasoconstriction. The arterioles that supply the skin are controlled almost entirely by the sympathetic nervous system. Usually the sympathetic nerves remain tonically active, causing continuous, slight constriction of these vessels. When the body comes in contact with cold, the sympathetic centers of the hypothalamus are stimulated and the blood flow to the skin can be reduced, almost stopped, as the body attempts to conserve heat.[24] A warm environment in the range of 21° to 22° C (70° to 72° F) should reduce sympathetic stimulation in persons with peripheral vascular deficiencies. In addition, the wearing of clothes suitable to maintaining body warmth is essential to prevent vasoconstriction. The most often neglected areas that are crucial to body heat maintenance are the head, face, hands, and feet. Hats, gloves, scarves, socks, and boots should be worn on chilly days, and a number of clothing layers appropriate to the temperature of the environment should cover the rest of the body. Persons with Raynaud's disease can be so sensitive to cold that must wear gloves when removing objects from a refrigerator.

A second major stimulator of the sympathetic nervous system is emotional stress. Persons with peripheral vascular deficiencies should learn how to relax both mentally and physically and should avoid emotionally stressful situations. Patients who have difficulty relaxing are often helped by relaxation techniques that provide biofeedback cues.

The elimination of smoking may be essential to the preservation of life and limbs of some patients with peripheral deficiencies. However, it is often difficult for patients to develop sufficient motivation to abstain permanently.

Indications that circulatory flow has been increased to tissues that have undergone structural changes but still have the potential to reverse the damage are reductions in serum enzyme levels and the nonspecific indicators of inflammation. As tissues regain energy production, their size, color, and firmness begin returning to normal. Levels of parenchymal function increase as evidenced by increased secretions and excretions and decreased body fatigue and part weakness. Episodes of numbness, tingling, and pain decrease in frequency as awareness of temperature and pressure increases. If ulceration or other tissue damage has occurred, healing progress will be evidenced by the filling in of tissue deficits and the appearance of granulation tissue and epithelialization.

Reduction of metabolic demands

The methods used to reduce the metabolic demands of ischemic tissues relate to both the parenchymal functioning level of the tissue and the functioning demands placed on other tissue or cell processes. When the parenchymal function of tissue can be consciously regulated, activity and rest can be patterned to keep metabolic demands at a level the circulation can meet. The patient with peripheral vascular deficiencies that cause intermittent claudication can use pain to govern activity levels. The pace of the activity can be slowed and resting initiated when the pain occurs. Cardiac demands can be monitored by pulse and recovery rates.

The metabolic demands of some tissues (e.g., cerebral tissue) are not governed by conscious control. When cerebral ischemia is experienced, the metabolic demands may be reduced temporarily by the administration of barbiturates and occasionally by hypothermia.[29,64]

In addition to managing or restricting activity levels of the involved tissues, increases in metabolic demands can also be forstalled by preventing additional trauma and infection. Healing of ischemic tissues can often increase metabolic demands past the circulation's ability even when the part is at rest.

The risk of trauma to ischemic tissues is often increased by decreased sensitivity of the part's nerves. Temperature extremes and pressure trauma are often not noticed until after damage has occurred. Persons with peripheral vascular deficiencies must take particular precaution. They should protect themselves from burns by checking the temperature of such things as bath water and hot water bottles with a thermometer instead of with the hand or toe. The temperature of these applications should not exceed 40.6° to 43.3° C (105° to 110° F). Skin should be kept clean and free of acids and dirt. The cleansing should be done with mild soaps to prevent drying of the skin. The skin of the extremities should be checked daily for dryness, cracks, blisters, and maceration. Daily application of water-based ointments or lanolin is often needed to reduce dryness. The nails should be kept smooth and trimmed straight across to prevent ingrown nails. Properly fitting socks and shoes should be worn during ambulation to avoid injury to the feet.

The skin of persons experiencing pressure ischemia should also receive special care. The skin should be cleansed to remove perspiration, urine, and feces. Lotion or lanolin can be used to moisten skin. Bedclothes should be kept clean and dry to prevent maceration.

Behavioral evidence that metabolic demands on an ischemic tissue have been reduced include the patient's identification that the pain precipitated by increased activity was relieved, the absence of signs of infection, progressive healing of injured tissues, and a return to normal size, color, and firmness in the ischemic tissues.

Relief of ischemic pain

One of the most effective ways to relieve ischemic pain caused by arterial deficiency is to rest the part to reduce demand levels, and to keep the part dependent to facilitate flow. The pain will subside when the circulation reduces the level of metabolites such as lactic acid. Nitrites are administered during anginal ischemia to relieve anginal pain. The deep aches caused by venous deficiency can often be quickly reduced or relieved by the use of gravity to increase venous outflow. In fact, all the previously identified measures to increase circulation should help alleviate ischemic pain. However, when the ischemia is caused by an infarct, the pain often must be controlled or relieved by administration of narcotics or other analgesics. Since severe pain can be such a frightening experience, it is essential that the pain be relieved to reduce the impact of emotional stress on the ischemic problem.

In addition to the patient's statement that the pain has been relieved, other behavioral evidence that this goal has been achieved includes a general relaxation of body musculature and resumption or increase in activity.

CONCEPT OUTLINE

I. *Conceptual definition:* Ischemia is a reduction in or absence of local or compartmental tissue perfusion that initiates and limits anaerobic metabolism.

II. *Antecedent conditions*
   A. Reduced vessel patency
      1. Restriction or obstruction of vessel lumens
      2. Reflexive vasoconstriction
      3. Extracorporeal mechanical pressure
      4. Intracorporeal mechanical pressure
   B. Increased metabolic demands

III. *Behavioral definition*
   A. Objective data
      1. Loss of function
         a. Muscle weakness and atrophy
         b. Interrupted consciousness and motor function
         c. Reduced excretions and secretions
      2. Changes in tissue structure
         a. Hyperemia
         b. Edema
         c. Loss of tissue firmness
         d. Necrosis
         e. Ulceration
         f. Increased serum enzyme (AST, LDH, CPK) levels
         g. Leukocytosis
         h. Elevated ESR
      3. Reduced vascular patency
         a. Reduced or absent pulse
         b. Hard, firm, tortuous, calcified vessels
         c. Rubor, cyanosis, and blanching
         d. Edema
         e. Brown pigmentation of lower extremities
         f. Reduced rate of healing
         g. Reduced pulse volume
         h. Reduced or absent sound of blood flow
         i. Reduced lumen size
   B. Subjective data
      1. Pain
      2. Diminished function
         a. Diminished sensitivity to pressure, temperature, and tissue trauma
         b. Numbness
         c. Tingling
         d. Fatigue

IV. *Intervening variables*
   A. Host factors
      1. Nutritional status and metabolic balance
      2. Tissue type and location
         a. Use of surface oxygen
         b. Dependence on aerobic metabolism
         c. Ability to store glucose and oxygen
         d. Metabolic rate of parenchymal cells
   B. Environmental factors
      1. Vasoconstrictors
         a. Emotional stress
         b. Cold
         c. Smoking
      2. Altered tissue integrity

V. *Nursing interventions—goals*
   A. Increase of arterial blood flow and venous return
      1. Facilitation of effects of gravity
         a. Use of body position
      2. Increase of structural support of vessels
         a. Program of moderate exercise and rest
         b. Mechanical support to veins
         c. Active and passive exercise and range of motion activity
         d. Buerger-Allen routine
         e. Manual massage of muscles
      3. Reduction of external compression
         a. Alteration of body position
         b. Limited use of modified Fowler's positions
         c. Increase of pliability of contact surface
         d. Contact surface kept clean and smooth
      4. Reduction of internal obstructions
         a. Application of heat
         b. Anticoagulant therapy
      5. Vasodilation
         a. Application of heat
         b. Manual massage
         c. Administration of nitrites
      6. Inhibition of vasoconstriction
         a. Environmental temperature kept in comfort range (not less than 21° to 22°C [70° to 72° F])
         b. Wearing of clothes appropriate to temperature of environment

c. Mental and physical relaxation
d. Elimination of smoking

B. Reduction of metabolic demands
   1. Pacing of activities and provision of rest periods
   2. Protection of tissues from trauma and infection
      a. Skin kept clean and soft
      b. Bed linen and clothes kept clean and dry
      c. Skin inspected daily for cuts, cracks, softness, and moisture
      d. Nails kept smooth and trimmed straight across
      e. Temperature of heat applications kept less than 40.6° to 43.3° C (105° to 110° F)

C. Relief of ischemic pain
   1. Use of measures to increase flow
   2. Use of measures to reduce metabolism
   3. Administration of narcotics or analgesics

VI. *Evaluation criteria*
   A. Normal tissue color and firmness
   B. Reduction of edema
   C. Increased secretions and excretions
   D. Decreased pain, numbness, tingling, and fatigue
   E. Increased sensitivity to pressure, temperature, and tissue trauma
   F. Reduced incidence of infection
   G. Normal enzyme levels, WBC levels, and ESR
   H. Increased level of activity

REFERENCES

1. Abramowicz, M., editor: On drugs and therapeutics, The Medical Letter 20(2, Issue 497): 11, 1978.
2. Ames, A., III, Wright, R. L., Kowada, M., Thurston, J. M., and Majno, G.: Cerebral ischemia. II. The no-reflow phenomena, Am. J. Pathol. **52**:437, 1968.
3. Armiger, L. C., and Gavin, J. B.: Changes in microvasculature of ischemic and infarcted myocardium, Lab. Invest. **33**:51, 1975.
4. Boley, S. J., Brandt, L. J., and Veith, F. J.: Ischemic disorders of the intestine, Curr. Probl. Surg. **15**:1, 1978.
5. Brosnan, J. T., Krebs, H. A., and Williamson, D. H.: Effects of ischaemia on metabolite concentrations in rat liver, Biochem. J. **117**:91, 1970.
6. Bylund, A.-C., Hammarsten, J., Holm, J., and Schersten, T.: Enzyme activities in skeletal muscles from patients with peripheral arterial insufficiency, Eur. J. Clin. Invest. **6**:425, 1976.
7. Chance, B., Schoener, B., Krejci, K., Rüssman, W., Weseman, W., Schnitger, H., and Bücher, T.: Kinetics of fluorescence and metabolite changes in rat liver during a cycle of ischemia, Biochem. Z. **341**:325, 1965.
8. Chiang, J., Kowada, M., Ames, A., III., Wright, R. L., and Majno, G: Cerebral ischemia. III. Vascular changes, Am. J. Pathol. **52**:455, 1968.
9. Clemmesen, T.: The early circulation of split skin grafts, Acta Chir. Scand. **124**:11, 1962.
10. Coffman, J. D., and Monnick, J. A.: Failure of vasodilator drugs in arteriosclerosis obliterans, Ann. Intern. Med. **76**:35, 1972.
11. DeLateur, B. J., Berni, R., Hongladarom, T., and Giaconi, R.: Wheelchair cushions designed to prevent pressure sores: an evaluation, Arch. Phys. Med. Rehabil. **57**:129, 1976.
12. DeLaurentis, D. A.,: How to evaluate and treat lower extremity ischemia in the diabetic, Geriatrics **31**:83, 1976.
13. Dinep, M.: Cold injury: a review of current theories and their application to treatment, Conn. Med. **39**:8, 1975.
14. Dinsdale, S. M.: Decubitus ulcers in swine: light and electron microscopy study of pathogenesis, Arch. Phys. Med. Rehabil. **54**:51, 1973.
15. Dinsdale, S. M.: Decubitus ulcers: role of pressure and friction in causation, Arch. Phys. Med. Rehabil. **55**:147, 1974.
16. Elson, R. A.: Anatomical aspects of pressure sores and their treatment, Lancet **1**:884, 1965.
17. Flores, J., DiBona, D. R., Beck, C. H., and Leaf, A.: The role of cell swelling in ischemic renal damage and the protective effect of hypertonic solute, J. Clin. Invest. **51**:118, 1972.
18. Frega, N. S., DiBona, D. R., Guertler, B., and Leaf, A.: Ischemic renal injury, Kidney Int. **10**:(suppl. 6):S-17, 1976.
19. Glaumann, B., Glaumann, H., Berezesky, I., and Trump, B. F.: Studies on the pathogenesis of ischemic cell injury. II. Morphological changes of the paraconvoluta (P1 + P2) of the proximal tubule of the rat kidney made ischemic in vivo, Virchows Archiv. [Cell Pathol.] **19**:281, 1975.

20. Goldblatt, H.: Reactive hypermia, Heart **12**:281, 1926.
21. Goodman, L. S., and Gilman, A., editors: The pharmacological basis of therapeutics, ed. 5, New York, 1975, Macmillan Publishing Co., Inc.
22. Groth, K. E.: Clinical observations and experimental studies of the pathogenesis of decubitus ulcers, Acta Chir. Scand. **87**:(suppl. 76):1, 1942.
23. Guttman, L.: Problem of treatment of pressure sores in spinal paraplegics, Br. J. Plast. Surg. **8**:196, 1955.
24. Guyton, A. C.: Textbook of medical physiology, Philadelphia, 1968, W. B. Saunders, Co.
25. Haljamäe, H., and Enger, E.: Human skeletal muscle energy metabolism during and after complete tourniquet ischemia, Ann. Surg. **182**:9, 1975.
26. Hamilton, T. R., and Angevine, D. M.: Fatal pulmonary embolism in 100 battle casualties, Milit. Surg. **99**:450, 1946.
27. Harman, J. W.: A histological study of skeletal muscle in acute ischemia, Am. J. Pathol. **23**:551, 1947.
28. Hills, C. P.: Ultrastructural changes in the capillary bed of the rat cerebral cortex in anoxic-ischemic brain lesions, Am. J. Pathol. **44**:531, 1964.
29. Hoff, J. T.: Resuscitation in focal brain ischemia, Crit. Care Med. **6**:245, 1978.
30. Hoper, J., Kessler, M., Ji, S., and Acker, H.: Disturbances of extracellular pK, pNa and pH during no-flow anoxia. In Silver, I. A., Erecinska, M., and Bicher, H. I., editors: III, Oxygen transport to tissue, Adv. Exp. Med. Biol. **94**:553, 1978.
31. Hoper, J., Kessler, M., and Starlinger, H.: Preservation of ATP in the perfused liver. In Bicher, H. I., and Bruley, D. F., editors: Oxygen transport to tissue: instrumentation, methods and physiology, Adv. Exp. Med. Biol. **37A**:371, 1973.
32. Hume, M., Sevitt, S., and Thomas, D. P.: Venous thrombosis and pulmonary embolism, Cambridge, Mass., 1970, Harvard University Press.
33. Husain, T.: An experimental study of some pressure effects on tissues with reference to the bedsore problem, J. Pathol. Bacteriol. **66**:347, 1953.
34. Jarrett, F.: Frostbite: current concepts of pathogenesis and treatment, Rev. Surg. **31**:71, 1974.
35. Johnson, M. L.: Problems involved in the prevention of pressure sores, Nurs. Mirror **135**:39, 1972.
36. Jussila, E., Niinikoski, J., and Inberg, M. V.: Tissue gas tensions in the calf muscle on patients with lower limb arterial ischemia, Scand. J. Thorac. Cardiovasc. Surg. **13**:77, 1979.
37. Kessler, M., Höper, J., and Krumme, B. A.: Monitoring of tissue perfusion and cellular function, Anesthesiology **45**:184, 1976.
38. Kessler, M., Höper, J., and Simon, W.: Methodology and application of a multiple ion selective surface electrode (pH, pK, pNa, pCa, pCl) for tissue measurements, Fed. Proc. **33**:279, 1974.
39. Koletsky, S.: Effects of temporary interruption of renal circulation in rats, Arch. Pathol. **58**:592, 1954.
40. Kosiak, M.: Etiology and pathology of ischemic ulcers, Arch. Phys. Med. Rehabil. **40**:62, 1959.
41. Kosiak, M.: Etiology of decubitus ulcers, Arch. Phys. Med. Rehabil. **42**:19, 1961.
42. La Celle, P. L., and Weed, R. I.: The contribution of normal and pathologic erythrocytes to blood rheology, Prog. Hematol. **7**:1, 1971.
43. Lewis, T., and Grant, R.: Reactive hyperemia in man, Heart **12**:73, 1925.
44. Lindan, O.: Etiology of decubitus ulcers: an experimental study, Arch. Phys. Med. Rehabil. **42**:774, 1961.
45. Luckmann, J., and Sorensen, K. C.: Medical-surgical nursing: a psychophysiologic approach, Philadelphia, 1974, W. B. Saunders Co.
46. Ludbrook, J.: Aspects of venous function in the lower limbs, Springfield, Ill., 1966, Charles C Thomas, Publisher.
47. Lundborg, G.: Ischemic nerve injury, Diss. Scand. J. Plast. Reconstr. Surg. Suppl. **6**:3, 1970.
48. Mergner, W. J., Marzella, L., Mergner, C., Kahng, M. W., Smith, M. W., and Trump, B. F.: Studies on the pathogenesis of ischemic cell injury. VII. Proton gradient and respiration of renal tissue cubes, renal mitochondrial and submitochondrial particles following ischemic injury, Beitr. Pathol. **161**:230, 1977.
49. Mergner, W. J., Smith, M. W., Sahaphong,

S., and Trump, B. F.: Studies on the pathogenesis of ischemic cell injury. VI. Accumulation of calcium by isolated mitochondria ischemic rat kidney cortex, Virchows Archiv. [Cell Pathol.] **26**:1, 1977.
50. Mergner, W. J., Smith, M. W., and Trump, B. F.: Studies on the pathogenesis of ischemic cell injury. IV. Alterations of ionic permeability of mitochondria from ischemic rat kidney, Exp. Mol. Pathol. **26**:1, 1977.
51. Mergner, W. J., Smith, M. W., and Trump, B. F.: Studies on the pathogenesis of ischemic cell injury. XI. P/O ratio and acceptor control. Virchows Archiv. [Cell Pathol.] **26**:17, 1977.
52. Metzler, M., and Silver, D.: Vasospastic disorders, Postgrad. Med. J. **65**:79, 1979.
53. Michenfelder, J. D., and Theye, R. A.: The effects of anesthesia and hypothermia on canine cerebral ATP and lactate during anoxia produced by decapitation, Anesthesiology **33**:430, 1970.
54. Modry, D. L., and Chu-Jeng Chiu, R.: Pulmonary reperfusion syndrome, Ann. Thorac. Surg. **27**:206, 1979.
55. Monies-Chass, I., Hashmonai, M., Hoerer, D., Kaufman, T., Steiner, E., and Schromek, A.: Hyperbaric oxygen treatment as an adjuvant to reconstructive vascular surgery in trauma, Injury **8**:274, 1977.
56. Munro, D.: Care of the back following spinal cord injuries: a consideration of bed sores, N. Engl. J. Med. **223**:391, 1940.
57. Pinel, C.: Pressure sores, Nurs. Times **72**:172, 1976.
58. Reichel, S. M.: Shearing force as a factor in decubitus ulcers in paraplegics, J.A.M.A. **166**:762, 1958.
59. Rhodes, R. S., DePalma, R. G., and Druet, R. L.: Reversibility of ischemically induced mitochondrial dysfunction with reperfusion, Surg. Gynecol. Obstet. **145**:719, 1977.
60. Robbins, S. L.: Pathologic basis of disease, Philadelphia, 1974, W. B. Saunders Co.
61. Romanus, M.: Microcirculatory reactions to local pressure induced ischemia, Acta Chir. Scand. [Suppl.] **479**:1, 1977.
62. Rossen, R., Kabat, H., and Anderson, J. P.: Acute arrest of cerebral circulation in man, Arch. Neurol. **50**:510, 1943.
63. Rusk, H. A.: Rehabilitation medicine, ed. 4, St. Louis, 1977, The C. V. Mosby Co.
64. Safor, P., Bleyaert, A., Nemoto, E. M., Mossy, J., and Snyder, J. V.: Resuscitation after global brain ischemia-anoxia, Crit. Care Med. **6**:215, 1978.
65. Santavirta, S., Luoma, A., and Arstila, A. U.: Ultrastructural changes in striated muscle after experimental tourniquet ischemia and short reflow, Eur. Surg. Res. **10**:415, 1978.
66. Scull, C. W.: Massage-physiologic basis, Arch. Phys. Rehabil. Med. **26**:159, 1945.
67. Sevitt, S.: Fatal road accidents: injuries, complications and causes of death in 250 subjects, Br. J. Surg. **55**:481, 1968.
68. Sevitt, S., and Gallagher, N.: Venous thrombosis and pulmonary embolism: a clinico-pathological study in injured and burned patients, Br. J. Surg. **48**:475, 1961.
69. Siesjo, B. K., Carlsson, C., Hagerdal, M., and Nordström, C.-H.: Brain metabolism in the critically ill, Crit. Care Med. **4**:283, 1976.
70. Sjostrand, T.: Volume and distribution of blood and their significance in regulating the circulation, Physiol. Rev. **33**:202, 1953.
71. Taylor, B. M., Jamieson, W. G., and Durand, D.: Preinfarction diagnosis of acute mesenteric ischemia by simple measurement of inorganic phosphate in body fluids, Can. J. Surg. **22**:40, 1979.
72. Todd, M. E., Thompson, J. H., Bowie, E. J. W., and Owen, C. A., Jr.: Changes in blood coagulation during pregnancy, Mayo Clin. Proc. **40**:370, 1965.
73. Trump, B. F. Croker, P. B., Jr., and Mergner, W. J.: The role of energy metabolism, ion and water shifts in the pathogenesis of cell injury. In Richter, G. W., and Scarpelli, D. G., editors: Cell membranes: biological and pathological aspects, Baltimore, 1971, Williams & Wilkins Co.
74. Trump, B. F., and Mergner, W. J.: Cell injury. In Zweifach, B. W., Grant, L., and McCluskey, R. T., editors: The inflammatory process, New York, 1974, Academic Press, Inc.
75. Wakim, K. G.: Physiologic effects of massage. In Licht, S., editor: Massage, manipulation and traction, New York, 1976, R. E. Krieger Publishing Co., Inc.
76. Wakim, K. G., Martin, G. M., and Krusen, F. H.: Influence of centripetal rhythmic compression on localized edema of an extremity, Arch. Phys. Med. Rehabil. **36**:98, 1955.
77. Wakim, K. G., Martin, G. M., Terrier, J. C.,

Elkins, E. C., and Krusen, F. H.: The effects of massage on the circulation in normal and paralyzed extremities, Arch. Phys. Med. Rehabil. **30**:135, 1949.
78. Wells, H. S., Youman, J. B., and Miller, D. G., Jr.: Tissue pressure (intracutaneous, subcutaneous and intramuscular) as related to venous pressure, capillary filtration and other factors, J. Clin. Invest. **17**:489, 1938.
79. Wilgis, E. F. S.: Observations on the effect of tourniquet ischemia, J. Bone Jt. Surg. (Am.) **53-A**:1343, 1971.
80. Williams-Kretschmer, K., and Majno, G.: Ischemia of the skin, Am. J. Pathol. **54**:327, 1969.
81. Wintroke, M. M., Thorn, G. W., Adams, R. D., Braunwald, E., Isselbacher, K. J., and Petersdorf, R. G., editors: Harrison's principles of internal medicine, New York, 1974, McGraw-Hill Book Co.

RITA A. FARREN FRANTZ

Chapter 15

SHOCK

CONCEPTUAL DEFINITION

Shock is a systemic state of rapidly decreasing tissue perfusion that produces multiple deleterious effects on the body's cells and vital organs and, if unabated, rapidly leads to death.

The cellular changes that occur during shock are initiated by decrease or cessation of circulating blood volume. The cellular changes precipitated by hypoxia and ischemia are present systemically during shock.[3,11,13] These changes are discussed in Chapters 13 and 14. Shock is differentiated from the concept of ischemia by its rapid systemic involvement, which causes cellular deterioration of the vital organs. If shock continues, the progressive impairment of major organ systems causes further reduction in systemic perfusion.

The most significant impairment occurs in the circulatory system, where decreased myocardial perfusion weakens myocardial contractility and reduces cardiac output. This results in a corresponding decrease in arterial blood pressure, reducing blood flow through the coronary arteries and further depressing myocardial contractility. The decreased blood flow to the brain causes systemic vascular dilation as a result of hypoxic injury of the autonomic vasomotor center.[7] The effects of this dilation are intensified by increased capillary permeability. Capillary permeability is caused by the diminishment of essential nutrients to the vessels and the release of lysosomal enzymes from ischemically injured cells. These enzymes appear to stimulate the release of vasoactive substances such as bradykinin, histamine, and acetylcholine that increase capillary permeability.[6] As a result, large amounts of fluid begin to transude into surrounding body tissues, markedly reducing total blood volume. As the amount of venous return to the right side of the heart decreases, cardiac output becomes progressively more inadequate.

The systemic ischemic impairment of cellular function leads to the deterioration of other major bodily functions.[5] Rapidly rising blood lactic acid levels precipitate hypercoagulability. If the slow-moving, acidic blood of shock comes in contact with bacterial toxins arising from uncontrolled sepsis or with thromboplastin released from hemolyzed red blood cells, widespread intravascular clotting occurs.[4] Minute clots begin to plug the microcirculation, markedly depressing and eventually completely blocking tissue perfusion. If this process cannot be reversed, tissue necrosis, organ failure, and death ultimately ensue.

The liver is particularly vulnerable to the effects of inadequate perfusion and often is one of the first organs to exhibit signs of deterioration. This occurs because of the liver's rapid exposure to the highly concentrated toxins, which normally come from the gut, and the liver's high rate of metabolism. Ischemic injury of the liver precipitates an elevation of serum enzyme levels in approximately 60% of the patients in shock.[12] Elevated serum levels of aspartate transaminase (AST, formerly GOT), alanine transaminase (ALT, formerly GPT) and lactic dehydrogenase (LDH) reflect significant cellular damage to the liver. As the liver deteriorates, it becomes less able to trap and dispose of toxic materials.

Decreased perfusion also results in mucosal congestion and ischemic necrosis of the intestinal mucosal barrier. The loss of mucosal integrity allows intestinal bacteria to escape into the bloodstream, producing septicemia. The loss of blood into the lumen also adds to the systemic perfusion problem.

The loss of the detoxifying capability of the liver and the reticuloendothelial system (RES) is particularly significant to the effects of shock on the gastrointestinal tract. Resistance to portal circulation is created by minute clots obstructing the small hepatic channels. This causes venous blood to be dammed back in the intestinal capillaries. The resulting slowed blood flow allows increased absorption of the endotoxins released from the gram-negative bacteria in the intestine. Decreased perfusion and loss of monitoring capability render the RES increasingly incapable of removing bacteria and shock-produced endotoxins from the bloodstream. The rising levels of endotoxin in the blood lead to extensive depression of myocardial contractility and to massive systemic vascular dilation.

Decreased tissue perfusion of the pancreas promotes activation of pancreatic enzymes. These enzymes give rise to degenerative processes in the pancreatic tissues, causing the release of toxic factors into the bloodstream. The most detrimental of these is the myocardial toxic factor (MTF). This toxin can decrease cardiac contractility by as much as 50%.[3] This cardiac depression appears to result from interference with the action of calcium ions on the excitation-contraction coupling process in the myocardial tissue.

As shock progresses, lesions occur in the kidneys, lungs, heart, and brain. When perfusion pressure through Bowman's capsule is reduced, glomerular filtration decreases. If this situation is not reversed, acute tubular necrosis and renal failure follow. The interstitium of the lungs becomes congested with edema because of inadequate venous return. Reduced blood flow decreases the production of lung surfactant, resulting in increased alveolar surface tension and alveolar collapse, further reducing gaseous exchange potential.[8] Gaseous exchange is further compromised by the microembolization of significant amounts of the pulmonary microcirculation.

Although the heart has tremendous reserves to withstand periods of impaired perfusion, ischemic changes ultimately occur in the myocardium. These often precipitate electrical conduction defects, which produce fatal arrhythmias. Eventually the brain is also affected by perfusion failure. Ischemic injury of cerebral cells leads to cerebral edema and increased intracranial pressure. When the brain stem is affected, vital autonomic functions are depressed and death ensues.

The failures in vital organ function are enhanced by accompanying increases in the degree of acidosis. Tremendous quantities of lactic acid flood the bloodstream as more and more cells revert to anaerobic metabolism in response to impaired perfusion. This state of acidosis is potentiated by the functional failure of the poorly perfused liver, heart, skeletal muscles, and other organs to remove lactic acid from the blood.[7] Acidosis is also intensified by the decreased removal of carbon dioxide from body tissues. The carbon dioxide combines at the cellular level with water to form high concentrations of carbonic acid. The rapidly deepening acidosis potentiates further vital organ injury, which in turn further reduces systemic tissue perfusion.

Ultimately the point of no return is reached. Large quantities of destructive enzymes flood the body fluids, and local tissue and systemic acidosis become profound. The function of vital organs becomes so deteriorated that even a return to adequate perfusion cannot reverse the continuing cellular destruction. When cellular impairment pervades the body, death ensues.

ANTECEDENT CONDITIONS

Major disruptions in homeostasis can precipitate the four shock syndromes categorized as hypovolemic, cardiogenic, neurogenic, and vasogenic.

Hypovolemic shock

Shock owing to hypovolemia results from an acute loss of a significant portion of the blood volume. A marked decrease in circulating blood volume can arise from hemorrhage, plasma loss, or fluid loss.

Hemorrhage. The most frequent precipitator of hypovolemic shock is hemorrhage. The amount of blood loss required to precipitate shock depends on the rate at which the blood is lost, the compensatory capability of the cardiopulmonary system, the degree of tissue injury associated with the hemorrhage, and the preinjury hemoglobin level. Regardless of the impact of these factors, if the loss of blood volume continues, the systemic filling pressure eventually will be reduced and venous return to the heart will decrease. When cardiac output is diminished and hypotension occurs, perfusion of all tissues is reduced.

Plasma loss. Severe plasma loss can also reduce blood volume to the point that tissue perfusion is affected. Common sources of extreme plasma loss are denudation traumas (e.g., severe burns) and intestinal obstruction. The outpouring of body fluids and proteins from burns or large denuding wounds can significantly reduce the plasma portion of the blood. This reduces the total blood volume available for tissue perfusion. An excessive loss of plasma volume also can accompany episodes of intestinal obstruction. It appears that the intestinal distention that occurs in response to an obstruction either injures the capillaries in the intestinal walls or stretches the veins on the intestinal surface, raising capillary pressure by increased resistance. In any case, intestinal distention can cause a large amount of plasma fluid to leak into the intestinal walls and lumen.

Fluid loss. Systemic fluid loss can also decrease blood volume to the point that tissue perfusion is compromised. Fluid deficits can arise from insufficient intake and/or excessive output of fluid. Inadequate intake levels often go unnoticed when output levels do not appear exaggerated. Such fluid deficits build gradually, and the body slowly becomes dehydrated. However, once fluid deficits initiate shock, changes occur rapidly.

Exaggerated fluid loss can occur from the gastrointestinal tract in the form of diarrhea and vomiting. When renal parenchyma becomes injured or destroyed, kidney diuresis can be a source of excessive fluid loss. Hormonal disorders also can cause marked fluid loss. Injury to the adrenal cortices reduces aldosterone levels, rendering the kidneys incapable of reabsorbing sodium, chloride, and water. Depression of antidiuretic hormone (ADH) secretion by the pituitary gland can reduce fluid volume dramatically through kidney diuresis, quickly diminishing the circulating blood volume. The osmotic diuresis produced by hyperglycemia can also reduce extracellular fluid volume sufficiently to cause a significant decrease in blood volume.

Cardiogenic shock

Impaired tissue perfusion caused by cardiogenic factors results from sudden and rapid failure of the heart to function as an effective pump. Pump failure can arise from cardiac tamponade, which causes rapid accumulation of pericardial effusion, thus depressing diastolic filling and reducing cardiac output. Severe myocardial damage such as that which occurs with acute myocardial infarction and/or myocarditis diminishes tissue perfusion by markedly depressing myocardial contractility. Weak, ineffective contractions of the myocardium such as those accompanying cardiac arrhythmias can lead to a rapid deterioration in blood supply to systemic tissues. Damage to cardiac valves also dramatically reduces the forward flow of blood.

Neurogenic shock

Neurogenic factors precipitate shock by decreasing the vascular tone of the systemic circulation. As a result of diminished peripheral resistance the normal blood volume becomes inadequate to fill the greatly increased vascular capacity. The resultant reduction in systemic filling pressure produces a corresponding decrease in venous return. The venous pooling that occurs can be accentuated by the upright position, which allows great quantities of blood to fill the distended peripheral veins.

It is theorized that the loss of systemic vascular tone arises from interruption of the neural control processes that are responsible for maintaining vascular tone.[10] Deep general anesthesia can precipitate a sudden loss of vascular tone by depressing the vasomotor center in the brain. Spinal anesthesia, most notably that which extends to the superior portions of the spinal cord, can precipitate vascular collapse by blocking the efflux of sympathetic stimuli from the nervous system. Craniocerebral trauma involving the basal regions of the brain can profoundly depress vasomotor activity, causing vascular collapse. Vascular tone may be compromised by excessive amounts of insulin reducing the blood glucose level so low that the metabolism of the central nervous system and the vasomotor center is depressed.

Vasogenic shock

Two major pathological processes that directly affect dilation of the systemic vasculature are anaphylactic reactions and uncontrolled sepsis.

Anaphylaxis. During anaphylactic reactions the whole body responds to the presence of an antigen in the bloodstream to which the individual was previously immunologically sensitized. The profound antigen-antibody reaction that ensues causes release of histamine or histamine-like substances. Histamine produces a strong systemic vasodilation, greatly increasing vascular capacity. The arterioles become markedly dilated, causing arterial pressure to drop and tissue perfusion to decrease. As capillaries become increasingly permeable, fluid leaks into the interstitial spaces, thus reducing the circulating blood volume. As venous return is reduced, a corresponding decrease in cardiac output occurs and tissue perfusion rapidly becomes inadequate.

Sepsis. Uncontrolled sepsis, most often caused by a gram-negative organism, is thought to precipitate shock through release of toxins from the invading bacteria. The mechanism by which these toxins alter tissue perfusion is not completely understood. Findings from animal research indicate that the presence of endotoxins in the blood activates the complement system and vasoactive substances such as histamine and kinins, producing widespread arteriole vasodilation.[15] Ultimately, large amounts of blood become trapped in the spleen and liver to undergo detoxifiction. This intensifies the hypotension precipitated by the vasodilation.

Research evidence also suggests that endotoxins may cause direct injury to cells and peripheral organs. Examination of liver tissue subjected to endotoxins showed impairment of mitochondrial respiration and cell membrane transport.[18] These findings indicate that uncontrolled sepsis may not directly impair tissue perfusion, but rather, may interfere with the cells' ability to use oxygen. The resulting cell injury leads to progressive deterioration of vital organ function.

BEHAVIORAL DEFINITION

Although the deleterious effects of shock occur initially at the cellular level, eventually the impaired tissue perfusion leads to progressive deterioration of the body's major organ systems. The objective signs of deterioration in vital organ functions signal the presence of shock.

Objective data

Altered cardiovascular function. The initial cues of imminent shock arise from sympathetic compensatory responses to impaired perfusion. The cardiac acceleration and myocardial irritability precipitated by the release of epinephrine increase the heart rate and potentiate cardiac arrhythmias. The increased peripheral resistance resulting from secretion of norepinephrine causes the blood pressure and central venous pressure to remain stable or to decrease transiently. The pulse pressure also remains unaltered as long as the stroke volume is maintained by high concentrations of epinephrine. The selective vasoconstriction in response to norephinephrine causes the peripheral pulses to become rapid and thready, and capillary refill is prolonged. Decreased blood supply to the skin results in pale skin that feels cool and clammy. As a result of the cooling effect of the peripheral vasoconstriction, pilomotor erection may occur.

As shock progresses, the impairment in myocardial perfusion and the injury to the vasomotor center in the brain result in depression of cardiovascular function. Mechanical failure of the heart leads to a progressive deterioration in hemodynamic function. The pulse rate decreases markedly and becomes weak and thready. The systolic blood pressure falls in response to decreasing stroke volume and loss of integrity of the arteries and arterioles. As vasomotor control is lost, decreasing peripheral resistance produces a reduction in diastolic blood pressure. However, this reduction is not as rapid as that of the systolic pressure. Of greater significance is the decrease in pulse pressure that accompanies shock. Pulse pressure provides the most direct noninvasive indication of decreased stroke volume resulting from loss of myocardial contractility.[9]

More precise indications of hemodynamic changes associated with shock can be obtained through invasive techniques. Arterial cannulation can provide intra-arterial blood pressure readings. This pressure drops as arteriolar dilation occurs, providing the most accurate indication of the perfusion deficit to vital organs. Central venous pressure decreases as the amount of circulating blood volume returning to the right side of the heart diminishes. Pulmonary artery and pulmonary wedge pressures, measured with a Swan-Ganz catheter, also decrease in response to diminished blood volume and reduced left ventricular end-diastolic pressure.

Physiological indicators of the adequacy of peripheral circulation provide additional evidence of shock. Peripheral pulses become weak and ultimately nonpalpable. Capillary refill is extremely sluggish. Superficial veins collapse with digital pressure caused by inadequate circulating volume. Decreased perfusion of the skin causes it to feel cold. The skin takes on an ashen pallor, which progresses to cyanosis as the perfuson deficit intensifies. This is caused by accumulation of deoxygenated hemoglobin in the peripheral capillaries. In addition, diaphoresis may occur because sodium and water are secreted through the sweat glands in response to impaired aldosterone secretion.[1] As a result, the skin feels clammy.

Although impaired myocardial perfusion initially causes mechanical failure of the heart with hemodynamic breakdown, electrical failure ultimately occurs. At this point the apical pulse becomes irregular, and ECG recordings indicate conduction defects resulting from ischemic changes in the myocardium.

Depressed kidney function. Lack of adequate perfusion of the kidney causes additional signs of shock or impending shock. Decreases in circulating blood volume reduce urine output because the body attempts to conserve fluid. Continued impairment of renal circulation leads to acute tubular necrosis and complete anuria. Anuria is present when kidney output drops below 20 ml/hour.

Depressed respiratory function. The cellular hypoxia that accompanies shock initially increases the respiratory rate and depth. However, when the perfusion deficit begins to affect the respiratory center, respirations become slow and shallow. Alveolar surface tension rises with decreased surfactant production, and atelectasis follows. This loss of functional pulmonary tissue causes PaO_2 to decrease and $PaCO_2$ to rise. The lack of ventilation in the shock-injured lung tissue results in an absence of breath sounds over the affected area. As permeability of the pulmonary capillaries increases, rales and rhonchi become evident.

Decreased cerebral function. Initially, the heightened sympathetic nervous system activity and increased secretion of epinephrine cause signs of accentuated cortical arousal. The individual appears apprehensive or even agitated, exhibiting an increased alertness to environmental stimuli. As impairments in cerebral perfusion and concurrent cerebral hypoxia progress, the level of alertness becomes reduced and confusion and restlessness may occur. When shock is precipitated by uncontrolled sepsis, drowsiness and stupor are the predominant signs. Regardless of the antecedent, unless cerebral perfusion is reestablished quickly, unconsciousness and coma ensue.

Acidosis. Arterial pH decreases markedly in response to rising levels of lactic acid and carbonic acid. Metabolic acidosis is also evidenced by a decreasing bicarbonate level. The degree of acidemia is further reflected in elevated blood lactate and pyruvate levels. Although lactate and pyruvate levels initially rise in proportion to impaired perfusion, as shock intensifies and hypoxia becomes pervasive, a greater increase in the blood lactate level occurs.[7] Lactate levels, which can be determined from arterial blood samples, provide the most reliable indication of metabolic deficiency caused by perfusion failure.[7,13,16] In a study of 142 patients who exhibited clinical signs of circulatory shock, the blood lactate levels provided a clear demarcation between survivors and nonsurvivors. As blood lactate levels increased from 2.1 to 8.0 mM, estimated probability of survival decreased from 90% to 10%.[14] Lactacidemia is the ultimate indicator of perfusion failure that characterizes shock. Hypoxia without impaired tissue perfusion does not increase arterial lactate levels.[17]

Electrolyte and enzyme changes. During the initial phases of shock, reduction in the energy available for the active transport process causes a shift of sodium and chloride ions into injured cells with a concomitant outward flow of potassium. As a result, urine sodium and chloride levels drop below normal, whereas potassium levels are elevated. As shock progresses and urinary output decreases, hyperkalemia and hyponatremia occur.

Glucose imbalance. As a result of increased hydrocortisone secretion and subsequent liver glycogenolysis and gluconeogenesis, blood glucose levels rise. The early rise in blood glucose level is one of the most constant findings associated with shock, regardless of the antecedent condition.[7] As shock progresses, the blood glucose level generally remains high until liver and muscle glycogen is depleted. At this late stage, hypoglycemia occurs.

Liver and gastrointestinal tract dysfunction. The ischemic changes and tissue necrosis that occur in response to lack of perfusion of the liver and gastrointestinal tract provide additional indicators of shock. Loss of integrity of the bowel causes excessive diarrhea that contains large amounts of occult blood. Serum levels of LDH, AST, and ALT rise in response to cellular liver damage precipitated by shock.

Decreased body temperature. The lack of adequate perfusion significantly reduces the amount of heat liberated by body cells. As a result of shock, the body's core temperature decreases. This fall in body temperature is exaggerated when the environmental temperature is low. When impaired cerebral perfusion disrupts the thermoregulatory center in the brain, the body cools more rapidly.

Subjective data

The earliest subjective indications of shock occur in response to a decreasing level of cellular metabolism throughout the body. Initially, shock produces extreme fatigue, marked muscular weakness, and, often, thirst. The individual may say, "Something is wrong," or "I'm not feeling good." However, the person may have difficulty specifically describing the feeling. Often feelings of restlessness accompany these sensations. The loss of heat production that accompanies the reduced cellular metabolism may cause complaints of feeling cold or "chilled to the bone." As peripheral circulation decreases, the individual may feel cold, tingling, or numbness in the extremities. When perfusion to the cerebrum diminishes, tinnitis, blurred vision, light-headedness, dizziness, and visual blackness may occur.

INTERVENING VARIABLES

The degree to which physiological compensatory mechanisms are able to maintain adequate perfusion of the vital organs determines the extent to which reduced tissue perfusion will progress to a state of shock.

Sympathetic compensatory vasoconstriction

Compensatory activity aimed at maintaining blood flow to vital organs is mediated by the sympathetic nervous system. Sympathetic stretch receptors are located in the baroreceptors of the aortic arch and carotid sinuses. When blood volume is reduced, these baroreceptors receive less stimultion. A depression in the number of stretch signals transmitted to the vasomotor center in the medulla oblongata stimulates the bilateral excitatory portion of the vasomotor center. This portion of the medulla transmits excitatory impulses through the sympathetic nerve fibers to the heart, causing an increase in heart rate and contractility. In addition, the sympathetic vasoconstrictor fibers distributed throughout the systemic circulation are activated. This activation produces powerful vasoconstriction in the kidneys, the gastrointestinal tract, the spleen, and the skin, where these vasoconstrictor fibers are more highly concentrated. Stimulation of these fibers causes secretion of norepinephrine in the postganglionic fibers of these sympathetic nerves. Norepinephrine acts directly on the alpha receptors of the arteriolar smooth muscle, causing pronounced vasoconstriction. This selective vasoconstriction enhances tissue perfusion to the brain and heart by emptying vascular reserves. At the same time that norepinephrine is exerting its vasopressor effect, sympathetic vasonconstrictor impulses are transmitted to the adrenal medulla, activating secretion of epinephrine and norepinephrine. This additional norepinephrine accentuates the already increased peripheral resistance. The epinephrine stimulates the heart, increasing the pulse rate and the stroke volume. Concurrently, beta receptors of skeletal and cardiac muscle are excited, producing vasodilation, a drop in peripheral resistance, and widening pulse pressure. The overall effect of these two catecholamines on the circulation is to promote tissue perfusion by increasing systemic peripheral resistance, heart rate, and myocardial contractility.

When this sympathetic compensatory mechanism responds during the initial phase of the insult, the rate of progression of the shock state is slowed. If the antecedent condition can be removed, corrected, or neutralized during this compensatory phase, shock may be averted. It is the alteration in cardiovascular function which occurs in response to sympathetic activity that provides the major objective manifestations of this compensatory response.

Body position

When shock is precipitated by a loss of vasomotor tone owing to depression of the vasomotor center or marked vasodilation arising from direct action of vasoactive substance on the vessels, the sympathetic compensatory mechanisms are not functional. In these situations body position can significantly affect venous return. When the body is in a supine position, pooled venous blood may flow back to the heart in quantities sufficient to maintain cardiac output.

Fluid shifts

In an effort to maintain blood flow to vital organs, compensatory adjustments occur in fluid distribution.[1] As cardiac output and the rate of blood flow in the arterial capillaries decrease, so does the hydrostatic pressure of the capillaries. This decrease in hydrostatic pressure combined with gradual dilation of the arterioles produces a further reduction in blood flow and a reduced filtration of fluid from the capillaries of the vascular compartment into the interstitial compartment. As a result, small plasma proteins are retained in the capillaries of the vascular compartment and fluid movement into the interstitial compartment is decreased. With the retention of plasma proteins, colloid osmotic pressure increases. The depressed rate of blood flow through the capillaries prolongs the effects of the increased colloid osmotic pressure. As a consequence of the increased colloid osmotic pressure and the decreased hydrostatic pressure in the vascular compartment, greater amounts of fluid leave the interstitial compartment at the venous end than enter at the arterial end. Thus large amounts of fluid from the interstitial compartment move into the vascular compartment. This increases blood volume and venous return to the right side of the heart. If cardiac output can be increased sufficiently by this mechanism, a return to adequate tissue perfusion may result. As fluid shifts from the interstitial compartment, tissue dehydration occurs. Mucous membranes become dry, thirst increases, and turgor decreases. The resulting interstitial sodium and chloride deficiency produces a clammy feel to the skin surface.

Fluid retention

Efforts to increase blood volume are augmented by compensatory hormonal influences on the kidneys. In response to the physiological stress of impaired tissue perfusion, corticotropin releasing factor (CRF) is secreted from the primary capillary plexus of the hypothalamus and carried to the anterior pituitary gland, where it induces adrenocorticotropic hormone (ACTH) secretion.[3] ACTH stimulates the adrenal cortex to produce mineralocorticoids. The most prominent of these, aldosterone and desoxycorticosterone acetate, act on the renal tubules to increase the resorption of sodium in exchange for potassium in the distal tubules. Fluid retention by the kidney is also enhanced by the effects of ADH. When the osmolarity of the blood increases; the osmoreceptors in the hypothalamus stimulate the posterior pituitary gland to secrete ADH, causing the kidney tubules to retain increasing amounts of water.

As a result of the influence of these hormonal compensatory mechanisms on the kidneys, urine output decreases, the urine sodium level decreases, and the serum sodium level increases. In response to renal arteriolar vasoconstriction resulting from initial compensatory secretion of epinephrine, the kidneys release renal pressor substance (RPS) into the bloodstream. RPS promotes arteriolar constriction by increasing arteriolar tone. The ischemia that occurs in the kidneys as a result of the renal arteriolar vasoconstriction causes the juxtaglomerular cells to produce the enzyme renin. Renin promotes the release of angiotensin I from a globulin fraction of the plasma, which is then converted to angiotensin II by plasma and tissue enzymes. Angiotensin II is a potent vasconstrictor that increases cardiac output with its vasoconstricting properties. The purpose of these compensatory mechanisms is to maintain a blood pressure that can provide adequate kidney perfusion.

Mobilization of energy resources

The release of ACTH from the anterior pituitary stimulates secretion of glucocorticoids from the adrenal cortex. The major glucocorticoid in humans, hydrocortisone, stimulates glycogenolysis and gluconeogenesis in the liver. As a result of glycogenolysis, hyperglycemia rapidly occurs. The hyperglycemia is accentuated by the inhibitory effect of epinephrine on insulin production. The rapid elevation in the blood glucose level is an attempt to provide a substrate that can be used during anaerobic metabolism.[2] However, in approximately 2 hours glycogen stores in a nutritionally healthy adult are depleted. Gluconeogenesis becomes a major source of energy supply. The resulting protein catabolism produces a negative nitrogen balance. It is suggested that during shock the better perfused organs, most notably the brain and heart, may use lactate as a source of energy.[2]

Other compensatory activities aimed at promoting an adequate supply of cellular energy occur in response to the cellular hypoxia. In response to the decreased tissue oxygenation resulting from the impaired tissue perfusion, the bone marrow produces additional red blood cells, which are released into the bloodstream and increase the oxygen-carrying capability of the blood. However, because of the rapid rate of red blood cell production, many reticulocytes are released into the blood. Because of their immaturity they lack a full complement of hemoglobin. Consequently, their oxygen-carrying ability is limited. In addition to increased release of red blood cells from the bone marrow, the liver and spleen also move extra red blood cells into the vascular space. These extra cells attempt to enhance oxygen delivery to the cells while perfusion is impaired.

NURSING INTERVENTIONS—GOALS AND EVALUATION CRITERIA

The primary goal of nursing intervention in shock states is to increase blood supply to tissues to a level sufficient to meet the metabolic demands of the cells. This general goal can be achieved through attainment of the following specific nursing care goals: (1) anticipation and prevention of shock, (2) maintenance of tissue perfusion, (3) promotion of cellular oxygenation, (4) decrease of cells' metabolic needs, and (5) prevention of further injury and infection.

Anticipation and prevention of shock

Early recognition of the antecedent conditions of shock and activation of compensatory mechanisms are essential to the prevention of shock progression. If increases in heart rate and respiration, decreases in hourly urine output, and cold extremities are recognized as compensatory activities, medical measures can be initiated to reverse or neutralize antecedent conditions before the situation becomes life-threatening.

Close monitoring of fluid balance permits early identification of insufficient intake or excessive loss. This provides the opportunity for fluid replacement before circulating blood volume dramatically decreases. Persistent monitoring of patients with hemorrhage risk can also provide the opportunity for replacement prophylaxis.

Systematic cardiac assessment for shock-producing cardiac arrhythmias and murmurs can facilitate the initiation of corrective treatment before arrhythmias become life-threatening. The individual who is recovering from deep general or spinal anesthesia requires consistent monitoring to ensure identification of the initial signs of neurogenic shock. Attention to subtle changes in levels of consciousness of the diabetic patient allows institution of glucose replacement before neurogenic shock occurs. Vasogenic shock may also be prevented by careful assessment and by avoidance of agents to which the patient is hypersensitive. Early identification of the initial signs of systemic anaphylaxis such as diffuse erythema, urticaria, pruritus, and chest tightness provides the opportunity to initiate counteractive therapeutic measures. Early recognition and aggressive treatment of systemic infections can effectively reduce the quantity of bacterial toxins released into the bloodstream, thereby preventing uncontrolled sepsis.

Behavioral indications that shock has been prevented arise from a reversal of the initial cardiovascular compensatory manifestations. The pulse rate and blood pressure return to the preshock level. The cold and pallor of the skin decrease, and the patient reports feeling less chilled and/or less fatigued.

Maintenance of tissue perfusion

Medical therapy attempts to maintain adequate perfusion to vital organs through the administration of fluid replacement in combination with vasopressor and/or vasodilator agents. Although these therapeutic regimens primarily involve medical management, the nurse needs to understand the purpose of these therapies and the vital importance of accurate and frequent monitoring of administration rates and the patients' response to the therapy. When an extensive amount of vascular fluid is pooled in the microcirculation, fluid replacement is essential to restore circulating blood volume. The choice of fluid used for replacement is dictated by the type and amount of fluid lost. When blood loss exceeds 1 L, blood transfusion usually is instituted to replace the lost volume. When the antecedent condition to shock causes excessive loss of plasma, solutions of plasma, dextran, or albumin may be used to expand vascular volume. Such solutions are preferable to crystalloid volume expanders, since their larger molecules are more readily retained in the vascular bed. These large-molecule solutions more effectively maintain colloid osmotic pressure and hold fluid volume in the vascular space. Liberal amounts of Ringer's lactate or a balanced saline solution may be incorporated with these volume replacements in an effort to correct the fluid and electrolyte imbalances that result from depressed cellular metabolism and altered cell membrane integrity. Bicarbonate solutions may also be administered in combination with fluid therapy in an attempt to correct metabolic acidosis. The amount of fluid replacement depends on the changes in the blood pressure, central venous pressure, pulmonary artery pressure, and pulmonary wedge pressure. One of the primary responsibilities of the nurse in replacement therapy is frequent monitoring of these fluid pressure indicators so that the fluid therapy can be adjusted to maintain adequate perfusion and correct hypovolemia, yet not precipitate fluid overload and pulmonary edema.

Volume replacement is often augmented with vasopressors or vasodilators in an effort to enhance tissue perfusion. The use of vasopressors remains controversial because of the accentuated vasoconstriction they produce. However, when cerebral blood flow is compromised by a drop in systolic blood pressure to less than 60 mm Hg, vasopressors may be used in combination with fluid therapy to preserve cerebral integrity. Commonly used vasopressor agents include epinephrine, norepinephrine, levarterenol (Levophed) bitartrate, dopamine, isoproterenol (Isuprel) hydrochloride, and metaraminol bitartrate (Aramine). These medications are generally administered intravenously at a rate titrated to maintain systolic blood pressure at 80 mm Hg. Since the vasoconstricting effect of these medications can precipitate dramatic changes, the rate of infusion and the patient's blood pressure should be assessed as frequently as every 5 minutes. The urinary output must also be carefully monitored. The kidney is profoundly affected by the combination of vasopressor drugs and autonomically occurring compensatory vasoconstriction. Diuretic therapy in the form of mannitol (Osmitrol) or furosemide (Lasix) may be required to maintain urine output of at least 25 to 30 ml/hour.

When tissue perfusion is significantly compromised by vasoconstriction, vasodilators may be administered concurrently with rapid fluid replacement in an effort to promote blood flow to tissues. Among the vasodilators commonly used for this purpose are phentolamine (Regitine), phenoxybenzamine (Dibenzyline), chlorpromazine (Thorazine), and sodium nitroprusside (Nipride).

Tissue perfusion can also be enhanced by positioning the patient in a manner that facilitates venous return. It was formerly thought that the Trendelenburg position would maximize this effect. However, this position can depress ventilation by inhibiting the downward movement of the diaphragm. Currently the supine position is preferred, with the legs elevated to a 45-degree angle from the hip and the head level with or slightly higher than the chest. This position facilitates venous return from the lower extremities without interfering with diaphragmatic excursion. It also reduces the possibility of stimulating the carotid and aortic baroreceptor reflexes, which activate vasoconstriction of cerebral vessels.

Tissue perfusion can be augmented through application of certain external devices. External counterpulsation devices, which enclose the patient's legs in tubular bags filled with water or air, increase venous return and diastolic pressure by applying pressure to the legs during diastole and relaxing during systole. A sustained pressure to the lower extremities can be maintained through use of the antishock trousers, more generally referred to as military antishock trousers (MAST). This device provides rapid restoration of fluid volume and mean arterial blood pressure in the patient with hypovolemic shock. However, because of the rapid fluid shifts that accompany its use, it is contraindicated in cardiogenic shock.

Behaviors that indicate that tissue perfusion has been maintained include the return to preshock levels of blood, central venous, pulmonary artery, and pulmonary wedge pressures. As perfusion to systemic tissues improves, heart rate returns to the preshock rate and becomes strong and regular. Peripheral pulses increase in amplitude, and the skin temperature gradually rises. A return of adequate cerebral blood flow is documented by increasing levels of consciousness and a decrease in agitated behavior. As improved perfusion reverses the anaerobic metabolism of cells, blood lactate levels decrease and arterial pH returns to the normal range.

Promotion of cellular oxygenation

Since systemic cellular hypoxia accompanies shock, it is crucial that measures to increase cellular oxygenation be rapidly implemented. A number of specific measures for achieving this goal are discussed in detail in Chapter 13. However, when shock causes a decrease in surfactant production and physiological shunting, it may be necessary to support respiration with endotracheal intubation and mechanical ventilation to maintain $Pa{O_2}$ above 60 mm Hg. To maintain the $Pa{O_2}$ level without precipitating alveolar damage with excessively high concentrations of forced inspiratory oxygen (FIO_2), ventilatory support in the form of positive end-expiratory pressure (PEEP) may be required. Positive pressure prevents collapse of the alveoli during expiration, thereby enhancing oxygen and carbon dioxide exchange across the alveolocapillary membrane. This increase in the functional residual capacity decreases physiological shunting and facilitates a higher $Pa{O_2}$ with lower concentrations of delivered oxygen (FIO_2).

Special cardiac support measures may also be needed to maintain delivery of the oxygen supply during the shock state. Antiarrhythmic therapy may be needed to control ventricular arrhythmias, which markedly reduce stroke volume. Cardiac glycosides (e.g., digitalis) are often administered to strengthen cardiac contractility. When shock is accompanied by profound left ventricular failure, an intra-aortic counterpulsation balloon pump may be used. The balloon-tipped catheter is inserted through the femoral artery to the level of the thoracic aorta. Blood is forced into the coronary arteries and into the periphery by inflation of the balloon during early diastole. When the balloon deflates just prior to systole, peripheral resistance in the aorta is decreased and ventricular ejection is enhanced. The overall effect is increased cardiac output, enhanced oxygen delivery to myocardial tissues, and decreased myocardial oxygen consumption.

Specific behaviors indicative of the effectiveness of the cellular oxygenation efforts include a return of heart and respiratory rates to preshock levels. Pulse pressure narrows as stroke volume increases. Anxiety behaviors decrease as breathing becomes less labored. With improved oxygenation, PaO_2 increases. Breath sounds return, and rales and rhonchi decrease.

Decrease of cells' metabolic needs

Since the oxygen and substrates needed for cellular energy production are limited during shock, measures to reduce general energy demands should be implemented. The patient should be kept warm because chilling and shivering increase the metabolic rate. However, the patient should not be overheated because this may stimulate hypoperfusion of the vital organs as a result of vasodilation and movement of blood to the body surface. Additional energy may be wasted on diaphoresis. Only the essential aspects of physical care should be attended to, and these actions should be carried out in a manner that requires the least expenditure of energy by the patient. Measures to relieve pain and increase general comfort should also be instituted. Since tissue perfusion is slowed during shock, analgesics are often administered intravenously to ensure maximum absorption and to decrease localized tissue accumulation.

The patient experiencing shock is often extremely fearful and hypervigilant. This heightened anxiety level, which is often accentuated by the unfamiliar critical care atmosphere, increases metabolic demands. Efforts to decrease anxiety must be incorporated in all aspects of the patient's care. A trusting relationship between the patient and the nurse is essential to anxiety control. Such a relationship is fostered by consistent anticipation of the patient's needs and provision of ongoing feedback regarding progress. All procedures and treatments should be explained, with emphasis on the sensations the patient will experience and the reason for the procedure. The patient's significant others should be familiarized with the events they are observing so that they do not communicate unnecessary anxiety to the patient. Nonessential talking, noise, and movement around the patient should be eliminated, since they may accentuate hypervigilance. Alternate means of communication should be provided for the patient who cannot verbalize owing to endotracheal intubation.

Behavioral indications that metabolic demands have been reduced include decreased restlessness and increased general muscular relaxation. The patient will verbalize an absence of pain or feelings of being chilled. Skin temperature is warm, and the patient has periods of restful sleep.

Prevention of further injury and infection

The major sources of avoidable injury and infection for the patient in shock are those arising from physical immobilization, infection from invasive procedures, and dislodgment of tubes and lines. Although conservation of energy by decreasing metabolic needs of the patient is important, it is also essential to prevent the serious complications of immobilization. The patient in shock is particularly susceptible to the complications of thrombophlebitis, accumulation of pulmonary secretions, atelectasis, and skin breakdown. When possible the patient should be turned every 2 hours, even if only for a few minutes. At this time the patient should deep breathe. Passive range of motion exercises should be performed on the extremities, especially the lower limbs. Exercise should progress to active range of motion when the patient's condition allows.

The loss of the detoxifying capability of the liver and RES makes the patient in shock highly susceptible to infection. The multiple invasive procedures required to monitor the patient in shock further increase the risk of infection. Broad-spectrum antibiotic therapy is often instituted to protect against both gram-positive and gram-negative organisms. Strict aseptic technique is essential during endotracheal suctioning as well as during the handling of all invasive tubes and lines. Intra-arterial and intravenous tubing should be changed at least every 72 hours. The dressings over the insertion sites should be kept dry and should be changed at least daily. The sites should be assessed regularly for signs of infection and infiltration. This is especially critical when vasopressors are being administered. Extravasation of certain vasopressors, particularly norepinephrine, causes marked tissue sloughing.

Accidental injury resulting from restlessness and confusion is an ever-present danger for the patient in shock. Side rails are essential. The irritation caused by arterial and venous lines and the endotracheal tube may cause the restless, confused patient to pull at them, possibly causing tissue injury. If the patient is unable to cooperate to prevent dislodgement, soft arm restraints may be necessary. Such restraints should be removed at least every 4 hours to facilitate inspection and movement of the extremities.

Criteria used to determine the effectiveness with which infections and injuries are prevented include absence of signs of infection at arterial and venous catheter sites. Clear urine and nonpurulent endotracheal secretions are further indications that infection has not occurred. The lack of injury from dislodgment of tubes and catheters substantiates that safety is being maintained.

CONCEPT OUTLINE

I. *Conceptual definition:* Shock is a systemic state of rapidly decreasing tissue perfusion that produces multiple deleterious effects on the body's cells and vital organs and that, if unabated, rapidly leads to death.

II. *Antecedent conditions*
  A. Hypovolemic shock
    1. Hemorrhage
    2. Plasma loss
    3. Fluid loss
  B. Cardiogenic shock
    1. Cardiac tamponade
    2. Myocardial ischemia
    3. Myocardial inflammation
    4. Cardiac arrhythmia
  C. Neurogenic shock
    1. Deep general anesthesia
    2. Spinal anesthesia
    3. Craniocerebral trauma
    4. Excess insulin
  D. Vasogenic shock
    1. Anaphylaxis
    2. Sepsis

III. *Behavioral definition*
  A. Objective data
    1. Altered cardiovascular function
      a. Increased heart rate, ultimately progressing to a weak, depressed heart rate
      b. Cardiac arrhythmia
      c. Rapid, thready peripheral pulses
      d. Prolonged capillary refill time
      e. Cold, clammy skin
      f. Diaphoresis
      g. Pilomotor erection
      h. Ashen pallor, progressing to cyanosis
      i. Decreased systolic and diastolic blood pressures
      j. Decreased pulse pressure
      k. Decreased central venous, pulmonary artery, and pulmonary wedge pressures
    2. Depressed kidney function
      a. Oliguria
      b. Anuria
    3. Depressed respiratory function
      a. Initial increase of respiratory rate and depth
      b. Ultimate appearance of slow, shallow respirations
      c. Reduced PaO_2
      d. Increased $PaCO_2$
      e. Absence of breath sounds
      f. Increased rales and rhonchi
    4. Decreased cerebral function
      a. Apprehension
      b. Agitation
      c. Increased alertness to environmental stimuli
      d. Unconsciousness and coma
    5. Acidosis
      a. Decreased arterial pH
      b. Elevated blood lactate and pyruvate levels
    6. Electrolyte and enzyme changes
      a. Decreased urine sodium and chloride levels
      b. Elevated urine potassium level
      c. Hyperkalemia
      d. Hyponatremia
    7. Glucose imbalance
      a. Hyperglycemia in early stage
      b. Hypoglycemia in late stage
    8. Liver and gastrointestinal tract dysfunction
      a. Diarrhea with occult blood
      b. Increased serum levels of AST, ALT, and LDH
    9. Decreased body temperature
  B. Subjective data
    1. Extreme fatigue
    2. Marked muscular weakness
    3. Thirst
    4. Malaise
    5. Cold or chilled feeling
    6. Tingling or numbness in extremities
    7. Impaired vision
    8. Light-headedness or dizziness

IV. *Intervening variables*
  A. Sympathetic compensatory vasoconstriction
  B. Body position
  C. Compartmental shifts of fluid
  D. Fluid retention
  E. Mobilization of energy resources

V. *Nursing interventions—goals*
  A. Anticipation and prevention of shock
    1. Early recognition of compensatory mechanisms
    2. Close monitoring of fluid balance and early replacement of losses

3. Identification of cardiac arrhythmias and initiation of early treatment
4. Identification of subtle changes in levels of consciousness
5. Identification of initial signs of anaphylaxis, followed by rapid treatment
6. Early recognition and treatment of systemic infections

B. Maintenance of tissue perfusion
1. Monitoring of rate of fluid replacement and patients' pressure response
2. Use of pharmacological agents
   a. Vasopressors
   b. Vasodilators
   c. Diuretics
3. Monitoring of urine output
4. Body positioning
5. Use of counterpulsation devices

C. Promotion of cellular oxygenation
1. Endotracheal intubation
2. Mechanical ventilation with PEEP
3. Antiarrhythmic therapy
4. Cardiac glycosides
5. Intra-aortic counterpulsation balloon pump

D. Decrease of cells' metabolic needs
1. Provision of warmth
2. Prevention of overheating
3. Physical care limited to essential activities
4. Provision of pain relief
5. Development of trust relationship to reduce patient's anxiety
   a. Anticipation of patient's needs
   b. Procedures and treatments explained to patient and significant others
   c. Provision of benchmarks of progress
   d. Reduction of environmental noises and activity
   e. Provision of alternative forms of communication for intubated patient

E. Prevention of further injury and infection
1. Prevention of complications of physical immobilization
2. Maintenance of strict aseptic technique
3. Protection of patient from hazardous therapy equipment

VI. *Evaluation criteria*

A. Cardiovascular changes
1. Return of pulse rate and blood pressure to preshock levels
2. Increased strength and regularity of peripheral pulses and rapid capillary refill
3. Return of central venous, pulmonary artery, and pulmonary wedge pressures to preshock levels
4. Return of pulse pressure to preshock level
5. Warm, dry skin with no pallor or cyanosis

B. Respiratory changes
1. Return of rate and depth of respirations to previous levels
2. Normal $Pa{O_2}$
3. Normal $Pa{CO_2}$
4. Return of breath sounds
5. Absence of rales and rhonchi

C. Cerebral changes
1. Increased level of consciousness
2. Decreased apprehension and agitated behavior
3. Decreased hypervigilance

D. Fluid and electrolyte changes
1. Return of urine output to preshock level
2. Normal serum and urine electrolyte levels
3. Normal blood glucose level

E. Acid-base changes
1. Normal arterial pH
2. Return of blood lactate and pyruvate to preshock levels

F. Liver and gastrointestinal changes
1. Return of bowel function to preshock pattern
2. Normal levels of AST, ALT, and LDH

G. Other changes
1. Reduction in fatigue
2. Increased muscular strength
3. Decreased thirst and feelings of being cold
4. Absence of tingling and numbness in the extremities
5. Improved vision
6. Absence of light-headedness and dizziness

REFERENCES

1. Brodicks, K. J.: Patterns of shock, New York, 1965, Macmillan Publishing Co., Inc.
2. Fritz, S. D.: Energy metabolism in shock, Heart Lung **4**:615, 1975.
3. Guyton, A. C.: Textbook of medical physiology, Philadelphia, 1976, W. B. Saunders Co.
4. Hardaway, R. M.: Intensive study and treatment of shock in man, J.A.M.A. **199**:779, 1967.
5. Janoff, A.: Alterations on lysosomes (intracellular enzymes) during shock: effects of preconditioning (tolerance) and protective drugs, Int. Anesthesiol. Clin. **2**:25, 1964.
6. Janoff, A., Weissman, G., Zweifach, B. W., and Thomas, L.: Pathogenesis of experimental shock. IV. Studies on lysosomes in normal and tolerant animals subjected to lethal trauma and endotoxemia, J. Exp. Med. **116**:451, 1962.
7. Levenson, S. M.: Metabolic considerations. In Weil, M. H., and Shubin, H., editors: Diagnosis and treatment of shock, Baltimore, 1967, Williams & Wilkins Co.
8. Motsay, G. J., and Lillehei, R. C.: Respiratory distress syndrome. In Shumer, W., and Nyhus, L. M., editors: Treatment of shock: principles and practice, Philadelphia, 1974, Lea & Febiger.
9. Nickerson, M.: Vasoconstriction and vasodilation in shock, Int. Anesthesiol. Clin. **2**:385, 1964.
10. Robbins, S. L., and Angell, M.: Basic pathology, Philadelphia, 1976, W. B. Saunders Co.
11. Schumer, W., and Sperling, R.: Shock and its effect on the cell, J.A.M.A. **205**:215, 1968.
12. Shubin, H., and Weil, M. H.: Acute elevation of serum transaminase and lactic dehydrogenase during circulatory shock, Am. J. Cardiol. **11**:327, 1963.
13. Walt, A. J., and Wilson, R. E.: The treatment of shock, Adv. Surg. **9**:1, 1975.
14. Weil, M. H., and Afifi, A. A.: Experimental and clinical studies on lactate and pyruvate as indicators of the severity of acute circulatory failure (shock), Circulation **41**:989, 1970.
15. Weil, M. H., and Shubin, H.: Shock associated with infection—bacterial shock. In Weil, M. H., and Shubin, H., editors: Diagnosis and treatment of shock, Baltimore, 1967, Williams & Wilkins Co.
16. Weil, M. H., and Shubin, H.: Monitoring and measurements during shock. In Schumer, W., and Nyhus, L. M., editors: Treatment of shock: principles and practice, Philadelphia, 1974, Lea & Febiger.
17. Weil, M. H., Shubin, H., Sacks, S., and Michaels, S.: Lactate concentrations during respiratory failure, Am. J. Cardiol. **26**:665, 1970.
18. White, R. R., Mela, L., Bacalzo, L. V., Olofsson, K., and Miller, L. D.: Hepatic ultrastructure in endotoxemia, hemorrhage, and hypoxia: emphasis on mitochondrial changes, Surgery **73**:525, 1973.

SANDRA R. POWELL
SONJA I. LIVELY

Chapter 16

PSYCHOLOGICAL CRISIS

Here I sit
no stranger to you
than to myself.

Here I sit
pieces of confusion
bits of pride.

Here I sit
on a chair, on a curb,
on a subway, on a plane.

Here I sit
screaming in my silence
yelling without words.

Here I sit
till I can sit no longer
till my silence becomes hoarse.

Then I rant
and I rave,
I scream
and I stomp,
Some say, "overworked,"
others say, "irresponsible,"
still others, "insane."

Yet I am none of these
I am your friend, your patient
I am the part of you that can
no longer cope.

PAULETTE R. Di ANGI

CONCEPTUAL DEFINITION

Psychological crisis is the response to a temporary failure of adaptation to a challenge. It is a critical phase that evolves from the perception of an overwhelming threat. A psychological crisis can develop at any point on the health-illness continuum. A crisis may occur in a person in good health or in one who has an acute or chronic illness. It can initiate an illness or precipitate the resolution of an illness. Psychological crisis is not an illness, but rather a phase or time when the usual patterns of coping are blocked or useless. Suddenly a potentially dangerous state of psychological disequilibrium is experienced.[9,14]

Psychological crisis begins when an individual encounters a stressor that threatens an aspect of the self-system such as self-esteem, life goals, or significant relationships. In response to the perceived threat, anxiety is initiated. These anxious feelings accelerate when attempts to remove or neutralize the threat through the use of previously successful coping mechanisms are ineffective. When the threat continues, behavioral responses shift from neutralization of the problem to reduction of anxiety. If the anxiety is not reduced, overwhelming feelings of helplessness and cognitive disruption lead to behavioral disorganization. In this crisis state the individual is vulnerable to accidents or suicide. The focus of attention is extremely narrow, so factors in the immediate environment may not be acknowledged. During this time the individual feels unable to handle the situation and becomes receptive to outside help.[15]

The response to psychological crisis consumes a high degree of energy, since emotional changes are rapid and intense. As the level of anxiety experienced during this state increases, the length of time that the crisis can be sustained decreases. A person whose anxiety remains just below the severe level may be able to meet this energy demand for as long as 8 weeks. The person experiencing panic, however, is able to meet energy demands only for periods of hours rather than days or weeks. A continued high expenditure of energy leads rather quickly to exhaustion.[3]

When the threat persists and the crisis is not resolved, an individual is protected from exhaustion by moving into a state of psychological disorganization to avoid continued confrontation with the threat. The resultant state of sustained disorganization leaves the individual unable to respond to short-term crisis intervention techniques. In this situation long-term assistance is often required.[3]

Psychological crisis is a transitional period that provides an individual with an opportunity for growth or the possibility of increasing psychological disorganization. When new and better ways to solve the problems are found, the person emerges healthier and better able to cope with life. When crisis is not adequately resolved, a major psychological disorganization may occur, leaving the individual less able to cope with future situations.[3]

Since psychological crisis is a subjective experience evolving from perceptions that an overwhelming threat has been encountered, its existence can be validated only by the person experiencing it. A person is in crisis only if that person thinks so, not because someone else believes it.

ANTECEDENT CONDITIONS

The situation that characteristically precipitates psychological crisis is a perceived loss that is sudden and unavoidable.[8,16] Being unprepared for the change and lacking the ability to accept the change appear to be crucial elements of crisis precipitation. Although all crisis situations stem from inadequate development of successful coping responses, specific situational crisis can be precipitated by negative or accidental events that result in losses such as the death of a loved one, loss of a body part, loss of property, or changes in body image or usual life patterns. Such events often precipitate a crisis not just because of their accompanying loss but because of their suddenness. The individual has not been able to prepare for the emotions experienced.[1,2]

The anniversary of a loss can also trigger a crisis for similar reasons. For example, a woman knows that in a week it will have been over 1 year since her husband died or her divorce became finalized. However, when that day arrives, she finds she had not anticipated the myriad feelings that begin to engulf her. She almost relives the experience of her loss and finds herself unprepared to handle such intense feelings. This anniversary may simply be the last of the accumulation of changes she has had to face. Her feelings about her loneliness and the unfairness of her situation intensify. Although the anniversary is anticipated, the feelings experienced when she focuses on the many changes (losses) she has lived through during the past year are not. The occurrence of these feelings is the last straw.[1]

Some loss is, of course, inherent in change of any type. All life's changes hold the potential for crisis precipitation. Socially positive events such as marriage, graduation, job advancement, or the addition of a new baby to the family can initate a crisis. The person is confronted with an unfamiliar role. The comfortable, old, secure life-style or behavior patterns no longer suffice. Even when the change is seen as an improvement, the loss of sameness and predictability in life patterns can be unsettling. Unexpected feelings suddenly appear. The individual finds there has been no time to think through these feelings. For example, the student preparing to graduate understands cognitively the events that will occur on graduation day. The gathering of relatives and friends, the commencement ceremonies, and the graduation party are all anticipated. This event may be perceived primarily as a celebration of victory, a societal noting of achievement. What may be unanticipated are the emotions experienced regarding the new life about to begin. School friends will be left behind. The threat of failure attached to the challenge of this new role can be unsettling. The greater the anticipated loss from changes in role, daily living activities, and support from significant others, the greater the threat. The situation's potential for crisis precipitation increases as the preparation for emotions and the ability to handle the change decrease.

Societal expectations of behavior at different developmental levels can also be the source of crisis.[11,15] The individual is to cast off old patterns of behavior and acquire new patterns. How one responds to these demands relates to the level of understanding of or preparation for the change and the ability to cope with the loss of the old behavior. Reactions to developmental advancement vary. What one individual perceives as an overwhelming threat, another may see as a challenge or a zestful experience. Another person may pass so smoothly through a developmental level as to appear unaware of any change.

Each developmental task is a stepping stone designed to prepare the individual with skills necessary for subsequent task mastery. Each new task is accompanied by behavioral patterns that carry new freedoms and responsibilities as the individual moves toward more independent stages. However, these new freedoms are accompanied by the loss of previously acceptable dependency behaviors.[5]

A person who has not mastered earlier developmental expectations is not equipped to deal with the progressively more sophisticated stages that follow. For example, it is impossible for an individual who has never learned trust to form a satisfying, sustaining, intimate relationship with another. Likewise, generativity cannot be perceived as a zestful challenge if the task of industry was never successfully mastered. The individual is both unprepared for new tasks and ill-equipped to cope with more advanced expectations because of inability to perceive and/or understand the dynamics of the new expectations.[5] This includes not only why, but how expectations have not been met. Crisis can be precipitated by the developmental dynamics when the new freedoms of the more advanced stages are accepted but the responsibilities neglected, or when old dependence patterns are maintained and used to meet new responsibilities. When old patterns are found wanting and the individual becomes aware of how unacceptable or unsuccessful these behaviors are, the situation may be perceived as overwhelming, precipitating crisis.[11,15]

BEHAVIORAL DEFINITION

Inherent in psychological crisis is an increase in the individual's anxiety level. By the time the crisis is acknowledged, the level of anxiety is usually approaching or past a severe state. The cognitive and affective manifestations of psychological crisis relate to the level of anxiety experienced. The behaviors exhibited are those the individual previously has found successful to reduce anxiety.

Objective data

The key and only valid indicator that a person is in a state of psychological crisis is that person's identification of its presence.[3,9] Persons in crisis are often first encountered when they seek or ask for help. The approach used to request help usually depends on past behavior patterns. In the community a person may directly call or go to a crisis center, minister's rectory, or friend's home. In the hospital the person may go to the nurse's station and state that help is needed, or the person may simply show up but remain quiet until approached by someone. The person may say, "I am having a crisis," but most often phrases such as "I'm in trouble," "I can't get it together," "I feel overwhelmed," "I'm having difficulty, (a problem)," "I am in distress," "I hurt," or "I don't know what to do" are used.[9]

Cognitive responses. The changes exhibited in the individual's cognitive ability relate to the level of anxiety being experienced. As anxiety increases, perceptual abilities decrease. The person's focus may narrow to only specific details, ignoring all other aspects of the situation. The person may relate to many scattered details of the situation without being able to connect them in a unified whole. In panic states, perceptions become further disorganized. Only one unimportant detail may be seen and its meaning distorted. The person in panic is unable to think through a problem without assistance. Specific aspects of the situation may not be identified, and facts related to previous problems may be intermixed with the current problem. The ability to organize thoughts and process them in a logical way is severely diminished. For these reasons the person may be confused about the problem and may appear to respond inappropriately to questions.

If the person's previous behavior is not known, changes in cognitive ability may need to be verified by the individual or by significant others. Changes in ability to solve problems and a decrease in decision-making ability and in job performance are key indicators of cognitive pattern changes.[9,15]

Motor-behavioral responses. The smooth and skeletal muscle tension as well as the energy expenditures that occur in high anxiety states account for the variety of the physiological changes that occur before and during psychological crises. Usually the most apparent of these, when the person first asks for help, is tension, or contraction, of the skeletal musculature. The increased tension promotes jerky, rigid movement and posturing. There may also be increased activity of a specific body part such as swinging of a leg or tapping of a foot or a hand while the rest of the body is rigidly immobile.

There may be an excess of body movements, with swinging arms and pacing back and forth. Increases in smooth muscle tension may precipitate urinary frequency, diarrhea, or vomiting. Sleeping and eating patterns may be disrupted.

The specific behavioral patterns the person exhibits usually relate to the type of coping behavior found successful in the past. Since these behaviors have not been observed by health personnel, verification by the person or significant others is necessary. For example, immobilization, agitation, or destructive behavior patterns may be exhibited. Specific descriptions of these behaviors can be found in Chapters 3 to 6.

Subjective data

Affective responses. The individual in psychological crisis is in a state of disequilibrium. Past coping skills are not helping, and feelings of loss of control over the cognitive, emotional, and even environmental aspects of life become overwhelming.[3] The anxiety this situation produces may be clearly perceived by the individual, that is, the person may be aware of the anxiety and the need for help. Sometimes these feelings are expressed as helplessness, loss of control, being overwhelmed, or inability to take action or to decide what to do. The anxiety may be camouflaged as guilt, shame, fear, or anger.[4] Usually the manner the individual uses to describe why help is being sought provides a cue to the individual's awareness of underlying anxiety. The person who is aware of these feelings is more apt to request help directly, specifically, and descriptively.[9]

Motor-behavioral responses. The muscular tensions experienced during crisis may precipitate subjective physiological complaints such as nausea, insomnia, anorexia, gastrointestinal pains, headache, backache, neck pain, and chest pain. Previous health problems may recur.

INTERVENING VARIABLES

Primary factors affecting how an individual survives a psychological crisis are the individual's ability to meet the energy demands of the situation, available assistance, and previous problem-solving success.

Ability to meet energy demands

The anxiety experienced during crisis produces a high energy demand. Any factors that reduce the body's ability to meet this demand will decrease the individual's ability to work through the crisis.[3,4,16] The body's nutritional state and metabolic balance are key factors affecting energy production. Job or family demands, physical illness, and the use of drugs place additional energy demands on the body. Disrupted sleep patterns reduce energy recovery capabilities.

Available assistance

At times the realization that help is available if it is needed is enough to support the person through the crisis. The idea of not being isolated may provide a great deal of stability. Accessibility of external assistance depends on its availability, the individual's knowledge about this availability, and the individual's ability to communicate the need for assistance.[1]

The types of available environmental assistance vary in urban and rural areas. Urban areas often provide a greater variety of institutional facilities (e.g., mental health centers, crisis centers, telephone crisis lines, and acute psychiatric care units in a variety of hospitals). Rural areas are often more limited in the number of institutional supports. The sources for help commonly available to rural populations are the clergy, the family physician, concerned neighbors, the county public health nurse, and the general community hospital. Although the number of resources may be less, the person needing them may be more aware of their availability than the city dweller with a wide variety of unknown resources.

Although the informality of the rural facilities may increase the ease of access, the level of intervention may be less sophisticated and varied than that in the urban setting. If one does realize the existence of a support facility (e.g., mental health center) in the urban area, one may still not know how to request assistance. However, once access to the system has been gained, the intervention may be more intense and inclusive.

Previous problem-solving success

If the person has been able to solve major problems in the past, this ability can be an asset. The skills gained in these previous experiences can be used in the current problem-solving task if the person can be helped to realize how to use them. Two skills that are of great assistance in working through a crisis are the ability to communicate and the ability to trust.

NURSING INTERVENTIONS—GOALS AND EVALUATION CRITERIA

Since psychological crisis is not an illness, but rather a time-oriented event or situation, the end goal of crisis intervention is the resolution of the individual's immediate crisis and the restoration of at least a precrisis level of functioning. The optimum goal is attainment of a more successful level of functioning, with the long-range goal of preventing further crises.[1,10]

Time is the prime factor that influences the techniques used in crisis intervention. It is unusual for an individual to meet the energy demands of a crisis for much longer than 6 to 8 weeks.[3] The time therefore available for effective interventions is usually limited to this period.

The four major guiding principles of crisis intervention emanate from this time limitation. First, the closer the intervention to the beginning of the crisis, the more apt is the individual in crisis to have the energy to respond to the assistance offered. Second, because of the time and energy limitations, the intervention must be actively focused on the current situation and address its resolution. History taking and diagnostic evaluation must be limited to the data relevant to the present problem. Third, since the client's focus is often narrowed, a direct approach must be used to increase awareness that the current crisis situation is being addressed. Fourth, the intensity of the techniques used in intervention should match the intensity and rate of change in the individual's emotional state. The higher the level of anxiety and the greater the rate of change, or increase, the more direct, frequent, and intense the methods must be. Contact in a crisis situation must be at least daily.[1,9,12,15]

Achievement of the following short-term goals will help the individual find ways to successfully deal with the crisis.

Provision of a safe and secure environment

As an individual's anxiety level increases, cognitive abilities reduce, attention spans shorten, and focus narrows. Awareness of the immediate environment may be limited. Accidents may be precipitated by inattention to the environment, ranging from small lapses in concentration resulting in cuts or abrasions to a preoccupation so intense that a person steps into traffic without realizing the danger. Another avenue of possile harm is the potential of the person perceiving suicide to be a final solution to the problem.[9]

One of the first decisions that one must make when working with someone in psychological crisis is whether specific environmental supports for physical safety are needed. Such supports could include having someone stay with the person or call or visit at scheduled times. Significant others or groups specific to the precipitating problem could provide this assistance. Examples of groups that could provide this type of support are church groups, Alcoholics Anonymous, and Make Today Count. Hospitalization is also an option when physical safety is threatened.

These types of external assistance convey security to the client. They relieve the person from worry about safety, so attention can be directed to resolution of the crisis. Behavior indicative of the achievement of this goal includes the absence of injury.

Maintenance of energy levels

Crisis response and resolution places high energy demands on the individual. Therefore methods of energy conservation, supply, and restoration must be supported. The individual may not be obtaining adequate rest or nutrition. If this deficit is a major detriment to the individual's condition and the individual has little or no support systems available, hospitalization may be necessary to supply these basic needs. If significant others are available, they can be mobilized to provide assistance needed to supply these basic needs. Contacting family, neighbors, friends, or employers to arrange for assistance with daily living activities such as food provision and/or temporarily relieving the individual of some family or job responsibilities can be done after obtaining the individual's permission.

The individual should be assisted in identifying the options available for relief from those tasks which require energy expenditure. The individual may need to consider alternatives for assistance with child care such as arranging for a spouse to give additional assistance, for a baby-sitter for some period (depending on financial resources), for children to help at home, or for assistance from relatives or neighbors. Depending on available finances, food preparation tasks might be reduced by eating out more often, food might be brought in by neighbors or relatives, or frozen prepared meals might be used. If reductions in job responsibility would help, necessary assistance might be sought from coworkers or the employer. Arrangements might be made to reduce the amount of time worked or to reduce job responsibilities for a brief time. These decisions must take into account not only energy expenditure levels but also the client's feelings about the task and the meaning attached to the function. Meal preparation may reduce the client's anxiety, or job delegation may increase feelings of incompetence. Spending time with one's child or at work may be a diversion that provides needed recovery time.

Behaviors indicative that these basic areas of energy maintenance are being supported include increased levels of food ingestion and increased rest or sleep. Also maintenance of the client's ability to focus and direct attention to the problem-solving task at hand indicates maintenance of an energy reserve.

Development of a trust relationship

An individual who is alone and overwhelmed in a psychological crisis needs human contact and concern. It is essential that a trusting, working relationship be developed so that this individual will accept help to work through the current situation. A sense of warmth and caring can be communicated to the individual from the onset of the relationship by using active listening skills and making the individual's world safer, more secure, and less energy consuming.[9]

Because an individual in crisis often has difficulty with decision making, a direct, positive approach communicates the message that there are things that can be done to help the situation and that the nurse is available to help with the problem. Early in intervention sessions a tentative agreement regarding sharing of activities should be identified. If the person's cognitive ability is only slightly impaired, a nondirective, open-ended question approach may help the person initiate a solution. When anxiety levels are higher, more directive, collaborative approaches may be needed, in which responsibility for developing a workable plan is shared equally. When thought processes are very disorganized, a third level of working relationship is necessary. Since the client is unable to take responsibility for the present situation, explicit directions must be given regarding the activities to be undertaken. In each instance the goal is to develop a working relationship in which the client begins to believe that it is possible to acquire help.[9]

The person in psychological crisis needs to believe that the person helping can do something concrete and that a practical, workable solution is possible. One method to promote this idea is to develop a working plan that identifies specific, concrete activities related to the most pressing aspects of the situation, for example, "From what you say, the most important thing to do right now is to find a baby-sitter so you can continue your job. Before we meet again tomorrow, you check on your work hours for the next 2 weeks, and I will check with the community day nursery." This working plan communicates that the individual is seen as a capable person able to work through the crisis if assistance is offered. A situation does not appear so overwhelming when help is available to approach each aspect one step at a time. In addition to these "homework assignments," immediate tasks can also consist of thinking tasks, for example, "Before we meet tomorrow, I would like you to think of the pros and cons of getting a divorce, and we will start with that."

It is essential to the maintenance of a trusting, working relationship that commitments be fulfilled. For example, if a person was to be contacted or information obtained before the next planned session, this must be done, or one must explain what prevented the task's completion and what alternatives are still available.[6]

Behavior indicative of the development of a trusting relationship includes the person arriving on time for sessions, sharing of information and feelings, and implementing agreed on activities. In addition, symptoms of anxiety are less evident during the contact time. However, when the person is working through difficult aspects of the problem, the muscular symptoms of anxiety may again increase temporarily.

Development of an intellectual understanding of the crisis situation

The first step toward solving a problem is identification of the problem. The diminished level of cognition that occurs in psychological crisis often necessitates assistance with reality orientation and structuring of events. Complete restructuring of events includes both cognitive sequencing and identification of emotional responses. To reduce anxiety, the initial reality orientation should address only the cognitive sequencing. Since cognitive disorganization is often extremely frustrating, the individual should be assisted in identifying as much data as can be tolerated without further increasing anxiety. The individual should be helped to identify the precipitating event, describe what happened, and identify why help was sought and what caused the problem.[7,13]

When events are being restructured, only small, manageable pieces of data should be addressed. Limited questions such as "Tell me what happened first" assist the client in systematically identifying relevant information about the problem. They also assist the client in gathering information into a unified whole without letting the situation become so overwhelming that problem identification is blocked.

Behavior indicating that an intellectual understanding has been achieved is the person's ability to state in a cohesive manner what problem caused the crisis and to describe the sequence of events.

Development of self-awareness

Once the problem can be intellectually addressed, the person is ready to become aware of emotional responses to the situation. One way to begin this process is to have the person state what emotions are currently being experienced. The next areas to be explored relate to the feelings that were experienced at the time of the event and the aspects of the event that were attached to emotional changes. It is also helpful to explore whether these types of feelings had been experienced in the past and, if so, what initiated them.[13]

Included in the development of self-awareness is the identification of what the person perceives to be an available support system. Who in the environment is perceived as supportive, available, and willing to help? In some instances such as that of the alcoholic who has lost family, jobs, and friends the client may need to be temporarily hospitalized while a support group is formed. Others may need only to validate that supportive friends are available to be asked for help.[9]

Behavior indicative of increased awareness of feelings and emotional supports is the ability to identify and describe feelings that relate to "here and now" events.

Development of skills to deal with current and future crisis situations

The following types of questions can assist in identifying the skills and methods the person has successfully used in the past to solve problems: Under what circumstances were specific skills used with success? Has there been an attempt to use these skills in the current situation? If the skills have been unsuccessful, how have they failed? Were any other methods used? Have others been asked for help? How could others by helpful—by listening, showing interest, assisting in procurement of daily needs such as food, providing relief from child care and other job responsibilities, or helping in decision making?

Benchmarking progress provides reinforcement of skills being learned. The accomplishment of short-term immediate tasks often carries its own reinforcement, thus increasing feelings of control. However, for complex skills such as developing self-awareness or improving communication abilities the patient often needs external assistance to accurately evaluate progress.

It is often helpful to spend the last few minutes of each meeting summarizing. Who assumes the summary activity depends on the level of the client's functioning. In the beginning the nurse usually reviews the progress made and identifies the agreements. A larger role in summarizing the session and identifying the progress made with problem solution and personal growth should be assumed by the individual as improvement occurs. Included in these evaluations are such things as the identification of interactions that have become more comfortable, of improvements in cognitive abilities or job performance, and of changes in feelings.

During the end of the crisis or during the end period of its resolution the person should be assisted in assessing the skills that were used to resolve the problem.

After identification of what helped in the current situation, the following type of questions can help the individual prepare for future problems: What can you do if something like this occurs in the future? How and when should you decide that outside help is needed? How can you activate and use your support system? How can you anticipate problems so they can be prevented or their impact minimized?[4,7]

It is often helpful to list and discuss problems that might occur in the same areas as the current problem. What might precipitate them and when they might be expected should be considered. For example, if the current situation related to a relationship with a child, the problems to be expected during the child's future developmental stages might be discussed. If the current situation was one of marital problems of a middle-aged couple, possible problems related to retirement changes might be discussed.

Behavioral indices that the psychological crisis is resolving relate to the changes in the behavior that the crisis disrupted or disorganized. In general, the individual should be returning to a precrisis level of functioning. However, as with the identification of the crisis, the cardinal sign of resolution is the individual's statement that the crisis has passed, things have changed, and the problem is being handled or can be coped with. The person, however, may still be anxious or display facets of maladaptive behavior used prior to the crisis. Conclusion of the psychological crisis simply means the situation is no longer overwhelming to the client.

At this point, if problems continue, the individual should be helped to decide whether to continue working on these problems. Options regarding where and how such assistance can be obtained should be examined.

CONCEPT OUTLINE

- I. *Conceptual definition:* Psychological crisis is a critical phase or time that evolves from the perception that an overwhelming threat is being encountered for which one's usual patterns of coping are useless.
- II. *Antecedent conditions*
  - A. Sudden, unavoidable loss
  - B. Anniversary of loss
  - C. Loss of predictable life pattern
  - D. Developmental expectations
- III. *Behavioral definition*
  - A. Objective data
    - 1. Cognitive responses
      - a. Decreased perceptual ability
      - b. Narrowing of focus
      - c. Thought disorganization
      - d. Changed ability to solve problems
      - e. Decreased ability to make decisions
      - f. Decreased job performance
    - 2. Motor-behavioral responses
      - a. Skeletal muscle tension
        - 1. Jerky, rigid movement
        - 2. Restlessness
        - 3. Constant movement of body part
      - b. Smooth muscle tension
        - 1. Urinary frequency
        - 2. Diarrhea
        - 3. Vomiting
  - B. Subjective data
    - 1. Affective responses
      - a. Feeling of being overwhelmed by problem
      - b. Helplessness
      - c. Loss of control
      - d. Anxiety
      - e. Guilt
      - f. Anger
    - 2. Motor-behavioral responses
      - a. Nausea

b. Insomnia
c. Anorexia
d. Gastrointestinal pains
e. Headache
f. Backache
g. Neck pain
h. Chest pain

IV. *Intervening variables*
A. Ability to meet energy demands
B. Available assistance
C. Previous problem-solving success

V. *Nursing interventions—goals*
A. Provision of safe and secure environment
1. Use of support groups for safety monitoring
2. Hospitalization
B. Maintenance of energy levels
1. Provision of adequate opportunity for rest and nutrition
2. Temporary relief from family and/or job responsibilities
3. Reduction in other energy demands
C. Development of trust relationship
1. Inclusion of patient in decision making
2. Communication that individual is seen as capable of working through problem
3. Fulfillment of commitments
D. Development of intellectual understanding of crisis situation
1. Factual sequence of problem event restructured by using piece-by-piece approach
E. Development of self-awareness
1. Identification of emotions currently experienced
2. Identification of past experience that initiated similar feelings
3. Identification of feelings experienced at different points during crisis event
4. Identification of individual's perceived support system
F. Development of skills to deal with current and future crisis situations
1. Identification of skills used in past successful problem solving
2. Identification of alternative skills to use in current problem
3. Evaluation of success of skills tried
4. Identification of accomplishments and progress
5. Review of skills used to solve problems
6. Discussion of possible future problems and available approaches to solution

VI. *Evaluation criteria*
A. Absence of injury
B. Increased ability to focus on problem-solving task
C. Decrease in restless movements
D. Sharing of information
E. Implementation of agreed on activities
F. Description of event sequence
G. Description of current and past emotional responses
H. Use of support system
I. Return to precrisis cognitive functioning
J. Patient's statement of own ability to handle problem

REFERENCES

1. Aguilera, D. C., and Messick, J. M.: Crisis intervention: theory and methodology, ed. 3, St. Louis, 1978, The C. V. Mosby Co.
2. Beck, J. C., and Worthen, K.: Precipitating stress, crisis theory, and hospitalization in schizophrenia and depression, Arch. Gen. Psychiatry **26:**123, 1972.
3. Caplan, G.: Principles of preventative psychiatry, New York, 1964, Basic Books, Inc., Publishers.
4. Carter, F. M.: Psychosocial nursing: theory and practice in hospital and community mental health, New York, 1976, Macmillan Publishing Co., Inc.
5. Erickson, E.: Childhood and society, New York, 1963, W. W. Norton & Co., Inc.
6. Golan, N.: Treatment in crisis situations, New York, 1978, The Free Press.
7. Hitchcock, J.: Crisis intervention: the pebble in the pool, Am. J. Nurs. **73:**1388, 1973.
8. Hitchcock, J.: Social and psychological crisis. In Kalkman, M. E., and Davis, A. J., editors: New dimensions in mental health psychiatric nursing, New York, 1974, McGraw-Hill Book Co.
9. King, J. M.: The initial interview: base for assessment in crisis intervention, Perspect. Psychiatr. Care **9:**247, 1971.
10. Langsley, D. and Yarvis, R.: Evaluation of crisis intervention, Curr. Psychiatr. Ther. **15:**274, 1975.
11. Maloney, E.: The subjective and objective definition of crises, Prespect. Psychiatr. Care **9:**257 1971.
12. Messick, J. M.: Intervention concept-implication for nursing practice, J. Psychiatr. Nurs. **10:**3, 1972.
13. Nelson, L., and Mowrey, D.: Contracting in

crisis intervention, Community Ment. Health J. **12**:37, 1976.

14. Parad, H. J., and Resnik, H. L. P.: The practice of crisis intervention in emergency care. In Resnik, H. L. P., Ruben, H. L., and Ruben, D. D., editors: Emergency psychiatric care: the management of mental health crises, Bowie, M., 1975, The Charles Press Publishers, Inc.
15. Rapoport, L.: The state of crisis: some theoretical considerations. In Parad, H. J., editor: Crisis intervention: selected readings, New York, 1965, Family Service Association of America.
16. Rosenbaum, C. P., and Beebe, J. E.: Psychiatric treatment: crisis/clinic/consultation, New York, 1975, McGraw-Hill Book Co.

INDEX

Q

R